Humanising Mental Health Care in Australia

Humanising Mental Health Care in Australia is a unique and innovative contribution to the healthcare literature that outlines the trauma-informed approaches necessary to provide a more compassionate model of care for those who suffer with mental illness. The impact of abuse and trauma is frequently overlooked in this population, to the detriment of both individual and society. This work highlights the importance of recognising such a history and responding humanely.

The book explores the trauma-informed perspective across four sections. The first outlines theory, constructs and effects of abuse and trauma. The second section addresses the effects of abuse and trauma on specific populations. The third section outlines a diverse range of individual treatment approaches. The final section takes a broader perspective, examining the importance of culture and training as well as the organisation and delivery of services.

Written in an accessible style by a diverse group of national and international experts, *Humanising Mental Health Care in Australia* is an invaluable resource for mental health clinicians, the community managed and primary health sectors, policy makers and researchers, and will be a helpful reference for people who have experienced trauma and those who care for them.

Dr Richard Benjamin is a public sector psychiatrist and psychotherapist. He is particularly interested in the long-term effects of child abuse, their manifestations in adults presenting with mental illness, and the benefits of incorporating an understanding of both trauma and relationship in therapeutic responses.

Dr Joan Haliburn is a child, adolescent and family psychiatrist and psychotherapist. She is also a Lecturer at the University of Sydney, Australia. She is the former President and Director of Training of the Australian and New Zealand Association of Psychotherapy (ANZAP) and a member of the board of the International Society for the Study of Trauma and Dissociation (ISSTD).

Serena King is a clinical psychologist. She has worked extensively in community mental health and the tertiary education sector. She has held senior roles as a clinician, manager, supervisor and training provider. She has a particular interest in trauma-informed and relational treatments when working with clients with complex mental health issues. She facilitates multidisciplinary training in trauma-informed and psychotherapeutic approaches.

Humanising Mental Health Care in Australia

A Guide to Trauma-informed Approaches

Edited by
Richard Benjamin, Joan Haliburn and Serena King

Routledge
Taylor & Francis Group
LONDON AND NEW YORK

First published 2019
by Routledge
2 Park Square, Milton Park, Abingdon, Oxon OX14 4RN

and by Routledge
52 Vanderbilt Avenue, New York, NY 10017

Routledge is an imprint of the Taylor & Francis Group, an informa business

British Library Cataloguing in Publication Data
A catalogue record for this book is available from the British Library

Library of Congress Cataloging-in-Publication Data
Names: Benjamin, Richard, 1963- editor. |
Haliburn, Joan, editor. | King, Serena, editor.
Title: Humanising mental health care in Australia : a guide to trauma-informed approaches / edited by Richard Benjamin, Joan Haliburn and Serena King.
Other titles: Humanizing mental health care in Australia
Description: Abingdon, Oxon ; New York, NY : Routledge, 2018. | Includes bibliographical references and index.
Identifiers: LCCN 2018041125| ISBN 9780367076580 (hardback) |
ISBN 9780367076603 (pbk.) | ISBN 9780429021923 (ebk.)
Subjects: LCSH: Psychic trauma--Treatment--Australia. | Traumatic neuroses--Treatment--Australia. | Mental illness--Treatment--Australia. |
Mental health services--Australia.
Classification: LCC RC552.T7 H86 2018 | DDC 362.19685/2100994--dc23
LC record available at https://lccn.loc.gov/2018041125

ISBN: 978-0-367-07658-0 (hbk)
ISBN: 978-0-367-07660-3 (pbk)
ISBN: 978-0-429-02192-3 (ebk)

Typeset in Bembo
by Taylor & Francis Books

To all those who have suffered
Your story deserves to be heard

Contents

Figures

A Plea

Tired, angry, sad.
Pain, fear, loss.

Can you sit with it?
Not fix it,
not react to it,
not control it.

Tiredness, angriness, sadness.
Grief-stricken, heart-broken,
loss, loss, loss...

Can you sit with it?
Not schedule it,
not medicate it,
not make plans, or change thoughts,
not brainstorm, examine or question,
not prescribe "breathe and relax".

Not judge.
Just sit.
Just feel.
Just flow.
Just be.

Can you listen?
Can you hear me?
Are you there?
With me
in this moment
now.

Anonymous

About the editors

Richard Benjamin is a psychiatrist with psychotherapy training who works in the public community mental health sector in Tasmania. Almost all people he sees would meet the definition of having a severe mental illness, including many with psychosis. In the 1990s he worked with two people who had been repeatedly diagnosed with Schizophrenia. Both had been severely abused at the hands of caretakers, and their symptoms were evidence of this, but only if the complex effects of trauma were considered. As a result, he is particularly interested in the relevance of early trauma to adult life and to psychiatric presentations, and of the potential of therapy to assist. However, taking a primarily medical perspective precludes such an approach. Time pressure in the public sector also tends to focus attention on acute symptom and risk management, which is often paradoxically ineffective. A more human approach requires clinicians to listen intently to those they treat, to understand them as unique individuals, and to work with them within a therapeutic relationship, often over many years. He believes that both the medical and the human approaches are necessary, although the balance is rarely seen.

Joan Haliburn is a child, adolescent and family psychiatrist and psychotherapist in private practice and a lecturer, University of Sydney. Her main areas of interest are the assessment and management of adolescents and young adults with major mental illness – Eating Disorders, Obsessive Compulsive Disorder, Depression, Psychosis, Personality Disorder and suicidal young people. Their attachment and developmental histories are of particular relevance, as Dynamic Psychotherapy is her main treatment modality, with or without the addition of pharmacotherapy when necessary. Trauma in her experience is highly prevalent in young people, irrespective of their socioeconomic status. She has been keenly interested in teaching and writing on the increasing need to adopt an empathic psychotherapeutic attitude not only in psychiatry but more broadly throughout the field of medicine. She lectures nationally and internationally and has written widely. Her latest book, *An Integrated Approach to Short-Term Dynamic Interpersonal Psychotherapy*, was published by Karnac in 2017.

Serena King is a clinical psychologist. She has worked extensively in community mental health and the tertiary education sector. She has held senior roles as a clinician, manager, supervisor and training provider. She has a particular interest in trauma-informed and relational treatments when working with clients with complex mental health issues. She facilitates multidisciplinary training in trauma-informed and psychotherapeutic approaches.

List of contributors

Jackie Amos, MBBS, FRANZCP, PhD

Children's Services Unit, Centacare

Adelaide, Australia

Toni Ashmore, MPH, BSW

Private Practice

Canberra, Australia

Valerie (Judy) Atkinson, BA, PhD

We Al-li Pty Ltd

Lismore, Australia

Josephine Beatson, MBBS, FRANZCP

Spectrum Personality Disorder Service for Victoria

Melbourne, Australia

Nicholas Bendit, MBBS (Hons), FRANZCP, MMed (Psychotherapy)

Centre for Psychotherapy

Newcastle, Australia

Richard Benjamin, MBBS, FRANZCP, Dip Adult Psychotherapy (ANZAP)

Clarence and Eastern Districts Adult Community Mental Health Service

Hobart, Australia

Sandra L Bloom, MD

Dornsife School of Public Health

Drexel University

Philadelphia, USA

Jackie Burke, BPsych (Hons), MAPS, FANZMHA

School of Social Sciences and Psychology

Western Sydney University

Sydney, Australia

Veronica Burton, BA, AGDPSY
Children and Youth Services
Burnie, Australia

John Cooper, MBBS, FRANZCP
Phoenix Australia
Department of Psychiatry
University of Melbourne
Melbourne, Australia

Christine A Courtois, PhD, ABPP, PLLC
Author and Consultant
Trauma Psychology and Treatment
Bethany Beach, Delaware, USA

Martin J Dorahy, DClinPsyc, PhD
Department of Psychology
University of Canterbury
Christchurch, New Zealand

Julian D Ford, ABPP, PhD
Department of Psychiatry
University of Connecticut
Farmington, Connecticut, USA

Timothea Goddard, BA, Dip Psychotherapy, Cert MBSR, Cert TCTSY
Private Practice
Openground and Mindfulness Training Institute
Sydney, Australia

Brin FS Grenyer, PhD
Illawarra Health and Medical Research Institute
School of Psychology
University of Wollongong
Wollongong, Australia

Joan Haliburn, MBBS, FRANZCP, MMed (Psychotherapy)
Division of Psychological Medicine
University of Sydney
Sydney, Australia

Mary-Anne Kate, PhD
School of Psychology and Behavioural Science
University of New England
Armidale, Australia

Marianne Kennedy, MA
Private Practice
Somatic Psychotherapy Institute of Australia
Sydney, Australia

Cathy Kezelman, AM, MBBS (Hons)
Blue Knot Foundation
Sydney, Australia

Ignatius Kim, BA, RN, Member ANZAP
Child and Adolescent Mental Health Service
Hobart, Australia

Anna Luise Kirkengen, MD, PhD
General Practice Research Unit
Department of Public Health and Nursing
Norwegian University of Science and Technology
Trondheim, Norway

Christopher W Lee, BSc (Hons), MSc, PhD
Faculty of Health and Medical Sciences
University of Western Australia
Perth, Australia

Johanna Lynch, MBBS, FRACGP, Grad Cert (Grief and Loss)
Primary Care Clinical Unit
The University of Queensland
Brisbane, Australia

Alexander McFarlane, AO, MBBS (Hons), MD, FRANZCP, Dip Psychotherapy

Centre for Traumatic Stress Studies

School of Medicine

Faculty of Health Science

University of Adelaide

Adelaide, Australia

Narelle McKenzie, MA (Hons)

Private Practice

Australian Radix Training Centre,

Radix Institute

Melbourne, Australia

Sarah Mares, MBBS, FRANZCP, Cert Child Psych, MMH

School of Psychiatry

University of New South Wales

Sydney, Australia

Russell Meares, MBBS, FRCPsych, FRANZCP, MD

Department of Psychiatry

University of Sydney

Sydney, Australia

Warwick Middleton, MBBS, FRANZCP, MD

Belmont Hospital

Brisbane, Australia

Katherine L Mills, PhD

National Drug and Alcohol Research Centre

University of NSW

Sydney, Australia

Janise Mitchell, MSW, BSW

Australian Childhood Foundation

Melbourne, Australia

Louise Newman, AM, MBBS, FRANZCP, PhD
School of Psychiatry
University of Melbourne
Melbourne, Australia

Agi O'Hara, BA Psych (Hons)
Private Practice
Sydney, Australia

Carolyn Quadrio, MBBS, FRANZCP, PhD
School of Psychiatry
University of New South Wales
Sydney, Australia

Sathya Rao, MBBS, FRANZCP, MD (Psych Med)
Spectrum Personality Disorder Service for Victoria
Melbourne, Australia

Nicole Sadler, MPsych (Clin)
Phoenix Australia
Department of Psychiatry
University of Melbourne
Melbourne, Australia

Leonie Segal, PhD
Health Economics and Social Policy Group
Centre for Population Health Research
University of South Australia
Adelaide, Australia

Elisabeth Shaw, FAPS (FCCLP, FCCOUNP), Dip Supervision, MProfEthics
Relationships Australia
Sydney, Australia

Derrick Silove, AM, MBChB (Hons I), FRANZCP, MD
Psychiatry Research and Teaching Unit
School of Psychiatry
University of New South Wales
Sydney, Australia

Matthew Spicer, BSc, AGDPSY

Sanctuary Institute Australia

Melbourne, Australia

Pam Stavropoulos, PhD

Blue Knot Foundation

Sydney, Australia

Maree Teesson, AC, FAAHMS, FASSA

National Drug and Alcohol Research Centre

University of NSW

Sydney, Australia

Joe Tucci, PhD

Australian Childhood Foundation

Melbourne, Australia

Carla J Walton, BSc (Psych), DClin (Psych)

Hunter New England Mental Health Service

Newcastle, Australia

Michael Williamson, MBBS, FRANZCP, MMed

Westmead Psychotherapy Program for Complex Traumatic Disorders

University of Sydney

Sydney, Australia

Acknowledgments

The editors extend their gratitude to the 44 authors who contributed to the chapters of this book. We cannot thank them enough for distilling their expertise and wisdom into the pages herein, or for their patience.

To Russell Meares, Australia's leading expert in the field of trauma, dissociation and unconscious traumatic memory, for his inspirational work in developing a profoundly compassionate model of therapy for those that others would not treat, and for the education, guidance and supervision he has offered, we are deeply indebted.

We would also like to acknowledge those who have mentored, nourished and worked alongside us over the years, particularly Kereth West, Judith Pickering, Warwick Ashley and Harvey Marrable. They showed us how important it is to think deeply about what we do, to be human with those we work with, and to advocate when, where and however necessary. Most importantly, they taught us to slow down, and to listen.

We thank Edward King, who provided IT support and advice, and Mary Fraser and Nigel Granger, librarians extraordinaire, who helped us with our research and delivered papers to us with incredible speed and regularity.

To our friends and families, who heard far too much about "the book", but supported us nevertheless, we also offer our heartfelt thanks.

Finally, to those of you who have shared your personal stories, we commend you for your courage and for your strength; a book such as this could not have been written without you.

Editors' notes

This book was written by a diverse group of experts who were engaged in the project for their academic and clinical excellence. The views expressed are those of the authors and each author or group of authors takes responsibility for chapter content. No contributor or editor will be paid for their work, and all royalties will be donated to relevant not-for-profit organisations or charities that work to support those who have experienced trauma.

Each chapter has been written so that it stands alone. Authors have sourced their own definitions and statistics. The term abuse however is usually used to refer to an event, whereas trauma can be seen as both an event or the result of an event. Complex Trauma refers to the effects of repeated trauma that usually begin in childhood. Such traumas are almost always of an interpersonal nature, and the effects long-lasting. Terms and definitions used in the area of child abuse can be particularly challenging. Australian statistics classically refer to four different types of abuse, some US data up to 10 different types of abuse, and in the preparation of this book at least 20 different types of child abuse were recognised.

It is useful to note that those working in the field may view several commonly used terms differently. "Patient", "client", "consumer", "survivor" and "victim" are examples of terms that carry a range of connotations. Authors were not asked, however, to favour a particular lexicon, but rather to maintain consistency. Though the term "patient" is used frequently throughout the book, this word has been associated with a patriarchal attitude in medicine which is especially problematic for those who have been traumatised, where every effort must be made to recognise, address and avoid power imbalances. It may be of assistance to note that the original definition of the term meant "one who suffers".

Authors were encouraged to provide clinical descriptions and vignettes, either real, composite or fictional. Where real, the author has the informed and written consent of the person described to publish. Personal details have been changed to ensure confidentiality.

The need for ongoing education, training and supervision for those working in the field is critical and resonates through several chapters. As such, it should be emphasised that this book has been written as an introduction to the paradigm of trauma-informed care and no technique suggested by the book should be used without reference to these principles.

Finally, it should be acknowledged that some of the information presented in this book may, by its very nature, be distressing, and that some readers may be disturbed by the content.

Foreword

Sexual abuse of a child is a terrible crime. It is but one of a number of ways in which a child or adult may be abused. Abuse may also be physical, emotional or occur by neglect. The Royal Commission into Institutional Responses to Child Sexual Abuse found that it was not uncommon for a child who is sexually abused to also suffer one, or more than one, of the other forms of abuse. Whatever be the nature of the abuse a victim suffers, the experience is commonly traumatic. Some victims will suffer Complex Trauma which may have wide ranging and long-term impacts.

Central to the work of the Royal Commission was to provide an opportunity for a survivor to speak confidentially with a Commissioner about their childhood experience. More than 8,000 people availed themselves of this opportunity. For each survivor, this was a deeply personal experience, many only disclosing for the first time that they had been abused. It was also essential for the Royal Commission to ensure that every survivor who made contact with it was supported by trained responders, led by a team of counsellors with knowledge and experience in trauma-informed care. Each survivor was supported both before and after their private session and, where appropriate, referred to qualified professionals for ongoing care. Although the Royal Commission was not required by its Terms of Reference to examine the available healthcare responses to survivors who had suffered sexual abuse as a child, it was inevitable that this would occur.

Our work was complemented by a comprehensive research program, which included consideration of the appropriate professional response to people who have been sexually abused as children. As part of the National Redress Scheme that the Royal Commission recommended, we identified the need to provide counselling and psychological care throughout a survivor's life. It is important, as the recommendations make plain, that counselling and psychological care should be provided by practitioners with appropriate training and experience to work with those who have Complex Trauma. The Royal Commission also recommended that counselling and psychological care should be provided to a survivor's family members if necessary for the survivor's treatment. We further recommended that a public register should be created to enable identification of practitioners with appropriate capabilities.

The acceptance of a trauma-informed approach to the treatment of survivors of child sexual abuse is a relatively recent development. As was made plain by the work of the Royal Commission, unless the origin of a patient's psychiatric condition is established, it may not be possible to provide an effective clinical response to the patient's problems. Although I understand that for some time abuse has been recognised as having a role in relation to major mental illness, unless a treatment regime is developed with an understanding of the patient's history of abuse, the response may prove less than optimal or ineffective.

The title chosen by the editors of this book reflects a significant step in the development of professional responses to individuals affected by Complex Trauma. Though not diminishing the significance of the biomedical paradigm of psychiatry, the Royal Commission was convinced that a better understanding of the role of trauma in psychiatric illness and the development of trauma-informed responses are essential.

In compiling this book, the editors have sought contributions from many experts who work in the area of trauma, to provide a resource for all practitioners who work with people who are suffering Complex Trauma. They have brought together senior clinicians and academics from many fields and disciplines. Some of the contributors are well-known to the Royal Commission. Some gave evidence before us. The work of others was considered by the Royal Commission when framing our conclusions and recommendations.

The primary audience for this book is diverse, although it is anticipated to be of greatest value to those who work with trauma survivors. I have no doubt it will become a fundamental reference for all those who seek to understand and to provide trauma-informed care. The learning from this book will also enable others to develop a greater understanding of the appropriate approach to the treatment of people suffering Complex Trauma.

I commend the editors and contributors and trust the book will receive a considered and informed response from both professionals and others who seek to help people suffering Complex Trauma.

The Honourable Peter McClellan, AM, QC,
Chair,
Royal Commission into Institutional Responses to Child Sexual Abuse.
Sydney,
June 2018.

Introduction

Richard Benjamin

> The lack of an accurate and comprehensive diagnostic concept has serious consequences for treatment, because the connection between the patient's symptoms and the traumatic experience is frequently lost. Attempts to fit the patient into the mold of existing diagnostic constructs generally result, at best, in a partial understanding of the problem and a fragmented approach to treatment. All too commonly, chronically traumatized people suffer in silence; but if they complain at all, their complaints are not well understood. They may collect a virtual pharmacopeia for remedies: one for headaches, another for insomnia, another for anxiety, another for depression. None of these tends to work very well, since the underlying issues of trauma are not addressed.
>
> Judith Herman, 1992, pp.118–119

A vignette – "Suzie"

In the mid-1990s, with limited experience in psychiatry, the author of this paper took a position at a community mental health centre where he met a patient, "Suzie". She was in her late 20s at the time, in an unstable relationship, with a three-year-old son. Having always had serious problems with her mental health, and substance abuse, her situation worsened shortly after she gave birth when she presented believing that her baby had put "barking dogs" into her head and that she could see her baby's face "change into the Devil". She also heard voices that "yell at me all the time, telling me to hurt my boy, telling me I'm going to die". Some of the voices, she said, "sounded like cartoon characters". Suzie suffered with high levels of distress and had required several admissions to the local mental health inpatient unit. On one occasion she had tried to abduct her son who had been boarding on the children's ward. Involuntary restraint and sedation had been used repeatedly.

The persecutory voices were serious symptoms which Suzie could have acted upon and would lead many, if not most, working in the field to consider the diagnosis of Schizophrenia. In fact, by the time the author met Suzie, her clinical record showed that eight different psychiatrists had already made that diagnosis. Following the prevailing paradigm of psychiatry, those presenting with significant auditory hallucinations and delusions are usually considered to have Schizophrenia, a brain disease, where antipsychotic medication is regarded to be the cornerstone of treatment. The natural history of Schizophrenia is highly variable, but with a range of other difficulties and a limited social support network, Suzie's prognosis would have been guarded, and it would have been expected that ongoing medication and public mental health sector input would be required.

When Suzie first presented to the community centre, the traditional case management model used for psychotic conditions was made available to her. Despite frequent review, continuing medication, and support, Suzie's symptoms continued unabated and her son was removed from her care by child services. Eventually Suzie met "Sandy", a clinical psychologist at the centre. A more detailed symptom history, taken with an awareness of trauma and its effects, revealed that Suzie was highly anxious and had trouble sleeping, was unable to identify her moods and "didn't know what feelings were", though she experienced considerable anger. Suzie also said that she had "never felt good" about herself, didn't trust anybody, and found relationships difficult. To look at, Suzie was agitated and had a marked startle response.

Subsequent exploration of Suzie's developmental history also revealed that she had experienced a very difficult childhood. Her first presentation was to the local child psychiatry service with "anger and attention-seeking behaviour". These problems were thought to be related to periods where she had been separated from her mother, who had difficulty caring for her, and Suzie's father leaving the family when she was only four. It was also recorded that her stepfather "may have aggravated her … she hates him and will not talk about him". As a teenager, she took multiple overdoses. She demonstrated violent behaviour as well and had been arrested approximately 90 times for verbal and physical outbursts; she spent more than two years in children's homes and detention centres as a result.

By the time she came to the community centre, Suzie had presented 35 times to the local emergency department for overdoses and self-harm and had been admitted for approximately 250 days to psychiatric wards. In addition, Suzie had spent several months in a drug withdrawal unit for a range of addictions. Her records at that time noted that she suffered constantly with nightmares, appeared confused, and needed to "block out emotional pain" through self-harming behaviour. A history of child abuse was also noted at this time, and she was referred to the local sexual assault service, although she did not attend.

Believing that Suzie's presentation was at least partially related to trauma, the community team decided that she might benefit from a more psychotherapeutic approach than that usually offered in a case management model, and, as Sandy had training and experience in Cognitive Behaviour therapy, she decided to offer it to her. Sandy began by developing a relationship, teaching relaxation techniques, looking for cause and effect connections, and working on cognitive restructuring. The team provided Sandy support with her work, as there were a range of significant risks involved, and Suzie eventually came to trust Sandy.

They met and talked frequently, often two or three times a week, in an office, or sometimes on a quiet veranda over a cup of coffee. It was in this safe and accepting therapeutic relationship that Suzie was able to tell her story of early and relentless trauma. Her mother had re-partnered when she was about seven, after which her stepfather began "spoiling" her, in an attempt to groom her. He maliciously referred to her as evil, and by the time she was nine years old he was sexually abusing her. By the time she was about 11 he began to involve others in the abuse, holding "parties" during which time she would be drugged and repeatedly raped. Her mother she described as cold and unprotective.

In therapy, Suzie eventually made significant connections between her symptoms and the abuse that she had endured. The first was to the voice of a television cartoon character that was known for rescuing others; in fantasy, he used to rescue Suzie. "He had his bag of tricks, he came everywhere with me, he blocked out the pain, just thinking about him" she said. "Numb a lot, it hurt so bad, I never thought about it. I left the abuse to visit him". The second connection she made was to the barking dogs, which she had both seen and heard in reality, but re-experienced in childbirth as a noise in her head; "they blocked out the pain". She remembered that she had heard the dogs one day, while she was being raped, "I listened to them, they were nice, they were better than the real stuff that was happening".

Both the voices of the cartoon character and the barking of the dogs had served to take her away from the pain that she was experiencing, by a process of dissociation which was protective and helped her to detach from the actual abusive experiences. Dissociation, an unconscious defence mechanism which separates the normally integrated processes of perception, memory, and identity, is helpful at first, but later becomes dysfunctional, resulting in the production of symptoms, as it did for Suzie.

After little more than two years of therapy, the "psychotic" symptoms resolved, her moods significantly stabilised, her ability to parent improved, and she was able to have her son returned to her care. She was also gradually weaned off antipsychotic medication, although she was occasionally prescribed anxiolytics to manage her agitation. She learnt that the abuse was not her fault, and that "love and closeness" were not only different from what she had experienced, but possible.

The author met Suzie again, 20 years after she first presented with psychotic symptoms. She was bright and spontaneous. She volunteered that she had a new partner, a part-time job as a support worker, and that she regularly travelled overseas. She reported having been admitted once to hospital seven years earlier for treatment of depressive symptoms in the context of family stressors. She stated that she had not experienced any further psychotic symptoms, she felt good in herself, and, unlike what she had been told, she no longer felt that she was "bad". She added that without therapy she was sure she would have killed herself or that she would still be "drugged to the eyeballs in an institution, with no hope".

This book has been written to highlight the need to take a trauma-informed approach with any person struggling with mental illness, but especially those with severe mental illness. To understand the need for such an approach, an appreciation of changing perspectives with respect to classification, diagnosis, and treatment within psychiatry is critical.

Paradigms within psychiatry

Diagnoses in psychiatry have always been made within the prevailing theories of the time and these theories have shifted dramatically over the last century. The biological perspective gained traction with the discovery in the early twentieth century of the syphilitic spirochaete, Treponema pallidum, in the brains of patients suffering with General Paralysis of the Insane (Noguchi and Moore, 1913), and obtained further credibility shortly thereafter when Julius Wagner-Jaurregg discovered that these patients, usually institutionalised with psychotic and neurological symptoms, could often have their conditions reversed and disease progress halted by inducing a fever with malaria (Shorter, 1997).

Similar discoveries relating definitive pathology to illness rarely followed, and, for the next 50 years, the psychoanalytic paradigm of Sigmund Freud and others held sway. Initially focusing on child sexual abuse as the root cause of neurotic illnesses, Freud moved away from this understanding to an intrapsychic theory of psychopathology based on instincts, drives, and internal conflict. Importantly, Freud wrote about the unconscious and its relevance to everyday life. Psychoanalysts in their practice placed emphasis on the meaning of symptoms, on life experience, on relationships, the effect of the past on the present, and on the work done in sessions with the analyst for treatment effectiveness. They focused on the unique individual in front of them and diagnosis was not seen to be of great importance. This paradigm remained in force until as recently as 1977, when almost two-thirds of visits to psychiatrists in the USA were exclusively for psychotherapy with no medication provided, although by 2002 this was the case for less than 10 per cent of psychiatrists (Eisenberg, 2010).

The challenges to psychoanalysis and psychotherapy that have affected psychiatric practice came from both the neuroscientists and the behaviourists and began in the middle of the twentieth century. Hans Eysenck started the behavioural debate by proclaiming that any psychotherapeutic successes were less than or equal to the rate of spontaneous remission and that psychotherapy may even be harmful (Eysenck, 1952). The conclusions drawn were heavily criticised but the "findings were damning", and well-publicised (Wampold, 2001: p.62). Proponents of behaviourism believed that what was in the mind, "the black box", could not be studied, so that only environmental stimuli and behavioural responses were worthy of review. Ivan Pavlov had previously focused on events that triggered responses, classical conditioning, and BF Skinner on modifications of behaviour via reward or punishment, or operant conditioning. In the context of trauma, Joseph Wolpe developed a treatment called Systematic Desensitisation, a variant of which is now used to treat some people with Posttraumatic Stress Disorder (PTSD), by increasingly exposing them to feared stimuli until their responses diminish.

Behaviour Therapy was followed by Aaron Beck's Cognitive Therapy in the 1960s and 1970s. Initially working psychoanalytically, Beck came to believe that the way his patients thought about themselves, the world, and the future, what he called the "cognitive triad", led to depressive symptoms, not unconscious conflicts. Treatment involved helping patients reappraise their thoughts. Cognitive and behavioural approaches came together in the 1980s, as Cognitive Behaviour therapy, or "CBT", and now comprises a wide array of therapy types. They are generally seen to be symptom and future focused, and action-oriented. CBT has been extensively studied and it has been shown to be efficacious in a wide range of disorders; it is generally seen as the gold standard, evidence-based psychotherapeutic treatment, especially for Anxiety Disorders (Hoffman et al., 2012). The CBT perspective is also becoming increasingly incorporated into classification systems (Borza, 2017). It is further important to note that some studies have raised concerns about the overall quality of the research into CBT and of effect sizes (Cuijpers et al., 2016), and that some investigators believe that there are very few differences between any of the schools of psychotherapy (Wampold, 2001; Beutler, 2009).

Biological perspectives began to make substantial contributions again after the discovery of several drugs effective for Schizophrenia and the Affective Disorders in the 1950s, starting with chlorpromazine and reserpine for Schizophrenia, and then imipramine for Depression and lithium for Manic-Depression. Chlorpromazine is particularly important to note; it was the first relatively safe antipsychotic medication that not only calmed patients and diminished their psychotic symptoms but also allowed for early discharge into the community. At around the same time as these drugs were discovered, serotonin and dopamine were identified as the first neurotransmitters implicated in mental illnesses, and the first theories regarding chemical imbalances of the brain causing mental illness were developed, including the relationship between dopamine and Schizophrenia, the "dopamine hypothesis" (Carlsson, 1977). Subsequent pharmacological studies led to a much greater emphasis on neuroscience, via brain receptors and neurochemistry, and neuroanatomy, as well as a new emphasis on classification and diagnosis; this latter area is of particular relevance for psychiatry as a branch of medicine.

A study by Rosenhan demonstrated that healthy volunteers, with no psychiatric history, complaining of voices just once, could be admitted to a psychiatric hospital for an extended period, despite wanting to leave; the average length of stay for eight patients was 19 days (Rosenhan, 1973). Another study involving psychiatrists from the USA and UK viewing videotapes of patients showed that there were very marked differences in practice, with the North

American psychiatrists diagnosing Schizophrenia much more broadly than the British, in lieu of conditions like Mania, Depression, Anxiety, and Personality Disorder (Kendell et al., 1971). As a result, it became apparent that specific diagnostic criteria for mental illnesses were simply not available. Controversy followed, and the American Psychiatric Association was pressured to revise its own classification system, the Diagnostic and Statistical Manual of Mental Disorders, or the DSM, previously highly psychoanalytic in focus in its first two editions.

Robert Spitzer was chosen as the Chair of the Taskforce in 1974, and the Third Edition, the DSM-III, was published in 1980 (American Psychiatric Association, 1980). This edition was written in the context of the new emphasis on science and scientific method, and the need for researchers and clinicians to agree, more closely, on a diagnosis; the concept of reliability. As such, it was almost completely atheoretical with respect to the aetiology of conditions, taking a primarily descriptive and criteria-based approach. Some conditions adopted came from work undertaken at the Washington University by Eli Robins, Samuel Guze, and George Winokur, the Feighner Criteria, that were later adapted to form the Research Diagnostic Criteria, and other conditions were arrived at by committee consensus. It is important to bear in mind that the system was initially designed to provide a common language for researchers and clinicians and that it was not designed as a guide for treatment. The manual has however become widely influential and in many jurisdictions is the dominant classification system in use; it is frequently referred to as the "Bible" of psychiatry. It is used by researchers, clinicians, managers, insurance companies, the justice system, and the general public. Importantly, diagnoses are often seen as equivalent to actual "diseases" requiring particular medical "treatments". Diagnoses are also used to determine funding and provision of services.

From the very beginning, however, the DSM system came under scrutiny. That diagnoses were determined by clustering of symptoms and signs of illness was questioned, as was their relationship to reliability and validity. Reliability is measured by the correlation coefficient kappa: a score of 1.0 indicates complete agreement between raters, 0.0 no agreement, and -1.0 complete disagreement. Field trials of the Fifth Edition of the DSM, the DSM-5 (American Psychiatric Association, 2013), have been of particular concern: the investigators lowered the reliability ranges used, with the likelihood of over-estimation of reliability (Vanheule et al., 2014). One reason given for the need for lower reliability scores included use of more real-world patients with fewer exclusions (Black and Grant, 2014). Even using the lower ranges, however, the correlation coefficients for many of the more commonly made diagnoses were low. The kappa for Major Depressive Disorder, was 0.28, or "questionable", and the kappa for Generalised Anxiety Disorder, 0.20, or "unacceptable". Even the kappa for Schizophrenia was only 0.46.

Thomas Insel, then Director of the US National Institute of Mental Health (NIMH), wrote in 2010 that diagnostic categories founded on clinical consensus were not likely to explain the underlying pathophysiology, were not predictive of treatment response, and were in fact hampering the development of targeted treatments; that is, they demonstrated little validity (Insel et al., 2010). As such, he explained that the NIMH would move away from the DSM criteria and instead utilise a new system based on neural circuitry and genomics, the Research Domain Criteria. The focus on the clustering of symptoms without consideration of the pathophysiological basis of disease is the fundamental problem of the DSM;

> Psychiatrists have gotten better at agreeing on which scattered particulars they will gather under a single disease label, but they haven't got any closer to determining whether those labels carve nature at its joints, or even how to answer that question. They have yet to figure out just exactly what a mental illness is, or how to decide if a particular kind of suffering qualifies.
>
> (Greenberg, 2013: p.20)

The DSM classification system has also been criticised for rendering normal human distress pathological. The number of categories has increased significantly over the decades, although there is little agreement in the literature regarding the exact number of diagnoses in each version. One comprehensive review of all the DSM iterations offered the following details: DSM-I, 128 different diagnostic categories, DSM-II 193, DSM-III 228, DSM-IV 383 and DSM-5 541 (Blashfield et al., 2014). Allen Frances, the Chair of the Task Force of the DSM-IV, has become a vocal critic of the system in this regard. Writing about his own edition, he said,

> Even though we had been boringly modest in our goals, obsessively meticulous in our methods, and rigidly conservative in our product, we failed to predict or prevent three new false epidemics of mental disorder in our children – autism, attention deficit, and childhood bipolar disorder.
>
> (Frances, 2013a: p.xiv)

In the case of Childhood Bipolar Disorder, in the 10 years after the DSM-IV was published, prevalence rates increased 40-fold, according to one study (Moreno et al., 2007).

Frances has been especially concerned with the expansion of diagnostic categories to include the "worried well", with overuse of psychotropic medication in these groups, at the expense of those with severe mental illness (Frances, 2013b). The expansion of diagnostic categories dovetails with the marketing arms of the pharmaceutical companies, who are said to spend twice as much on promotion than they do on research and development (Gagnon and Lexchin, 2008). In the field of psychiatry, medication sales have increased as a result, with expenditure on antipsychotics and stimulants approximately tripling between 1997 and 2004 (Stagnitti, 2007), and antidepressant use nearly quadrupling from 1998–2008 (National Center for Health Statistics, 2011) in the USA. Similar trends have been observed in Australia, with antipsychotic use increasing more than four-fold, antidepressant use increasing more than three-fold, and psychostimulant and memory enhancing drugs increasing over 57-fold between 1992–1993 and 2016–2017 (Australian Institute of Health and Welfare, 2018). With respect to antidepressants, per capita Australian consumption is now the second highest in the OECD group of countries (Organisation for Economic Co-operation and Development, 2015).

It is particularly important to note in making diagnoses by referring to clusters of symptoms that the individuality of the person is substantially diminished. More than a quarter of a century after the DSM-III was published, Robert Spitzer acknowledged this with respect to depressive symptoms (Spitzer, 2007). He noted that the DSM affects how individuals interpret their own experiences, and that "its criteria specified the symptoms that must be present to justify a given diagnosis but ignored any reference to the context in which they developed" (p.viii). He also suggested that those constructing the DSM-5 ought to take note of these issues. In contrast, the DSM-5 removed the bereavement exclusion from the diagnosis of Major Depressive Disorder, such that some of those experiencing normal grief may now be diagnosed with a medical condition.

The combined effect of classifying patients using the DSM system, the increasing use of psychotropic medications, and the rise of evidence-based therapies has been described as the "pax medica" of psychiatry: a broken model of mental illness, erroneously founded upon theories of chemical imbalance in the brain, with an inappropriate emphasis on symptom-based diagnoses and on specialised treatments and techniques, which together have, "medicalized psychology and psychiatry in a way that has become so pervasive it's almost invisible, like the air we breathe" (Linford and Arden, 2009: p.16).

Trauma-informed care

The 1990s saw progress in the fields of psychiatry and mental health in three different areas. "The Decade of the Brain" saw further advances in the neurosciences, which included increasingly sophisticated functional imaging techniques and the introduction of a range of antidepressants and antipsychotics with different modes of action. The concept of neural plasticity, which is the ability of the brain to change and adapt throughout life, and particularly during critical periods of neural development, especially childhood, also came to be seen as increasingly important to an understanding of both normal development and psychopathology. This new perspective proposes that the human brain is socially constructed, and that psychiatry is "all biological and social" (Eisenberg, 1995: p.1571). In the USA, the 1990s also saw the advent of a related paradigm in psychiatry, mental health, and the human service sector more broadly, that of trauma-informed care.

This new paradigm involves an understanding that those who are in receipt of mental health services have experienced particularly high rates of abuse and trauma and that such trauma has a wide range of biological, psychological, and social effects. One study revealed that 98 per cent of those with a severe mental illness, usually seen as Schizophrenia, Bipolar Disorder, and Depression, have been exposed to a traumatic event, and 43 per cent had PTSD, although only 2 per cent had this diagnosis recorded in their charts (Mueser et al., 1998). A later study in a more diverse population revealed a lifetime trauma exposure rate of 87 per cent, with 19–30 per cent suffering PTSD (Cusack et al., 2006). This later study also revealed that only 28 per cent had a trauma history recorded, and only 3 per cent had been given a diagnosis of PTSD. Psychiatric patients who have experienced child sexual or physical abuse also have earlier first admissions, are admitted more frequently to hospital and for longer, receive more medication, spend longer periods in seclusion, and are more likely to self-harm and to attempt suicide (Read et al., 2004). The paradigm also aims to provide education about what is reported to be a very common finding in health systems, namely an insensitivity by staff to patients who have been traumatised; most especially in inpatient units and in larger, institutional settings with patriarchal hierarchies. It further encourages working collaboratively with patients whenever possible and attempting to avoid shaming and humiliation at all times.

The immediate background of the trauma-informed care paradigm involved increasing awareness of the effects of abuse on women seen by public mental health services, and of the re-traumatising, and sometimes fatal effects of sedation, seclusion, and restraint on such patients (Weiss et al., 1998). But the history stretches back much further, to the late nineteenth century, when the eminent French neurologist, Jean-Martin Charcot, demonstrated in "hysterical" patients – those presenting with physical complaints where the cause was emotional – that symptoms could be both removed and reinstated by hypnosis, revealing that unconscious forces were at play. Also working at this time, Freud heard repeatedly of incest and sexual assault from his own patients and he described his belief in a causative relationship between incest and the symptoms of hysteria, his "Seduction Theory" (Freud, 1896/1966). Freud however retracted his theory the following year, unable to incorporate the immense social implications of his findings. Herman, among others, has been very critical of Freud with respect to this:

> The dominant psychological theory of the next century was founded in the denial of women's reality … . Psychoanalysis became a study of the internal vicissitudes of fantasy and desire, dissociated from the reality of experience. By the first decade of the twentieth century, without ever offering any clinical documentation of false complaints, Freud had concluded that his hysterical patients' accounts of childhood sexual abuse were untrue … . The study of psychological trauma came to a halt.
>
> (Herman, 1992: pp.14–15)

It was not until the wars of the twentieth century that psychological trauma was once again investigated. Under the horrific conditions of trench warfare in World War I, men broke down in large numbers, often complaining of physical symptoms, like headache, dizziness, and hypersensitivity to noise. The term "shell shock" came into use as medical staff thought that symptoms were due to lesions in the brain, resulting from the shock waves of bursting shells. Men would also display psychological symptoms, calling out, panic, freezing, hysterical blindness, gait or paralysis, and, particularly, amnesia. When it was realised that symptoms could occur in those who had not been exposed to artillery fire, shell shock came to be seen as the result of primarily emotional causes; when men presented with psychological symptoms their moral character was often questioned. During World War II it was discovered that illness could be predicted by the amount of combat exposure, 200 to 240 days in aggregate enough to break almost any man (Appel and Beebe, 1946). Interest in the effects of war resurfaced again particularly with Vietnam, where the soldiers themselves were the major force driving understanding and change, setting up their own "rap groups" in which they retold their experiences after their return home. The US Government responded with research and treatment programs, and in 1980 the diagnosis of psychological trauma was finally validated by the creation of the concept of PTSD in the DSM-III.

Interest in the abuse of children in the twentieth century was particularly ignited by Henry Kempe's description of childhood physical abuse, "The Battered Child Syndrome" (Kempe et al., 1962). As a result of this study it was recognised that child abuse was both a regular and a recurring pattern of family life, and that health practitioners had a central, and eventually mandated, role in the recognition and management of such abuse. The momentum generated was further advanced by the Women's Liberation movements of the 1970s where it was recognised that the most common psychological traumas occurred not to men in war but to women and children in civilian life. Research into rape began, and long and intimate personal interviews became the source of knowledge, just as they had been 80 years before, when hysteria was being intensively studied. Importantly, rape was redefined as a crime of violence and of control, enforcing the subordination of women through terror (Brownmiller, 1975). Other critical works included descriptions of the "Rape Trauma Syndrome" (Burgess and Holmstrom, 1974) and the "Battered Woman Syndrome" (Walker, 1979). The Women's Movement also brought about a treatment response: the creation of rape crisis centres. The initial focus on the rape of adult women led to a rediscovery of the sexual abuse of children. It was only after the creation of PTSD as a diagnostic category did it become clear that the psychological syndromes seen in the survivors of abuse were similar to those seen in the survivors of war.

Post-abuse sequelae

Abuse and trauma have been linked with a range of post-abuse syndromes, and child abuse, in particular, has been linked with many, if not most, psychiatric disorders, including more recently with psychotic symptoms and psychosis (Read et al., 2004; Moskowitz et al., 2008). Community surveys clearly demonstrate a relationship between child abuse and "hard" psychotic symptoms, or "Schneiderian" first-rank symptoms, usually indicative of Schizophrenia; symptoms including hearing voices talking with each other or feeling that your body or thoughts are not under your own control (Ross and Joshi, 1992). Gerald Ellenson, a social worker, noted frequent psychotic symptoms in 40 women aged 16 to 50 who presented to a community centre who had also disclosed sexual abuse histories (Ellenson, 1985). Their psychotic symptoms included a frightening feeling that there was an evil or malevolent entity in the home or in their body, recurrent auditory hallucinations including hearing a child cry out, or sounds of "intruders" and recurrent visual hallucinations involving movement of figures in peripheral vision. In addition, a range of other symptoms including nightmares, obsessions, phobias, and dissociation were described. Ellenson noted that the women involved rarely associated their symptoms with their abuse, and that the grouping of symptoms together might even constitute a useful diagnostic syndrome that would predict a history of incest. Ellenson also described incest survivors suffering with more persecutory voices that, "Condemned the survivor in sexual terms, calling her whore, bitch and slut. They told her that she was no good, that she was garbage" (Ellenson, 1986: p.153). Others experienced more "directive" voices goading them toward aggression, self-harm or suicide attempts.

Not long after Ellenson described his post-incest syndrome, Judith Herman published her seminal textbook on the after-effects of trauma more broadly, including her concept of a "Complex Post-Traumatic Stress Disorder", or C-PTSD (Herman, 1992). She wrote that survivors often presented with a wide array of symptoms which often led to misdiagnosis. Furthermore, the survivor is often blamed, and the treatment provided by the medical system often replicates the behaviour of the abusive family. The syndrome that Herman outlined was a result of repeated trauma, with effects across many domains. The first criterion includes a history of "subjection to totalitarian control" over prolonged periods, for example in prisoners of war or cult survivors, but also in sexualised family settings.

C-PTSD can occur after repeated trauma at any age but most often follows lengthy abuse in childhood. The effects include changes in affect or mood regulation, depression, anger, suicidal ideation, and self-harm; changes to consciousness including frequent remembrance of events as intrusive memories, or not remembering at all, dissociation, and nightmares; changes to self-view, shame, guilt, self-blame, and a sense of defilement; changes to beliefs about the abuser; changes to relationships including withdrawal and a lack of trust; and changes to "systems of meaning", including a loss of hope. The myriad nature of the effects also helps explain the "co-morbidity" that presents in abused people who are often diagnosed with multiple disorders that the DSM system promotes. More importantly, appropriate diagnosis helps both the clinician and the person who has been abused understand the origin of the difficulties.

Because of the diagnostic and treatment importance, attempts have been repeatedly made by proponents to have C-PTSD included in one of the major classification systems. C-PTSD was not included in the latest version of the

DSM, but, very importantly, it was included in the recently released 11th version of the International Classification of Diseases (World Health Organization, 2018); a watershed moment in psychiatry akin to the official diagnostic recognition of PTSD in 1980.

Purpose of the book

The main aim of this book is to draw attention to the all too often devastating effects of abuse and trauma on both children and adults, effects that are not always linked to the trauma by patient or clinician, particularly in those suffering with severe mental illness. When Suzie was found to experience voices and delusions, a diagnosis of Schizophrenia was made according to the primarily criteria-based DSM classification system, taken out of context, and because organic and psychotic illnesses trump all others, following the historical principle of Foulds' hierarchy in psychiatry (Foulds and Bedford, 1975). Several years of standard management for that condition followed, with no beneficial effects. However, when a trauma-informed history-taking process revealed symptoms of PTSD (anxiety, hypervigilance, nightmares, insomnia) and a history of child abuse along with the disparate nature of Suzie's difficulties were evident (emotional pain, anger, overdosing, self-harm, psychotic symptoms, dissociation, low self-esteem, difficulties with trust and intimacy, and substance abuse), a diagnosis of C-PTSD was strongly suspected; the wide variety of symptoms alone should be seen as suggestive of a trauma background. The trauma literature, indicating a relationship between incest and a range of psychiatric symptoms, including psychotic symptoms, further suggested the possibility of child sexual abuse being an important component of her presentation.

Although it is clear that biological conditions such as Schizophrenia, Bipolar Disorder, and Depression, present frequently, and require biological treatments, it is also readily apparent that the relationship between child abuse, psychotic symptoms, dissociation, and psychosis is complex, that there are multiple pathways to psychotic symptoms, and that in some cases abuse and trauma may explain all of a patient's symptoms or they may be an important contributor to the presentation. Of paramount importance then, in the context of the prevailing biomedical paradigm in psychiatry, is the need for clinicians to sensitively enquire about abuse and trauma in all people who present with severe mental illness as this group have often experienced high levels of such events and as routine enquiry "can reveal important links between psychotic symptoms and real traumatic events in a person's life" (Larkin and Read, 2008). Indeed, many affected by sexual or other abuse and trauma may present with a wide array of symptoms and as a result may be diagnosed with a primary Anxiety or Depressive disorder, Bipolar Disorder, Schizophrenia, Personality Disorder, Substance Abuse Disorder, or may be given a range of medical diagnoses, including Irritable Bowel Syndrome, Fibromyalgia, and Chronic Pain, with no reference to their history of trauma; clinicians must always have a high index of suspicion about this potential relationship. Confusion is more likely to occur when there is insufficient training in and understanding of the effects of early or preverbal trauma, when assessments are not comprehensive, when the focus is more on the needs of the system than those of the patient, and where there is inadequate organisational support. Importantly, the earlier the trauma, the less likely is it to be remembered.

A further objective of this book is to highlight the negative responses that those individuals who have been traumatised may be confronted with and to promote a more compassionate response. Suzie's experiences within a range of systems over many years involving frequent, lengthy incarcerations, numerous and repeated restrictive practices, including involuntary use of medication, could be likened to a repetition of Suzie's childhood abuse. On the contrary, empathic understanding on the part of a trauma-informed community mental health team supported a therapist to work closely with Suzie, who for the first time learned to trust and to talk about her own story, which helped her to make sense of her symptoms, and then to make sense of herself. The turn-around for Suzie was, indeed, remarkable. Those who have been traumatised are amenable to psychotherapy, as Suzie was; those who have been broken in relationship can only be healed in relationship. Despite Eysenck's assertion, psychotherapy is highly effective, with the average patient in therapy better off than 79 per cent of untreated patients, while the therapeutic relationship and the therapists themselves are significantly more important than the type of therapy delivered (Wampold, 2001; Wampold and Imel, 2015).

Outline of the book

The book represents the work of a cross-section of experts – senior clinicians, therapists, academics, theorists, researchers, consumer advocates and system managers – from many fields and disciplines. Most authors are from Australia although others hail from New Zealand, Europe, and the USA. They were consulted for their specialist knowledge of the area and for their diverse and extensive experience.

Authors were asked to write their chapters from first principles and to increasingly incorporate more complex concepts, so that each paper could be accessed by a broad audience, although clinicians and support workers are the main target population. Each author was requested to situate their chapter in its historical context, to give appropriate background to their contributions, as well as to focus on clinical constructs and issues. The use of illustrative vignettes was encouraged.

The book itself is organised into four sections. The first outlines theory, constructs, and effects of abuse and trauma, and is designed to orient the reader. The second section addresses the effects of abuse and trauma on specific populations. The third section outlines a diverse range of individual treatment approaches. The final section consists of a group of papers that look at a broader perspective and the organisation and delivery of services. Much of the material in the book reflects the situation as it currently stands in Australia, the last section particularly so, illustrating what has been done and what can be done across a range of different settings. It is hoped that this section particularly encourages the reader to further research abuse and trauma and its effects, and to instigate change in their own workplaces.

Conclusion

Just before his death, the eminent American psychiatrist Leon Eisenberg wrote about the impact of the biomedical paradigm on psychiatry, with its contemporary focus on the brain, with the result that the personhood of the patient was frequently lost. Whilst always sceptical of psychoanalysis as a science, he said it

> taught trainees to listen to patients and to try to understand their distress, not simply to classify their diseases or sedate them or lock them away. It highlighted the importance of memory, its vulnerability to distortion, and its centrality to patients' life narratives, the stories we tell ourselves and others. It made clear how those narratives can be self-defeating and defined the task of therapy as helping patients to reconstruct their autobiographies to permit growth. Psychoanalysis helped psychiatry preserve an abiding interest in the individuality of patients while other medical specialties were losing sight of the patient in their preoccupation with the biology of the disease. It connected the symptoms of mental illness to the psychopathology of everyday life.
>
> (Eisenberg, 2010: p.90)

Such an interest in the care of the those suffering with mental illness has been lost, particularly within the specialty of psychiatry. The system's negative and uninformed responses to Suzie's difficulties are an all too frequent occurrence. The perspective of trauma-informed care transforms our understanding that those with severe mental illness may be significantly affected by abuse and trauma. This insight, coupled with the ready availability of a range of therapeutic options, and the necessary training, funding and research, might just help us find the way back to a more humane model of care.

References

American Psychiatric Association (1980) *Diagnostic and Statistical Manual of Mental Disorders, Third Edition*. Washington, DC: American Psychiatric Publishing.

American Psychiatric Association (2013) *Diagnostic and Statistical Manual of Mental Disorders, Fifth Edition*. Arlington, VA: American Psychiatric Publishing.

Appel JW and Beebe GW (1946) Preventive psychiatry: An epidemiologic approach. *The Journal of the American Medical Association* 131(18): 1469–1475.

Australian Institute of Health and Welfare (2018) *Mental Health Services in Australia: Mental Health-related Prescriptions*. Government of Australia. Available at: aihw.gov.au/reports/mental-health-services.

Beutler LE (2009) Making science matter in clinical practice: Redefining psychotherapy. *Clinical Psychology: Science and Practice* 16(3): 301–317.

Black DW and Grant JE (2014) *DSM-5 Guidebook*. Arlington, VA: American Psychiatric Publishing.

Blashfield RK, Keeley JW, Flanagan EH, et al. (2014) The cycle of classification: DSM-I through DSM-5. *Annual Review of Clinical Psychology* 10: 25–31.

Borza L (2017) Cognitive behavioural therapy for generalised anxiety. *Dialogues in Clinical Neuroscience* 19(2): 203–207.

Brownmiller S (1975) *Against Our Will: Men, Women and Rape*. New York, NY: Simon and Schuster.

Burgess AW and Holmstrom LL (1974) Rape trauma syndrome. *American Journal of Psychiatry* 131: 981–986.

Carlsson A (1977) Does dopamine play a role in schizophrenia? *Psychological Medicine* 7(4): 583–597.

Cuijpers P, Cristea IA, Karyotaki E, et al. (2016) How effective are cognitive behaviour therapies for major depression and anxiety disorders? A meta-analytic update of the evidence. *World Psychiatry* 15(3): 245–258.

Cusack KJ, Grubaugh AL, Knapp RG, et al. (2006) Unrecognised trauma and PTSD among public mental health consumers with chronic and severe mental illness. *Community Mental Health Journal* 42(5): 487–500.

Eisenberg L (1995) The social construction of the human brain. *American Journal of Psychiatry* 152(11): 1563–1575.

Eisenberg L (2010) Were we all asleep at the switch? A personal reminiscence of psychiatry from 1940 to 2010. *Acta Psychiatrica Scandinavica* 122: 89–102.

Ellenson GS (1985) Detecting a history of incest: a predictive syndrome. *Social Casework: The Journal of Contemporary Social Work* 66(9): 525–532.

Ellenson GS (1986) Disturbances of perception in adult female incest survivors. *Social Casework: The Journal of Contemporary Social Work* 67(3): 149–159.

Eysenck HJ (1952) The effects of psychotherapy: An evaluation. *Journal of Consulting Psychology* 16: 319–324.

Foulds GA and Bedford A (1975) Hierarchy of classes of personal illness. *Psychological Medicine* 5: 181–192.

Freud S (1896/1966) The Aetiology of Hysteria. In: Strachey J (ed and trans) *Standard Edition of the Complete Psychological Works of Sigmund Freud, Volume Three*. London, UK: Hogarth Press.

Frances A (2013a) *Saving Normal: An Insider's Revolt Against Out-of-control Psychiatric Diagnosis, DSM-5, Big Pharma, and the Medicalization of Ordinary Life*. New York, NY: William Morrow.

Frances A (2013b) The past, present and future of psychiatric diagnosis. *World Psychiatry* 12(2): 111–112.

Gagnon MA and Lexchin J (2008) The cost of pushing pills: A new estimate of pharmaceutical promotion expenditure in the United States. *PLoS Med* 5(1): e1.

Greenberg G (2013) *The Book of Woe: The DSM and the Unmaking of Psychiatry*. New York, NY: Scribe.

Herman J (1992) *Trauma and Recovery*. New York, NY: Basic Books.

Hoffman SG, Asnaani A, Vonk IJJ, et al. (2012) The efficacy of cognitive behavioural therapy: A review of meta-analyses. *Cognitive Therapy and Research* 36(5): 427–440.

Insel T, Cuthbert B, Garvey M, et al. (2010) Research Domain Criteria (RDoC): Toward a new classification framework for research on mental disorders. *American Journal of Psychiatry* 167(7): 748–751.

Kempe CH, Silverman FN, Steele BF, et al. (1962) The battered child syndrome. *Journal of the American Medical Association* 181: 17–24.

Kendell RE, Cooper JE, Gourlay AJ, et al. (1971) Diagnostic criteria of American and British Psychiatrists. *Archives of General Psychiatry* 25(2): 123–130.

Larkin W and Read J (2008) Childhood trauma and psychosis: Evidence, pathways, and implications. *Journal of Postgraduate Medicine* 54: 287–293.

Linford L and Arden JB (2009) Brain-based therapy and the "Pax Medica". *Psychotherapy in Australia* 15(3): 16–23.

Moreno C, Laje G, Blanco C, et al. (2007) National trends in the outpatient diagnosis and treatment of bipolar disorder in youth. *Archives of General Psychiatry* 64(9): 1032–1039.

Moskowitz A, Schafer I and Dorahy MJ (2008) *Psychosis, Trauma and Dissociation: Emerging Perspectives on Psychopathology.* West Sussex, UK: Wiley-Blackwell.

Mueser KT, Goodman LB, Trumbetta SL, et al. (1998) Trauma and posttraumatic stress disorder in severe mental illness. *Journal of Consulting and Clinical Psychology* 66(3): 493–499.

National Center for Health Statistics (2011) *Health, United States, 2010: With Special Feature on Death and Dying. Table 95.* Hyattsville, MD: National Center for Health Statistics.

Noguchi H and Moore JW (1913) A demonstration of Treponema pallidum in the brain in cases of general paralysis. *The Journal of Experimental Medicine* 17: 232–238.

Organisation for Economic Co-operation and Development (2015) *OECD Health Statistics.* Available at: dx.doi.org/10.1787/health-data-en.

Read J, Goodman L, Morrison AP, et al. (2004) Childhood trauma, loss and stress. In: Read J, Mosher LR and Bentall RP (eds) *Models of Madness: Psychological, Social and Biological Approaches to Schizophrenia.* East Sussex, UK: Routledge, pp.223–252.

Rosenhan DL (1973) Being sane in insane places. *Science* 179: 250–258.

Ross CA and Joshi S (1992) Schneiderian symptoms and childhood trauma in the general population. *Comprehensive Psychiatry* 33: 266–273.

Shorter E (1997) *A History of Psychiatry: From the Era of the Asylum to the Age of Prozac.* New York, NY: John Wiley and Sons.

Spitzer R (2007) Foreword. In: Horwitz AV and Wakefield JC *The Loss of Sadness: How Psychiatry Transformed Normal Sorrow into Depressive Disorder.* New York, NY: Oxford University Press.

Stagnitti MN (2007) *Trends in the Use and Expenditures for the Therapeutic Class Prescribed Psychotherapeutic Agents and all Subclasses, 1997 and 2004. Statistical Brief #163.* Rockville, MD: Agency for Healthcare Research and Quality.

Vanheule S, Desmet M, Meganck R, et al. (2014) Reliability in psychiatric diagnosis with the DSM: Old wine in new barrels. *Psychotherapy and Psychosomatics* 83: 313–314.

Walker L (1979) *The Battered Woman.* New York, NY: Harper and Row.

Wampold BE (2001) *The Great Psychotherapy Debate: Models, Methods and Findings.* Mahwah, NJ: Lawrence Erlbaum Associates.

Wampold BE and Imel ZE (2015) *The Great Psychotherapy Debate: The Evidence for What Makes Psychotherapy Work*. New York, NY and East Sussex, UK: Routledge.

Weiss EM, Altimari D, Blint DF, et al. (1998) Deadly restraint: A Hartford Courant investigative report. October 11–15. *Hartford Courant.*

World Health Organization (2018) *International Classification of Diseases, 11th Revision (ICD-11).* Geneva, Switzerland: World Health Organization.

Part I

Theory and constructs

1 Trauma theory

Sandra L Bloom

Introduction

Across the millennia, the human brain has evolved to function as an integrated whole, with mind and body acting in concert, constantly adapting to a wide range of ecological challenges. The complex physiological mechanisms that have developed to accommodate this enormous flexibility are generically known as the human stress response. In the last several decades, the study of traumatic stress – capturing the most extreme mobilisation of the stress response – has garnered a significant body of knowledge and research.

For many years, the word "homeostasis" has been used to describe the exquisite balancing act that keeps human bodies functioning within an optimal range and in a state of equilibrium. This primarily involves the autonomic nervous system as it constantly responds to demands for activation or relaxation. More recently, researchers have been substituting the word "allostasis", a term that indicates variability in this balancing responsiveness. The sympathetic nervous system is activated as a stressor indicates the need for greater response, including an increased utilisation of energy. Powerful neurochemicals and neurohormones released by the brain stimulate end organs in turn to release adrenaline, cortisol, beta-endorphin, glucagon and others. When the need to respond to the stressor has passed, the parasympathetic nervous system calms that response down, so the organism can return to restoring energy and growth, and to repair any damage. The variable response to a stressor is influenced by the three levels of the brain: automatic responses to survival threats in the brainstem, emotionally-based responses originating in the limbic system, and more complex and even conscious responses that originate in the cortex.

Inadvertently, a linguistic problem has developed in that the word "trauma" is being used to describe reactions and results that emanate from events that may not be routinely understood as traumatic. It is not possible to coherently understand traumatic stress and the complex problems associated with it without also considering the other gradations of the stress response: positive stress, tolerable stress, relentless stress (increased allostatic load), and toxic stress. Positive stress is characterised by moderate, short-lived increases in heart rate, blood pressure, serum glucose and circulating levels of stress hormones, and occurs when the body adapts to any change, such as leaving home and getting into a car to drive to work. Tolerable stress refers to responses that could affect brain architecture, but generally occur for briefer periods that allow time for the brain to recover and thereby reverse potentially harmful effects. An increased allostatic load, or relentless stress, are the terms being used to describe the wear-and-tear on the body and brain resulting from chronic over-activity of the same physiological systems that are normally involved in adaptation to environmental challenge (McEwen, 2012). Toxic stress is the term employed to describe the strong and prolonged activation of the body's stress management systems that becomes particularly problematic when it occurs during critical developmental periods, because of the multiple ways that this activation affects the progressive unfolding of basic brain architecture (Shonkoff et al., 2012b).

This extensive variation in control mechanisms tells us a great deal about the problems that can arise for human beings in our modern world. We are still quite capable of responding as our ancestors did to survival threats. But we respond similarly to anything we perceive as emotionally threatening as well as threats to our status, our individual and group identities, and our ideological frameworks. Therefore, to understand the multiple ways in which stress affects people, there is a need to simultaneously understand basic physiology, human development, emotional processing, and cognitive processing, as well as group behaviour and moral systems, and the way each of these critical components of human existence interact with each other. This complexity requires the need for a more thorough understanding of stress, trauma, and human physiology in health and disease or dysfunction.

Stress, adversity, and trauma affects everyone, and the earlier it starts in life, the longer it lasts, the more frequently it happens, and the more distrust develops, the more challenging and long-lasting the effects will be. It is because of this complexity and the intersection with so many other dimensions of science and the humanities that it has become possible for a unified field theory of human behaviour to begin to emerge. A paradigm shift is finally occurring after several hundred years of advancing knowledge that can integrate and unite the varied schools of thought about trauma and the human condition.

Physical responses

Fight–flight

The physical response to danger referred to above is best known as the "fight–flight–freeze" response, the basic mammalian survival response. "The sympathetic nervous system kicks into action during emergencies, or what you think are emergencies. It helps mediate vigilance, arousal, activation, mobilization" (Sapolsky, 1998: p.22). This results in increases in blood pressure, heart rate, breathing, accelerated delivery of nutrients to muscles, blunted pain perception, increased blood clotting, activation of the immune system, and a brain that is on alert. At the same time, long-term digestion, growth, tissue repair, and reproduction are all turned off.

The amygdala, an almond-shaped structure found in both the right and left temporal lobes of the brain, is like a "central switchboard" for danger, so that when threat is perceived, the amygdala is activated and sends signals that trigger the full fight–flight response, all of which occurs at an unconscious level. As a result, the amygdala can be "hijacked", so that a response to non-dangerous stimuli can occur before there is a chance to think or evaluate a situation (Goleman, 1995). The right amygdala appears to be more influenced by early childhood experiences than the left.

Joseph LeDoux has described a "low road" and a "high road" of arousal, demonstrating that the low road from perception of potential danger to immediate arousal of the autonomic nervous system is unconscious and fast, while the high road, involving the appraisal process of the cortex, takes twice as long to be activated (LeDoux, 2002). Anyone who drives is aware of this; braking occurs before any conscious decisions can be made.

Chronic stress can result from living in chronically dangerous situations: war zones, domestic violence, incarceration, refugee status, child abuse. But chronic stress can also occur under conditions that are not actually physically dangerous but that are psychologically threatening, including events that are anticipated to happen. It is the generalisation of the stress response that sets humans apart from other animals; humans can elicit a fight–flight–freeze response in situations that are not physically threatening.

Chronic hyperarousal

Under conditions of chronic stress, something goes wrong as the body repeatedly attempts to mount the necessary physiological responses. The effectiveness of the response diminishes and the body becomes desensitised to the effects of some neurohormones, and hypersensitive to others. The entire system can become dysregulated in multiple ways. This results in a set of highly dysfunctional and maladaptive brain activities (Perry and Pate, 1994). The person experiences this as a state of chronic hyperarousal – a hallmark characteristic of Posttraumatic Stress Disorder (PTSD). Essentially, the baseline level of arousal for the person has changed, with a loss of control of their own responses to stimuli.

Once severely or repeatedly traumatised, people lose the capacity to modulate their level of arousal, they stay hyper-aroused and guarded, and they are unable to calm themselves down, even when there is no danger. They may feel embarrassed by their response, while at the same time they may also be irritable, angry, and frightened for no apparent reason. They may still be prepared to fight or to flee and they may also become flooded with memories, images, and sensations that are overwhelming. As a result, they are likely to feel that they are "going crazy." These reactions can be triggered by internal or external cues.

Fear-conditioning

Once a fear-evoking stimulus has been experienced, "fear-conditioning" occurs; a state that is very powerful and difficult for the logical centres of the brain to override (LeDoux, 1992, 1994). Because of the vast associational network of the human brain, fear can pair with virtually any stimulus. This happens very quickly at the time of the frightening event, and beyond conscious control. Later, the person is usually not consciously aware of the connection between the fear-provoking stimulus, since the fear-response has become completely automatic. Each episode of danger connects to every other episode of danger, so that the more danger a person is exposed to, the more sensitised that person becomes. This hypersensitivity is known as "kindling" and has been associated with not only PTSD but also with episodes of Mania and Depression (Monroe and Harkness, 2005). With each fight-or-flight experience, the mind forms a new network of connections that is triggered by every subsequent threatening experience or stimulus.

Since most individual cell growth and specialisation in the brain occurs after birth in response to complex and critical neurohormonal cues, chronic hyperarousal in childhood means that children are more likely to develop a panoply of destructive symptoms and behaviours in attempts to diminish this unsupportable state. Failure to provide children with sufficient protection from overwhelming stress appears to cause actual impairment in normal brain development. A growing body of evidence suggests that this exposure has long-term detrimental effects on basic brain architecture as well as cognitive, emotional, and social function, and moral development. Researchers studying childhood posttraumatic stress and adversity believe that childhood stress and trauma may be the common link between many medical and psychiatric conditions related to the immune system, the cardiovascular system, and the neuroendocrine system. These findings have been strongly supported by the landmark Adverse Childhood Experiences study (Anda et al., 2010).

Freeze and dissociation

The freeze component of the stress response is strikingly different. If there is no chance for survival by either fight or by flight, the freeze response may automatically occur. The freeze response activates a very different sequence of autonomic nervous system arousal, slowing the heart rate, preserving blood flow, and even simulating death so that a predator loses interest, since predatory behaviour is triggered by movement (Levine, 1997). The dissociative response, the "temporary breakdown in continuous, interrelated processes of perception, memory, or identity" (Brewin, 2011: p.211), has much in common with the freeze component of the stress response, although the difference between what happens to prey animals in the wild who do not get caught, and what happens to humans who dissociate at the time of a trauma is significant. Animals who enter the freeze state and who come out of that state of immobility spontaneously are far more likely to survive than animals who are forced to come out of that state. Apparently, the spontaneous recovery of the animal, often through repetitive almost seizure-like motor discharge, is associated with survival after the immediate source of danger has passed (Scaer, 2001). But humans frequently do not spontaneously come out of the acute dissociative state known as "shock", and, instead, fragments of the experience may become locked into that dissociative state, unavailable to full biographical narrative. These become the substrates for flashbacks, nightmares, and behavioural re-enactments.

Similarly, animals exposed to inescapable shock "learn" to be helpless so that even when they could escape they do not do so. This phenomenon of uncontrollability has been used as a model for chronic dissociation and the freeze response in humans who cannot control the trauma they are experiencing. A viable hypothesis is that the failure of the person to adequately discharge the state of immobility and the dissociative state accompanying it may lie at the heart of the memory disturbances and arousal symptoms of PTSD (Levine, 1997); it is well established that people who dissociate at the time of a traumatic event are more likely to develop PTSD (Van der Kolk and Van der Hart, 1989).

Tend and befriend

More recently, a different form of the human stress response has been captured in the phrase, "tend and befriend". It has been proposed that one of the most striking aspects of the human stress response is the tendency to affiliate, that is, to come together in groups to provide and receive joint protection in threatening times. This form of the stress response would have supported survival by arousing the need, particularly in females, to tend to the young and vulnerable, and could be served by circuitry involving the parasympathetic system with the release of oxytocin that then triggers the release of serotonin and dopamine, all of which supports affiliation (Taylor et al., 2000; Taylor, 2006). Differing gender-based strategies would have served evolutionary needs but may now help to explain gender differences in longer-term physical outcomes (Wang et al., 2007; Verma et al., 2011).

Cognitive responses to danger

Information processing

Human beings have two distinct ways of processing information: one under calm, low-arousal states termed "rational-thinking mode", and the other occurring during high stress and high arousal, given the term "the experiential-thinking mode". The experiential-thinking mode is automatic, rapid, occurs outside of conscious awareness, and takes precedence under life-threatening conditions. When danger is perceived, humans are physiologically geared to act, not to ponder and deliberate. In situations of acute danger, it is better that humans respond immediately without taking the time for complicated mental processing, so that responses can be more immediate, to save lives and to protect family. Calm rational thinking takes time and when faced with, for instance, a hungry predator, the deliberate and time-consuming nature of rational thought processes can cost one's life (Epstein, 1994).

As a result, under conditions of danger, perceptions are radically altered. As heart rate goes up, cognitive processes change radically (Grossman and Christiansen, 2008). First, there is a narrowing of the perceptual field, so that only information relevant to the immediate threat can be absorbed. Diminished or altered sound, tunnel vision or the loss of peripheral vision may also be experienced. Heightened visual clarity about some details of the event may occur, along with a sense of temporary muscle paralysis. There may also be perceptual distortion of time so that everything seems to be in slow motion, and intrusive or distracting thoughts about loved ones or other personal matters may occur. Similarly, flashbulb memories may be experienced, where the individual has a series of vivid images burned into memory, with the rest of the event somewhat confused, out of order, or even missing. Distance distortions, colour distortions, face recognition distortions and lighting distortions may also occur (Artwhol, 2002). These perceptual distortions and fragmentary memories later manifest through the intrusive flashback experiences that are so characteristic of PTSD.

Hemispheric specialisation

Another dimension of the challenges posed by information processing is the fact that the two cerebral hemispheres are functionally very different from each other, and these differences probably have significant implications for understanding what goes wrong in the processing of traumatic events, while supplying keys to understanding innovative forms of treatment (Joseph, 1992, 2012; McGilchrist, 2009, 2012).

Consciousness, language, and linguistic thought are intimately interrelated, and are supported and maintained by the left hemisphere of the brain. It is the left brain that generally controls the ability to talk and think in words, and it is the left brain that analyses spoken and written language. This is the brain that is associated with linguistic consciousness.

In contrast, the right brain cannot generally read, spell, or write, and cannot understand many aspects of human speech except for a few simple words, particularly those which are emotional. However, it can vocally express itself through singing, swearing, crying, praying, mimicking, or cooing sounds of love and sorrow. The right brain subserves a different kind of intelligence and may be the site of what is historically referred to as the "unconscious mind". The right brain is thought to be the antecedent of the left, an ancient form of consciousness that dominated millions of years of human hunter-gatherer existence (Joseph, 2012). The right brain communicates through feelings, valuation, and actions, and is the undercurrent of all human social interaction.

The structure that connects the two hemispheres is the corpus callosum. These large interconnected fibre tracts are not matured until age ten, and even in young adults the corpus callosum is only partially myelinated. This may be the reason that makes childhood memories, and most importantly, traumatic childhood memories, so difficult to put into words and to fully integrate into narrative form. Children are quite likely to dissociate in the face of overwhelming negative emotion, which deactivates the right hemisphere and interferes with right hemisphere processing (Lanius et al., 2005). The right hemisphere is vital in attention, maintaining a coherent sense of our bodies, pain processing, and ultimately a coherent, continuous, and unified sense of self, so events that interfere with interhemispheric communication are likely to interfere significantly with healthy brain development (Schore, 2017). Recent research has shown that there is diminished corpus callosum volume in adults with PTSD, suggesting that this may be at least one of the impairments in posttraumatic integration of verbal and nonverbal information (Saar-Ashkenazy et al., 2014).

This growing body of evidence suggests that the unliquidated memories, images, sensations, and bodily experiences associated with the intrusive symptoms of PTSD and other dissociative disorders may be related to deficits in interhemispheric communication (Schiffer et al., 1995; Teicher et al., 1997, 2000). Such an understanding helps to explain why many kinds of nonverbal approaches may be key to helping the survivor fully integrate their experience into a biographical narrative that allows it to be part of the past, rather than the living present.

Attention and focus

During a threatening situation, attention is riveted on the threat. But after the threat goes away, attentional problems may continue, and, in fact, research has shown that combat veterans with PTSD have attentional deficits. It has also been demonstrated that general memory and attention provide the best predictors of PTSD symptoms (Gilbertson et al., 2001). It is thought that attentional changes are related to exposure to extreme stress and the tendency to be biased from that point on toward threat stimuli. If this happens in childhood, children's capacities to study, to pay attention in the classroom, and to achieve academically may be severely compromised (Shonkoff et al., 2012b). Perceptual problems extend to the social environment as well. Child maltreatment teaches children – and the adults they become – to attend to environmental cues that indicate the possibility of danger, and systematically ignore those that do not. As a result, such children may develop what one investigator has called "negative social maps", so that they become hypersensitive to negative social cues and oblivious to positive social cues (Garbarino, 1999).

Decision-making and judgment

Decision-making and judgment can become very impaired under conditions of chronic stress. Cognition is likely to become overly simplistic, making it difficult to think about little else other than the immediate present, impairing the ability to consider the long-range consequences of an action. In such a state, decisions tend to be based on impulse and the need to self-protect (Janis, 1982). Many of those who have been traumatised have long-term problems with various aspects of thinking that impede decision-making and the exercise of good judgment. An intolerance of mistakes, denial of personal difficulties, anger as a problem-solving strategy, hypervigilance, and absolutistic thinking are other problematic thought patterns that have been identified (Alford et al., 1988).

State-dependent learning

Given the problems with attention, it is not surprising that learning is also affected by acute and chronic stress. Learning is dependent on the ability to categorise incoming material, but this can only happen optimally in a state of calm attentiveness. Learning is dependent on the state that one is in when the learning occurs, and fear creates a very special state of consciousness. Fear conditioning happens very rapidly in animals and humans – a single pairing is sufficient – and once established, the fearful reaction is relatively permanent. Higher brain centres may inhibit and control the fear response, but the "emotional memory" remains (LeDoux, 1994).

Once fear is learned, it is likely that it can never be "unlearned" at a basic physiological level. Later, when people are triggered by reminders of past trauma, they become hyper-aroused, and only the learning gained during past experiences with hyperarousal and danger will be available to them. Because of this, state-dependent learning can interfere with the efforts of others to help the victim. Strategies designed in the calm surroundings of a therapist's office may bear little relationship to the level of arousal the same person is in when confronted by a perceived danger. State-dependent learning combined with learned helplessness and experienced lack of control over one's own physiological states associated with a traumatic experience leads then to a diminished sense of self-efficacy, so that even when the person could take constructive action to prevent further harm, they seem unable to do so.

Memory

Memory is often profoundly altered by overwhelming stress. There are at least two different kinds of memory. Memory for details and events is called declarative or explicit memory. This memory system is grounded in the use of language. The human brain automatically categorises every new experience. This process begins at birth and continues making new categories of information throughout life. These categories comprise a system of mental schemata that are verbally encoded and become integrated into the already existing knowledge base. Most of this activity occurs in the part of the brain known as the hippocampus. The declarative memory system is open to change and distortion, both by previous experience, by new information, and by the state of arousal that the person is in at the time of recall.

The non-declarative, implicit, or procedural memory system does not require words or even thoughts (Squire, 1987; Southwick et al., 1994; Van der Kolk, 1994, 1996b; Van der Kolk et al., 1997). This is the memory of habits, skills, conditioned emotional and sensorimotor responses, intuition and "gut" responses. This is the memory automatically drawn upon when driving a car, or when riding a bicycle, even if not practised for many years. This memory system is not language-based and appears to be controlled largely by areas of the brain separate from normal memory, most importantly by the right hemisphere. The implicit memory system developed earlier in evolution than the more recently evolved verbal, explicit memory system, and may also be operational far earlier in development than the verbal system which does not become available until the child begins to understand speech (LeDoux, 1994; Van der Kolk, 1994). Children may, in fact, have nonverbal memories long before they have memories that can be given any kind of verbal form. The implicit memory system also functions much faster than the verbally based memory system and has been called a "quick and dirty" reaction mechanism (LeDoux, 1994).

It is the amygdala that appears to attach emotional meaning to experience, even before it can recognise what the reaction is in response to, or even what feelings are being experienced. It is only later that the higher cortical areas elaborate that experience and imbue it with meaning. This aspect of memory is especially important in the processing of "fear conditioning", and how fear is managed. This is important because many psychiatric disorders, including PTSD, appear to involve some malfunction in the brain's ability to control fear (LeDoux, 1994).

Under normal conditions, both memory systems are available for optimal functioning. Individuals can freely access information and draw upon biographical material. Emotional experience is attached to these memories, but day-to-day life is not dominated by powerfully emotionally charged memories or intrusive experiences from the past; the past remains in the past, and it is not experienced as the present. These two memory systems work in parallel, and their activities are seamlessly interconnected. There is a conscious awareness of the information held within the hippocampal system, but the implicit system remains unconscious, and is always exerting a powerful influence (LeDoux, 1994).

For the past century, many observers have noticed that the imprint of traumatic experiences is very different from the memories of normal events. Bremner and his colleagues reviewed the differences between "normal forgetting" and traumatic amnesia (Bremner et al., 1995). They point out that, from an evolutionary point of view, the efficient recall of memories associated with previous danger is crucial for survival. But it is difficult to explain how the over-remembering of danger associated with PTSD is adaptive, or why so many people develop under-remembering, or amnesia, in the face of danger. People who have experienced a variety of differing traumas are noted to have a wide range of memory problems with vivid intrusive memories of a past event, or flashbacks, often alternating with partial or total amnesia for the traumatic events. These intrusive experiences appear to be triggered in the present by emotions and sensations that are associated with the traumatic past, and the person often has amnesia for both the flashbacks and the original trauma.

People under severe stress also secrete neurohormones that affect the way their memories are stored. In animals and humans, high levels of glucocorticoids secreted during stress impair the functioning of the hippocampus. Neuroimaging techniques indicate that changes in the structure of the hippocampus may be secondary to prolonged stress (Bremner et al., 1995; Van der Kolk et al., 1997). This may partially or totally disable the ability of the brain to verbally categorise incoming information. At the same time, during states of high fear, the amygdala is extremely active, and interferes with hippocampal functioning (Van der Kolk, 1996b). The result is a partial or complete loss of the ability to assign words to incoming experience, the biological equivalent of "speechless terror" (Van der Kolk, 2000). Dependent upon words, the capacity to logically think through a problem is diminished or entirely shut down, and the mind shifts to a mode of consciousness that is characterised by visual, auditory, kinaesthetic images, and physical sensations, as well as strong feelings.

Evidence also exists that the over-secretion of neurohormones at the time of the trauma may deeply imprint the traumatic memory (Van der Kolk, 1994, 1996b). LeDoux has termed this "emotional memory" (LeDoux, 1992). In studying the influence of fear, he has shown that emotional memory appears to be permanent and quite difficult, if not impossible, to eliminate, although it can be suppressed by higher centres in the brain. This "engraving" of trauma has been noted by many researchers studying various survivor groups (Van der Kolk and Van der Hart, 1991; Van der Kolk, 1994).

Traumatic memory often poses the greatest problem for people who have suffered repeated or severe traumatic experiences. The intrusive symptoms of PTSD – nightmares, and the sensory, emotional, and physical flashbacks – all appear to be a result of disordered memory functioning. The alternation between flashbacks and amnesia is one of the most problematic aspects of stress disorders. Traumatic memories are vivid, state-dependent, do not fade, nor do they seem to be altered by ordinary experiences. Flashbacks are likely to occur when people are upset, stressed, frightened, or aroused, or when triggered by any association to the traumatic event (Van der Kolk, 1996b).

There are now data available from positron emission tomography (PET) scanning that provide more information about these intrusive phenomena. Traumatic memories "happen" principally in the emotional areas of the brain's right hemisphere, and are accompanied by an increase in activity in the visual areas of the brain, signifying that people with PTSD actually "see" their flashbacks, while there is a decrease in the area of the brain responsible for the translation of emotional states into language (Van der Kolk and Fisler, 1995; Rauch et al., 1996; Van der Kolk et al., 1997). This is experienced by the person as a total or partial reliving of the traumatic experience. It can be a sensory fragment of the trauma or the entire traumatic sequence, running like a virtual reality movie. In such a state, the traumatised person has difficulties distinguishing reality from flashback. The sensory experience is often quite vivid, feeding a vicious cycle of autonomic arousal that increases the sense of reality of the flashback even more. When people experience intrusive flashbacks as visual, olfactory, affective, auditory, or kinaesthetic sensations, it bears little if any relationship to the normal process of remembering.

Emotional responses to danger

The role of emotion

Under normal conditions, emotions serve as a "sensitive mental radar", alerting people to the significance of things around them (Harber and Pennebaker, 1992). Individuals cease having an emotional response when they have realigned their expectations of what is supposed to happen with what is actually happening, either by taking action that adjusts the given situation to their expectations, or by changing their expectations to fit better with what is happening. Traumatised individuals cannot predictably rely on their emotions to provide accurate evaluative information (Van der Kolk, 1996a). Incoming information is given emotional meaning by the amygdala. The amygdala mediates both inborn and acquired emotional responses and appears to be involved in mediating both conscious and unconscious emotional feeling.

This kind of emotional memory is likely to function completely outside of conscious awareness and be stored in the right hemisphere. When the event is recalled, or triggered by some association, the cognitive memories in the left hemisphere may be recalled in parallel with the emotional memories, not as a recognised memory but as a state of being, sensations in the body or feeling states that the person may not consciously connect to the cognitive memories of something from the past (LeDoux, 1994). When this has occurred, those who have been traumatised can no longer use their emotional states as directional signals or as warning signals to take adaptive action (Krystal, 1978).

In PTSD, emotional arousal and goal-directed action are often disconnected from each other. People with PTSD either have too much emotional arousal, inappropriate to the circumstances they are in, or they develop a sense of emotional numbness, an under-reactivity that leaves them feeling depressed, empty, unable to relate to other people and even to life. They respond to reminders of a previous traumatic event as if it were happening in the present, not the past, with increases in heart rate, skin conductance, and blood pressure (Van der Kolk, 1996a). People who have been traumatised lose the capacity to "modulate arousal". They tend to stay irritable, jumpy, and on edge. This loss of the ability to modulate internal emotional states means that people may become very labile, with rapidly shifting, easily triggered, and powerful negative emotions that are beyond their control.

These changes are particularly problematic when the traumatic exposure begins in childhood. Over the course of normal development and with the responsive and protective care of adults, the child's brain develops the ability to modulate the level of emotional arousal based on the importance or relevance of the stimulus. The capacity of adults to soothe frightened children is essential to their development: they cannot soothe themselves until they have been soothed by adults. In the absence of such soothing, as many as 80 per cent of abused infants and children develop disorganised attachment patterns which are associated with an inability to utilise care givers for soothing, resulting in pathological self-regulatory behaviours (Carlson et al., 1989). A substantial body of research has shown that early and prolonged trauma in childhood affects the capacity to regulate the intensity of emotional responses, problems that continue into adolescence and adulthood (Shonkoff et al., 2012a).

Emotional numbing and avoidance

Under conditions of extreme stress, dissociation spontaneously and unconsciously occurs, serving to buffer the central nervous system against the life-threatening aspects of overwhelming arousal. One common form of dissociation is the splitting off or separation of feelings from the actual experience. Alexithymia, the inability to identify specific emotions and put those emotions into words that can be shared, was first described in concentration camp survivors (Krystal, 1988). The incomplete emotional processing that is typical of PTSD and manifested by alexithymia appears to be closely associated with the somatisation that is a typical accompaniment of PTSD and Complex PTSD (Lumley and Norman, 1996). Engaging the emotions has been shown to be a vital ingredient in the successful emotional processing of traumatic experiences, while emotional numbing and alexithymia may interfere with the success of treatment (Harber and Pennebaker, 1992; LeDoux, 1996).

Those who have been traumatised will also try to avoid traumatic reminders, which may substantially limit the activities they undertake, the experiences they allow themselves to have, the places they go, and the relationships they engage in. There is often a gradual withdrawal from everyday life that has been variously called, "dead to the world", "a deterioration not dissimilar to that in schizophrenia", and "posttraumatic decline", so that any stimuli pleasant or unpleasant are avoided (Van der Kolk, 1996a).

Emotional contagion and social rejection

People who have been traumatised often have extreme difficulties with emotional control and they frequently give disturbing signals to others. They either signal too much emotion, too little, or emotion that is inappropriate to the given situation. Internally numbed, they may maintain an external mask of blankness that is confusing to the observer. Often, however, this confusion on the part of the other is not conscious. Most of what is registered about another's emotional state occurs at a level below consciousness, although it profoundly affects interactions. Since this experience is unconscious, it is not usually open to spontaneous exchange, which could at least lead to the possibility of explanation and understanding on the part of both persons.

Instead, the signals given off by the traumatised person have a strong tendency to evoke unconscious distancing and rejecting responses on the part of others. Researchers have studied listeners' responses to the disclosures of those who have been traumatised. What they found is very disturbing: listeners just "don't want to hear it". They tend to disrupt trauma stories by switching the topic of conversation away from the trauma, they attempt to press their own perspective of the trauma upon the victims, or they simply avoid contact with the person altogether. It is proposed that listeners have a difficult time listening because the stories of the victims' traumas threaten the listeners' assumptive world views about justice. Therefore, they tend to exaggerate the role of personal responsibility, and often end up blaming the person for a traumatic experience that they could not avoid (Coates et al., 1979).

Ultimately, those who have been traumatised recognise that people are withdrawing from them or avoiding them, and consequently begin to inhibit their own emotional expression and avoid discussion of the trauma. This presents powerful negative consequences, since the tendency to avoid disclosure of emotions is associated with increased risks for physical illness, impaired information processing, and a loss of social support, and therefore opportunities for healing and recovery.

Behavioural responses to danger

Traumatic re-enactment and the compulsion to repeat

Why do we repeat the past, particularly when the patterns of behaviour that we are repeating are, at best, unfulfilling and often traumatic? The philosopher Santayana observed that, "Those who cannot remember the past are condemned to repeat it" (Santayana, 2017: p.188), and this is as true in the lives of individual trauma survivors as it is for societies. Both Janet and Freud claimed that the crucial factor that determines the repetition of trauma is the presence of mute, unsymbolised, and unintegrated experiences (Van der Kolk and Ducey, 1989). Freud termed this the "repetition-compulsion" and wrote that in order for feelings to be experienced and become conscious, words had to be linked to them. It was the linkage with word representations that allowed the affect to cross the repression barrier and become conscious (Sashin, 1993).

Human beings are designed to function at a maximal level of integration, and any barrier to this integration will produce some innate compensatory mechanism to overcome it. Splitting off traumatic memories and feelings into nonverbal images and sensations by the mechanism of dissociation is life-saving in the short-term, but a barrier to full integration in the long-term. The memories of the traumatic experience remain dissociated, nonverbal, and unintegrated, possibly lodged in the right hemisphere. Traumatic re-enactment occurs when people repeatedly find themselves in situations that recapitulate earlier trauma, lacking any awareness of how this occurred or how to prevent it from recurring. The lack of conscious awareness may be secondary to the dissociative blockade between the left and right hemisphere integration that places the behaviour out of context of the left hemisphere's verbal, linear and conscious control. Since words are not available to sufficiently explain the experience, rational mode thinking cannot occur.

People will usually develop explanations for their strange behaviour, because the rational part of their mind is struggling to make sense of the situation. But without access to the dissociated material, the rational mind interprets behaviour in a simplistic, often naïve and punitive way, while the person helplessly re-exposes himself or herself to further trauma. This represents the psychodynamic idea that symptoms are nonverbal "cries for help" from the right hemisphere, that can only communicate with actions. It is this level of communication that underlies all modern cultures and forms the most basic medium of human communication, and is central to all the arts (Donald, 1991; Bloom, 2010, 2011).

The communication that the right hemisphere is attempting with the left hemisphere and the representatives of the social group – including the therapist – becomes a type of intermediary translator, helping to overcome the left hemisphere's unwillingness or resistance to incorporate the entire story of the past, a story that may severely contradict the left hemisphere's previous definitions of reality and self. The re-enactment behaviour cannot stop until the meaning in the message is heard, responded to, and integrated.

Self-harming behaviour and addiction

Traumatic re-enactment is often disguised by a wide variety of self-harming and addictive behaviours. Since the "language" of the right brain is concrete, metaphorical, and emotional, the signs and behaviours that are frequently noted as symptoms are actually "cries for help" from the right brain. Intrusive memories and flashbacks are likely to disrupt the emotional numbing that has become protective. Under such circumstances, people frequently turn to substances, like drugs or alcohol, or behaviours like sex, over-eating, gambling, engagement in violence, and self-injury, all of which help them to calm down, at least temporarily, in part because of the major, self-induced shift in internal body chemistry that accompanies Substance Abuse and self-harming behaviour. There are very good reasons why PTSD and chronic substance abuse often appear simultaneously in the same individual and diagnosis may depend entirely on the level of expertise of the diagnostician or the system to which they present. Similarly, it is important to consider what a person might be re-enacting with sexually compulsive behaviour but is unable to have close supportive and intimate relationships.

Addiction to drugs, alcohol, food, sex, and other compulsive behaviours may also be more comprehensible if seen as unconscious strategies to manage internal distress arising from the split-off and unmetabolised traumatic experiences. Individuals exposed to repetitive stress are more likely to abuse alcohol and other drugs and to relapse. This is supported by research with animals showing that stress increases the tendency of animals to self-administer drugs that are defined as illicit substances for humans. Research has shown that there is an overlap between the neurocircuitry that responds to drugs and those that respond to stress, and that it is these same neurocircuits that are involved in the development of PTSD and related syndromes (National Institute on Drug Abuse, 2002).

Those who are addicted to alcohol or other drugs also may be more sensitive than those who are not. This hypersensitivity may exist before the use of drugs, and may contribute to their initial drug use, or could result from the impact of chronic drug abuse on the brain. Studies have demonstrated that the nervous system of those who are addicted is hypersensitive to chemically-induced stress and, therefore, an addict may use drugs like heroin, morphine, and cocaine to alleviate the noxious aspects of the stress experience. But the constant on-and-off switching of the stress systems in the body when withdrawal begins heightens any hypersensitivity the person already may have had before starting to take drugs (Stocker, 1999).

In the case of self-mutilation it is important to consider what part of the body the person is hurting and why that might be. As a form of traumatic re-enactment, those who have been traumatised frequently wound themselves at the same real or symbolic place that their perpetrator hurt them. The visible gashes, burns and scars are bodily expressions of a much deeper inward pain that is visible only to the sufferer, but for whom any association with the experiences of the past is not usually consciously available. In their desperate and largely unconscious attempt to communicate their distress to the world that lies beyond the boundary of their skin, they re-enact the trauma by inflicting more trauma upon themselves. They have learned that if they hurt their bodies they will experience a temporary relief from a noxious state of hyperarousal and acute distress, or numbed emptiness, probably mediated chemically by the endorphins that are released whenever the stress response is mobilised.

Clinical reports consistently show that those who self-harm and suffer from addictions have childhood histories of physical or sexual abuse and/or other kinds of trauma, and that the earlier and more extensive the abuse or neglect, the more likely their aggression would be turned toward self-harming behaviour. In circumstances of betrayal trauma, when children are violated by the same person upon whom they are dependent for survival, it creates for many children and adults a major barrier to recovery (Freyd, 1996).

Risky behaviour and addiction to trauma

The endorphins produced by human bodies are not just painkillers. They reduce anxiety, rage, depression, and fear. They are vital to attachment behaviour from birth to death. They increase when social support increases and decrease when social support is withdrawn. Lack of early care in animals effectively reduces endorphins and may do so in people as well. Not surprisingly, given their powerful analgesic and calming effects, large amounts of endorphins are released as an integral part of the fight-or-flight response (Van der Kolk et al., 1985; Van der Kolk and Greenberg, 1987; Bremner et al., 1993; Van der Kolk, 1996b). It is particularly important to understand what happens to the normal endorphin response when people are exposed to chronic and repeated stress, when brains and bodies are repeatedly exposed to these powerful agents. Along with the other components of the flight–fight–freeze response, stress-induced analgesia has been described in animals following exposure to inescapable shock. In severely stressed animals, signs of opiate withdrawal can be triggered by stopping the stress or by giving the animal a drug that counteracts the effects of the endorphins.

One theory is that some chronically stressed people may become addicted to their own circulating endorphins because of overexposure and impaired regulation of the endorphins because of chronic stress. Whenever the stress is relieved, they feel worse, not better. They go into an opiate withdrawal syndrome that is like heroin withdrawal. They feel anxious, irritable, depressed, and miserable (Van der Kolk et al., 1985). To feel better, they must do something to get their endorphin level back up, and that means doing something stressful. What they end up doing is determined by what works, their own experience, and their own inclinations (Stanley et al., 2010).

Violence is "exciting" and stressful, and repeated violent acting out, gang behaviour, fighting, bullying, stealing, breaking and entering, and many other forms of criminal activity have the additional side effect of producing high levels of stress in people who have grown addicted to such risk-taking behaviour. Many people appear to seek out high-risk jobs or forms of recreation and talk about the "high" they feel, even while risking their lives. Others become addicted to sexual behaviours, some of which may involve potentially dangerous sadistic or masochistic behaviours. An important element of risk-taking involves control: whilst undertaking these behaviours, people can overcome and defeat helplessness by taking control.

Revictimisation and trauma-bonding

One of the two key survival strategies common to the human species are caretaking and attachment (Valent, 2007). When the person to whom one has become attached is also the source of danger, the result is increased attachment to the abusing person. This is called "trauma-bonding" and is part of the complicated picture for battered spouses, abused children, prisoners and victims of torture, hostages, and any other situation in which the abuse is prolonged and repeated (Herman, 1992).

As a result, highly untrustworthy and destructive relationships come to be considered normal (Dutton and Painter, 1981; Van der Kolk, 1989; Herman, 1992; James, 1994). The natural, innate protective mechanism of turning to people to whom an individual is attached for safety is reversed. If these same persecutors also provide intermittent nurturance in the form of food, shelter, relief from pain, or even affection, then the situation is even more confusing, cognitively, emotionally, and at a basic biological adaptive level. The combined effects of chronic hyperarousal, dissociation, and tend-and-befriend can help make sense of the otherwise confusing signs associated with captivity and the likelihood that captives will affiliate with their captors, known as the "Stockholm Syndrome". It has become clear that the traumatised person's pre-existing personality is not a major factor in explaining this behaviour, it is instead a result of the experience of helpless, prolonged captivity (LaViolette and Barnett, 2000; Bloom, 2009).

From victimisation to victimiser

Many perpetrators of criminal violence have had serious childhood traumatic experiences. This population is less well-studied because they do not present frequently to psychiatric services, they do not elicit sympathy from others, and they do not tend to be compliant with treatment or research. Gilligan, after spending much of his professional career working with violent offenders, has stated, "The violent criminals I have known have been objects of violence from early childhood" (Gilligan, 1996: p.45). In such cases, their early experiences have done such damage to them that they have become detached from other humans, and they have become incapable of empathy, often on a permanent basis. Because they are so severely impaired in their capacity to form and maintain attachment bonds, they are unable to attach to other people, or to a civilised system of laws and beliefs. They are unable to love and care for life other than their own, and even their capacity to love and respect themselves is severely impaired or missing on all levels other than that of pure survival (Strueber et al., 2007). It is very possible, and by clinical experience probable, that the damage done to some of these children in early childhood is irreversible by any means presently known to psychiatric science.

The challenge of habits

Traumatised people cope as best they can, as in the multiple ways described above, and the immediate survival responses can pose problems of their own. People are, after all, creatures of habit. Much of what is done each day is based on habits. Life would be unendurable if every day, in every way, all was brand-new. This tendency to form habits easily, to repeat behaviours and thought patterns that have guaranteed survival, constitute a way to order existence and make sense of the world. Forming habits is the brain's way of calming itself down. Making behavioural routines automatically saves valuable energy. The problem is that once a behavioural routine becomes a habit, it is governed by a part of the brain that is beyond conscious control known as the basal ganglia (Duhigg, 2012).

This may be the reason why changing habits is so difficult, and why habit change is so clinically challenging. The more powerfully life-saving the reason for the habit, the more anxiety victims experience if they try to alter that habit. Any attempt to alter or eradicate habits can lead people to re-experience the initial fear that created the need for the habitual routine in the first place. The strength of the fear will influence the strength of the habit. This creates the seemingly paradoxical symptom of hurt people who are unable to stop hurting themselves.

Personality distortions in response to trauma

To early workers such as Freud and Janet, it became obvious that traumatic experience had the effect of halting development.

> Unable to integrate the traumatic memories, they seem to have lost their capacity to assimilate new experiences as well. It is … as if their personality definitely stopped at a certain point and cannot enlarge any more by the addition or assimilation of new elements.
>
> (Van der Kolk and Van der Hart, 1989: p.1533)

The personality development of those who have been traumatised does not really stop, but it can certainly become distorted, veered away from a healthy trajectory and onto a new and often more destructive course. This change in life trajectory can occur to virtually anyone if the circumstances are sufficiently injurious. But when the traumatic experience occurs in childhood or adolescence, before the personality has fully developed, the person is more likely to develop severe personality problems; this might lead to the development of any of the Personality Disorders, or even Multiple Personality Disorder (Herman et al., 1989; Perry et al., 1990; Herman, 1992), now referred to as Dissociative Identity Disorder. The complexity of posttraumatic developmental challenges in these cases is best understood as Complex PTSD characterised by: alterations in ability to modulate emotions, alterations of identity and sense of self, alterations in ongoing consciousness and memory, alterations in relations with the perpetrator, alterations in relations with others, alterations in physical and medical status, and alterations in systems of meaning (Herman, 1992; Cloitre et al., 2011, 2013; Courtois and Ford, 2013; Ford and Courtois, 2013, 2014).

Intergenerational transmission and epigenetics

Intergenerational trauma has been best studied in research on the offspring of Holocaust survivors (Freyberg, 1980; Kestenberg, 1980; Sigal, 1989; Danieli, 1997). The effect has been concisely summarised in these words, "The children of survivors show symptoms which would be expected if they actually lived through the Holocaust" (Barocas and Barocas, 1979: p.331). War experience has also shown to be problematic for the next generation. It has been noted repeatedly that many of the symptoms of PTSD have a severe, ongoing, and disruptive effect on marital and family life (Figley and Sprenkle, 1978; Rosenheck, 1986; Matsakis, 1988). Studies on the intergenerational transmission of child maltreatment show extensive evidence that parents who were maltreated are more likely than non-maltreated parents to abuse their own children. About one-third of parents who were abused as children continue a pattern of seriously inept, neglectful, or abusive parenting. One-third do not. Another third remains vulnerable to the effects of social stress and are more likely to become abusive under such influences (Oliver, 1993).

This intergenerational transmission happens in various ways. A growing body of evidence demonstrates that one mechanism is through the attachment relationship. Mothers who have been rejected by their mothers tend to be rejecting of their own infants (Main and Goldwyn, 1984). In a large study of the intergenerational transmission of corporal punishment, social learning, passed from one generation to the next, appeared to be the most important factor (Muller et al., 1995), although the effect of establishing a family norm which then gets passed on from one generation to the next may also play a role (Simons and Wurtele, 2010). Other research focuses on the damage that child abuse does to the brain which interferes with normal parenting of the next generation (Teicher et al., 1993).

It is now thought that there are two modes of genetic change. One is slow and a result of natural selection, and another is more rapid and responsive to environmental changes. The epigenetic markers serve the latter system and are thought to influence the intergenerational transmission of trauma in ways that science is only just beginning to understand (National Scientific Council on the Developing Child, 2010). Research is now beginning to accumulate evidence showing how environmental cues can stimulate epigenetic changes that could contribute to many medical and psychiatric problems (Steinberg, 2006). There is a growing scientific consensus that the nature versus nurture controversy is over, and that nature and nurture are complexly interactive.

Moral and group responses to danger

Destroying the assumptive world

People who suffer profound trauma may no longer feel that they are alive. Instead, they feel like, "Zombies, the walking dead wandering in the wilderness". Trauma sets people outside the bounds of the normal human community (Bloom, 2013: p.76). Most people can get out of bed and leave the house in the morning because they make basic and unconscious assumptions that the world is safe and meaningful, and that one can function adequately in it (Janoff-Bulman, 1992). They assume that there is benevolence in the world around justice and meaning, and comfort from others allows people to go through their daily lives, do their work, tend to their families, and have reasonable expectations of what tomorrow will bring. Most people rarely if ever think about these underlying assumptions because they are premises that are just taken for granted.

Trauma shatters these assumptions upon which people's sense of safety and freedom in the world is based. The world may be perceived as no longer meaningful, or kind, and themselves as worthless, helpless, and hopeless (Janoff-Bulman, 1992). If this happens when one is a child it may sabotage the development of moral intelligence, which is the central intelligence for all human beings that binds us to our social group, culture, and moral system, and defines how our other forms of intelligence are used to give our lives purpose and meaning (Lennick and Kiel, 2005).

Many victims of trauma also come to believe that they are not worthy, because if they were, the trauma would not have occurred. They become deeply ashamed of whatever imagined fault has caused the trauma to have befallen them and stolen from them a sense of mastery. When other people scapegoat them it is a further confirmation of their blameworthiness. Burdened by such a sense of shame, sufferers often cast themselves into the wilderness, outside of the realm of human community.

For people who have held firm religious or spiritual beliefs, traumatic experiences may also shatter their faith. Abuse suffered at the hands of others may pose significant difficulties with the issues of forgiveness, particularly if there is no real remorse on the part of the perpetrator. Whatever a person's belief system is preceding a traumatic event, they will inevitably question the previous foundations of their moral existence and must search for meaning to make some sense of what has happened to them.

Group affiliation, xenophobia, and moral injury

Humans are the most social of all species and our individual existence emerged out of our primary group identities. There is then a social response to danger that historically preceded our individual responses. When danger is signalled, people who are attached to each other feel compelled to draw together. This makes sense from an evolutionary perspective, because human safety is so dependent on the protection of the group. This behaviour originates in the infant–mother bond, and proximity-seeking behaviour on the part of both is innate. This increased attachment behaviour in the face of danger or threat and in the service of survival has been noted in all social species. We learn as children that safety is to be found in the protection of others and, therefore, whenever fear is aroused, children and adults seek protection from others. But under such circumstances, humans also become more obedient and more open to suggestion, including the suggestions of charismatic leaders (Eibl-Eibesfeldt, 1989; Schumaker, 1995).

In situations of danger, the sense of stranger anxiety also increases, and bonding to an "in-group" escalates, along with the perception of threat from an out-group, a phenomenon known as xenophobia. The behaviour of other people has a significant effect on the behavioural responses of everyone to situations of danger. This relational aspect of dangerous situations has been studied intensively by the military. It is well-recognised that people tend to come together to seek aid and comfort. This finding has been borne out in field studies of infantry platoons, air crews, and disaster control teams, as well as through social psychological experiments with college students (Janis, 1972). This heightened need for affiliation leads to greater dependency on the group and an enhanced tendency to conform to group norms, even when they contradict one's own individual norms. In seminal work on World War II, it was noted that,

> The impersonal threat of injury from the enemy, affecting all alike, produces a high degree of cohesion so that personal attachments throughout the unit become intensified. Friendships are easily made by those who might never have been compatible at home and are cemented under fire. Out of the mutually shared hardships and dangers are born an altruism and generosity that transcend ordinary individual selfish interest.
>
> (Grinker and Spiegel, 1945: p.21)

This group affiliative behaviour may however place people in highly compromising moral situations. The term "moral injury" was first used by Shay as a descriptor for some of the profound experiences of combat veterans who experience a betrayal of what is right in a high-stakes situation by someone who holds power (Shay, 2003). But all people who have been intentionally hurt by others upon whom they must depend contend with the abuse of power that inevitably is a part of the sense of fundamental betrayal, while their normal need to affiliate may lead them to be influenced by highly destructive and even dangerous groups. Moral injury when it occurs in childhood may influence moral preferences away from altruism and mutuality and toward self-protection and self-interest (Bloom, 2017).

Conclusion – posttraumatic growth, the survivor mission, and trauma transformation

A traumatic experience, by definition, changes people. What is inspiring about the human species is how so many survivors struggle to make sense out of violence, transcending its effects, and transforming the energy of violence into something powerfully good for themselves and for their communities, developing what Herman has called "a survivor mission" (Herman, 1992). It is often a mission that encompasses the remainder of one's life. Confrontation with the spiritual, philosophical, and/or religious context – and conflicts – of human experience is impossible to avoid if recovery is to be ascertained.

With so much trauma worldwide and the innate human tendency toward xenophobia and violence, and the enormously complex problems that face humans as a species, there is a need to think about ways that larger groups of people can have transformative experiences. The author Tina Rosenberg has studied traumatised populations in Latin American and Eastern Europe and has stated, "Nations, like individuals, need to face up to and understand traumatic past events before they can put them aside and move on to normal life" (Rosenberg, 1995: p.xviii). But how does a group overcome the powerful dynamic pull of traumatic re-enactment to transform the trauma into something better for the group and the individuals within the group? Individuals and groups have searched throughout time for the means to turn adversity into strength. An individual's personal traumatic experience can serve as the basis for the creation and transformation of a group when the traumatised individual serves as the inspirational leader for the group. Alternatively, a group trauma occurs and must be transformed for the group-as-a-whole, frequently through the mediation or inspiration of a leader who arises out of the group and becomes the delegate for the group, giving voice to the conscious and unconscious aspirations of the group. Additionally, the witnessed traumatisation of others can cause a group response, even when the trauma has not been experienced directly by the group members. The interaction between the individual and the group, the leader and the led, is an interactive, dynamic one in which all of these elements can be found (Bloom, 1998).

There are many ways that human groups, led by inspiring leaders, have transformed traumatic personal and political experience into movements that change the world for the better, whether they are bearing witness to awful events and seeking justice; or rescuing people, animals, or the Earth; or providing mutual self-help; or doing what they can to educate and prevent more tragedy; or taking political action to stop extremist and destructive political behaviour: they all represent examples of positive transformation. But they all appear to have at least one thing in common – a sense of moral commitment, a sense that personal and group trauma must be converted into a community asset, not just a personal asset or catastrophe.

From such traumatic origins springs the co-construction or reconstruction of civilisation. In this sense, there is a "moral maturity" about these transformations. Trauma transformations hinge upon a moral position that is often implicit, but which is the guiding hand in such social transformations, and individuals who epitomise this moral position become the "moral exemplars" for entire cultural systems (Damon and Colby, 2015). This moral position hinges on a generalised sense of respect, compassion, and concern for all life, and a willingness to risk one's self-interest for the sake of these values. Ultimately, all positive transformation is rooted in the attempt to make sense out of inherently senseless acts of violence. The transformation of trauma is not a possible option, it is a moral necessity; we cannot heal as individuals or as groups, or as a species, without striving for something more whole, more loving, and more ethically coherent than our individual selves.

References

Alford JD, Mahone C and Fielstein EM (1988) Cognitive and behavioral sequelae of combat: Conceptualization and implications for treatment. *Journal of Traumatic Stress* 1 (4): 489–501.

Anda RF, Butchart A, Felitti VJ, et al. (2010) Building a framework for global surveillance of the public health implications of Adverse Childhood Experiences. *American Journal of Preventive Medicine* 39: 93–98.

Artwhol A (2002) Perceptual and memory distortion during officer-involved shootings. *FBI Law Enforcement Bulletin* 71: 18–24.

Barocas H and Barocas C (1979) Wounds of fathers: The next generation of holocaust survivors. *International Review Psychoanalysis* 6: 331–340.

Bloom SL (1998) By the crowd they have been broken, by the crowd they shall be healed: The social transformation of trauma. In: Tedeschi R, Park C and Calhoun L (eds) *Post-Traumatic Growth: Theory and Research on Change in the Aftermath of Crises*. Mahwah, NJ: Lawrence Erlbaum, pp.179–213.

Bloom SL (2009) Domestic violence. In: O'Brien P (ed) *Encyclopedia of Gender and Violence*. Thousand Oaks, CA: Sage, pp.216–221.

Bloom SL (2010) Bridging the black hole of trauma: The evolutionary significance of the arts, Part 1. *Psychotherapy and Politics International* 8: 198–212.

Bloom SL (2011) Bridging the black hole of trauma: The evolutionary necessity of the arts. Part 2: The arts and evolution – what is art for? *Psychotherapy and Politics International* 9: 67–82.

Bloom SL (2013) *Creating Sanctuary: Toward the Evolution of Sane Societies, Revised Edition*. New York, NY: Routledge.

Bloom SL (2017) The Sanctuary Model: Through the lens of moral safety. In: Cook J, Dalenberg CJ and Gold S (eds) *Handbook of Trauma Psychology*. Washington, D.C.: American Psychological Association, pp.499–513.

Bremner J, Southwick S, Johnson D, et al. (1993) Childhood physical abuse and combat-related posttraumatic stress disorder in Vietnam veterans. *American Journal of Psychiatry* 150: 235–239.

Bremner JD, Krystal H, Southwick SM, et al. (1995) Functional neuroanatomical correlates of the effects of stress on memory. *Journal of Traumatic Stress* 8: 527–553.

Brewin CR (2011) The nature and significance of memory disturbance in Posttraumatic Stress Disorder. *Annual Review of Clinical Psychology* 7: 203–227.

Carlson V, Cicchetti D, Barnett D, et al. (1989) Disorganized/disoriented attachment relationships in maltreated infants. *Developmental Psychology* 25: 525–531.

Cloitre M, Courtois CA, Charuvastra A, et al. (2011) Treatment of Complex PTSD: Results of the ISTSS expert clinician survey on best practices. *Journal of Traumatic Stress* 24: 615–627.

Cloitre M, Garvert DW, Brewin CR, et al. (2013) Evidence for proposed ICD-11 PTSD and Complex PTSD: A latent profile analysis. *European Journal of Psychotraumatology* 4(1): 20706–20712.

Coates D, Wortman CB and Abben A (1979) Reactions to victims. In: Frieze IH, Bar-Tal D and Carroll JC (eds) *New Approaches to Social Problems: Applications of Attribution Theory*. San Francisco, CA: Jossey Bass: pp.21–52.

Courtois CA and Ford JD (2013) *The Treatment of Complex Trauma: A Sequenced, Relationship-Based Approach*. New York, NY: Guilford.

Damon W and Colby A (2015) *The Power of Ideals: The Real Story of Moral Choice*. New York, NY: Oxford University Press.

Danieli Y (ed) (1997) *International Handbook of Multigenerational Legacies of Trauma*. New York, NY: Plenum Press.

Donald M (1991) *Origins of the Modern Mind: Three Stages in the Evolution of Culture and Cognition*. Cambridge, MA: Harvard University Press.

Duhigg C (2012) *The Power of Habit: Why We Do What We Do in Life and Business*. New York, NY: Random House.

Dutton D and Painter S (1981) Traumatic bonding: The development of emotional attachments in battered women and other relationships of intermittent abuse. *Victimology: An International Journal* 6: 139–155.

Eibl-Eibesfeldt I (1989) *Human Ethology*. New York, NY: Aldine de Gruyter.

Epstein S (1994) The integration of the cognitive and psychodynamic unconscious. *American Psychologist* 49: 709–723.

Figley CR and Sprenkle DH (1978) Delayed stress response syndrome: Family therapy indications. *Journal of Marital and Family Therapy* 4: 53–60.

Ford JD and Courtois CA (2013) *Treating Complex Traumatic Stress Disorders in Children and Adolescents: An Evidence-Based Guide*. New York, NY: Guilford.

Ford JD and Courtois CA (2014) Complex PTSD, affect dysregulation, and Borderline Personality Disorder. *Borderline Personality Disorder and Emotion Dysregulation* 1: 9.

Freyberg J (1980) Difficulties in separation-individuation as experienced by offspring of Nazi Holocaust survivors. *American Journal of Orthopsychiatry* 50: 87–95.

Freyd JJ (1996) *Betrayal Trauma: The Logic of Forgetting Childhood Abuse*. Cambridge, MA: Harvard University Press.

Garbarino J (1999) *Lost Boys: Why Our Sons Turn Violent and How We Can Save Them*. New York, NY: The Free Press.

Gilbertson MW, Gurvits TV, Lasko NB, et al. (2001) Multivariate assessment of explicit memory function in combat veterans with Posttraumatic Stress Disorder. *Journal of Traumatic Stress* 14: 413–432.

Gilligan J (1996) *Violence: Our Deadly Epidemic and its Causes*. New York, NY: GP Putnam's Sons.

Goleman D (1995) *Emotional Intelligence: Why It Can Matter More Than IQ*. New York, NY: Bantam Books.

Grinker RR and Spiegel JP (1945) *War Neuroses*. Philadelphia, PA: The Blakiston Company.

Grossman D and Christiansen L (2008) *On Combat: The Psychology and Physiology of Deadly Conflict in War and in Peace*. Millstadt, IL: Warrior Science Publications.

Harber KD and Pennebaker JW (1992) Overcoming traumatic memories. In: Christianson SA (ed) *The Handbook of Emotion and Memory: Research and Theory*. Hillsdale, NJ: Lawrence Erlbaum, pp.359–387.

Herman J (1992) *Trauma and Recovery*. New York, NY: Basic Books.

Herman JL, Perry JC and Van der Kolk BA (1989) Childhood trauma in borderline personality disorder. *American Journal of Psychiatry* 146: 490–495.

James B (1994) *Handbook for Treatment of Attachment Trauma Problems in Children*. New York, NY: Lexington Books.

Janis IL (1972) *Victims of Groupthink: A Psychological Study of Foreign-Policy Decisions and Fiascoes*. Boston, MA: Houghton Mifflin Company.

Janis IL (1982) Decision making under stress. In: Goldberger L and Breznitz S (eds) *Handbook of Stress: Theoretical and Clinical Aspects*. New York, NY: Free Press, pp.69–87.

Janoff-Bulman R (1992) *Shattered Assumptions: Towards a New Psychology of Trauma*. New York, NY: Free Press.

Joseph R (1992) *The Right Brain and the Unconscious: Discovering the Stranger Within*. New York, NY: Plenum.

Joseph R (2012) *The Right Brain and the Limbic Unconscious: Emotion, Forgotten Memories, Self-Deception, Bad Relationships*. Electronic publication: University Press Science Publishers.

Kestenberg J (1980) Psychoanalysis of children of survivors from the Holocaust: Case presentations and assessment. *Journal of the American Psychoanalytic Association* 28: 775–804.

Krystal H (1978) Trauma and affects. *Psychoanalytic Study of the Child* 33: 81–116.

Krystal H (1988) *Integration and Self Healing: Affect, Trauma, Alexithymia.* Hillsdale, NJ: Analytic Press.

Lanius RA, Williamson PC, Bluhm RL, et al. (2005) Functional connectivity of dissociative responses in posttraumatic stress disorder: A functional magnetic resonance imaging investigation. *Biological Psychiatry* 57: 873–884.

LaViolette AD and Barnett OW (2000) *It Could Happen to Anyone: Why Battered Women Stay, Second Edition.* Thousand Oaks, CA: Sage Publications.

LeDoux J (1994) Emotion, memory, and the brain. *Scientific American* 270: 50–57.

LeDoux J (1996) *The Emotional Brain: The Mysterious Underpinnings of Emotional Life.* New York, NY: Simon and Schuster.

LeDoux J (2002) *Synaptic Self: How Our Brains Become Who We Are.* New York, NY: Viking.

LeDoux JE (1992) Emotion as memory: Anatomical systems underlying indelible neural trances. In: Christianson SA (ed) *The Handbook of Emotion and Memory: Research and Theory.* Hillsdale, NJ: Lawrence Erlbaum Associates: pp.269–288.

Lennick D and Kiel F (2005) *Moral Intelligence: Enhancing Business Performance and Leadership Success.* Upper Saddle River, NJ: Wharton School Publishing.

Levine P (1997) *Waking the Tiger: Healing Trauma: The Innate Capacity to Transform Overwhelming Experiences.* New York, NY: North Atlantic Books.

Lumley MA and Norman S (1996) Alexithymia and health care utilization. *Psychosomatic Medicine* 58: 197–202.

Main M and Goldwyn R (1984) Predicting rejection of her infant from mother's representation of her own experience: Implications for the abused-abusing intergenerational cycle. *Child Abuse and Neglect* 8: 203–217.

Matsakis A (1988) *Vietnam Wives: Women and Children Surviving Life with Veterans Suffering Posttraumatic Stress Disorder.* Kensington, MD: Woodbine House.

McEwen BS (2012) Brain on stress: How the social environment gets under the skin. *Proceedings of the National Academy of Sciences* 109: 17180–17185.

McGilchrist I (2009) *The Master and His Emissary: The Divided Brain and the Making of the Western World.* New Haven, CT: Yale University Press.

McGilchrist I (2012) *The Divided Brain and the Search for Meaning: Why Are We So Unhappy?* New Haven, CT: Yale University Press.

Monroe SM and Harkness KL (2005) Life stress, the "kindling" hypothesis, and the recurrence of depression: Considerations from a life stress perspective. *Psychological Review* 112: 417–445.

Muller RT, Hunter JE and Stollak G (1995) The intergenerational transmission of corporal punishment: A comparison of social learning and temperament models. *Child Abuse and Neglect* 19: 1323–1335.

National Scientific Council on the Developing Child (2010) *Early Experiences Can Alter Gene Expression and Affect Long-Term Development.* Working Paper No. 10. Available at: developingchild.net.

National Institute on Drug Abuse (2002) *Stress and Substance Abuse: A Special Report.* Available at: nida.nih.gov/stressanddrugabuse.html.

Oliver J (1993) Intergenerational transmission of child abuse: Rates, research, and clinical implications. *American Journal of Psychiatry* 150: 1315–1324.

Perry BD and Pate JE (1994) Neurodevelopment and the psychobiological roots of post-traumatic stress disorder. In: Koziol L and Stout C (eds) *In the Neuropsychology of Mental Disorders: A Practical Guide*. Springfield, IL: Charles C Thomas, pp.81–98.

Perry JC, Herman JL, Van der Kolk BA, et al. (1990) Psychotherapy and psychological trauma in borderline personality disorder. *Psychiatric Annals* 20(1): 33–43.

Rauch SL, Van der Kolk BA, Fisler RE, et al. (1996) A symptom provocation study of posttraumatic stress disorder using positron emission tomography and script-drive imagery. *Archives of General Psychiatry* 53: 380–387.

Rosenberg T (1995) *The Haunted Land: Facing Europe's Ghosts After Communism*. New York, NY: Vintage Books.

Rosenheck R (1986) Impact of post-traumatic stress disorder of World War II on the next generation. *Journal of Nervous and Mental Disease* 174: 319–327.

Saar-Ashkenazy R, Cohen JE, Guez J, et al. (2014) Reduced corpus-callosum volume in Posttraumatic Stress Disorder highlights the importance of interhemispheric connectivity for associative memory. *Journal of Traumatic Stress* 27(1): 18–26.

Santayana G (2017) *The Life of Reason*. New York, NY: Open Road Integrated Media.

Sapolsky RM (1998) *Why Zebras Don't Get Ulcers: An Updated Guide to Stress, Stress-related Disease, and Coping*. New York, NY: WH Freeman and Company.

Sashin J (1993) Duke Ellington: The creative process and the ability to experience and tolerate affect. In: Ablon SL, Brown D, Khantzian EJ, et al. (eds) *Human Feelings: Explorations in Affect Development and Meaning*. Hillsdale, NJ: The Analytic Press: pp.317–332.

Scaer RC (2001) The neurophysiology of dissociation and chronic disease. *Applied Psychophysiology and Biofeedback* 26: 73–91.

Schiffer F, Teicher MH and Papanicolaou AC (1995) Evoked potential evidence for right brain activity during the recall of traumatic memories. *Journal of Neuropsychiatry and Clinical Neuroscience* 7: 169–175.

Schore A (2017) Modern attachment theory. In: Gold SN (ed) *APA Handbook of Trauma Psychology*. Washington, D.C.: American Psychological Association, Volume 2, pp.389–406.

Schumaker JF (1995) *The Corruption of Reality: A Unified Theory of Religion, Hypnosis, and Psychopathology*. Amherst, NY: Prometheus Books.

Shay J (2003) *Odysseus in America: Combat Trauma and the Trials of Homecoming*. New York, NY: Scribner.

Shonkoff JP, Garner AS, Siegel BS, et al. (2012a) The lifelong effects of early childhood adversity and toxic stress. *Pediatrics* 129: e232–e246.

Shonkoff JP, Richter L, van der Gaag J, et al. (2012b) An integrated scientific framework for child survival and early childhood development. *Pediatrics* 129: e460–e472.

Sigal J (1989) *Trauma and Rebirth: Intergenerational Effects of the Holocaust*. New York, NY: Praeger.

Simons DA and Wurtele SK (2010) Relationships between parents' use of corporal punishment and their children's endorsement of spanking and hitting other children. *Child Abuse & Neglect* 34(9): 639–646.

Southwick SM, Bremner D, Krystal JH, et al. (1994) Psychobiologic research in post-traumatic stress disorder. *Psychiatric Clinics of North America* 17: 251–264.

Squire LR (1987) *Memory and the Brain*. New York, NY: Oxford University Press.

Stanley B, Sher L, Wilson S, et al. (2010) Non-suicidal self-injurious behavior, endogenous opioids and monoamine neurotransmitters. *Journal of Affective Disorders* 124: 134–140.

Steinberg D (2006) Determining nature vs. nurture. *Scientific American Mind* 17: 12–14.

Stocker S (1999) Studies link stress and drug addiction. *National Institute on Drug Abuse Notes: Research Findings* 14(1): 12–14.

Strueber D, Lueck M and Roth G (2007) The Violent Brain. *Scientific American Mind* 17: 20–27.

Taylor SE (2006) Tend and befriend. *Current Directions in Psychological Science* 15: 273–277.

Taylor SE, Klein LC, Lewis BP, et al. (2000) Female responses to stress: Tend-and-befriend, not fight-or-flight. *Psychological Review* 107: 411–429.

Teicher MH, Glod CA, Surrey J, et al. (1993) Early childhood abuse and limbic system ratings in adult psychiatric outpatients. *Journal of Neuropsychiatry and Clinical Neurosciences* 5: 301–306.

Teicher MH, Ito Y, Glod CA, et al. (1997) Preliminary evidence for abnormal cortical development in physically and sexually abused children using EEG coherence and MRI. *Annals of the New York Academy of Sciences* 821: 160–175.

Teicher MH, Andersen SL, Dumont NL, et al. (2000) Childhood neglect attentuates development of the corpus callosum. *Society of Neuroscience Abstracts* 26: 549.

Valent P (2007) Eight survival strategies in traumatic stress. *Traumatology* 13: 4–14.

Van der Kolk BA (1989) The compulsion to repeat the trauma: Reenactment, revictimization, and masochism. *Psychiatric Clinics of North America* 12: 389–411.

Van der Kolk BA (1994) The body keeps the score: Memory and the evolving psychobiology of posttraumatic stress. *Harvard Review of Psychiatry* 1: 253–265.

Van der Kolk BA (1996a) Trauma and memory. In: Van der Kolk B, McFarlane A and Weisaeth L (eds) *Traumatic Stress: The Effects of Overwhelming Experience on Mind, Body and Society*. New York, NY: Guilford Press, pp.279–302.

Van der Kolk BA (1996b) The body keeps the score: Approaches to the psychobiology of posttraumatic stress disorder. In: Van der Kolk B, McFarlane A and Weisaeth L (eds) *Traumatic Stress: The Effects of Overwhelming Experience on Mind, Body and Society*. New York, NY: Guilford Press, pp.214–241.

Van der Kolk BA (2000) Posttraumatic stress disorder and the nature of trauma. *Dialogues in Clinical Neuroscience* 2: 7–22.

Van der Kolk BA and Ducey CP (1989) The psychological processing of traumatic experience: Rorschach patterns in PTSD. *Journal of Traumatic Stress* 2: 259–274.

Van der Kolk BA and Fisler R (1995) Dissociation and the fragmentary nature of traumatic memories: Overview and exploratory study. *Journal of Traumatic Stress* 8: 505–525.

Van der Kolk BA and Greenberg M (1987) The psychobiology of the trauma response: Hyperarousal, constriction, and addiction to traumatic reexposure. In: Van der Kolk B (ed) *Psychological Trauma*. Washington, D.C.: American Psychiatric Press, pp.63–88.

Van der Kolk BA and Van der Hart O (1989) Pierre Janet and the breakdown of adaptation in psychological trauma. *American Journal of Psychiatry* 146: 1530–1540.

Van der Kolk BA and Van der Hart O (1991) The intrusive past: The flexibility of memory and the engraving of trauma. *American Imago* 48: 425–454.

Van der Kolk BA, Burbridge JA and Suzuki J (1997) The psychobiology of traumatic memory: Clinical implications of neuroimaging studies. *Annals New York Academy of Sciences* 821: 99–113.

Van der Kolk BA, Greenberg M, Boyd H, et al. (1985) Inescapable shock, neurotransmitters, and addiction to trauma: Toward a psychobiology of posttraumatic stress. *Biological Psychiatry* 20(3): 314–325.

Verma R, Balhara Y and Gupta C (2011) Gender differences in stress response: Role of developmental and biological determinants. *Industrial Psychiatry Journal* 20: 4–10.
Wang J, Korczykowski M, Rao H, et al. (2007) Gender difference in neural response to psychological stress. *Social Cognitive and Affective Neuroscience* 2: 227–239.

2 The interpersonal construction of the human brain–mind system

Russell Meares

Introduction

This chapter is about relational trauma and its effect upon the development of self. Relational traumata are of immense importance. They are an aspect not only of nearly every clinical encounter but also of daily life. Most people will have had an experience, a moment of misery perhaps, a wave of desolation, or merely a flicker of such a state, triggered by something said or remembered. The moment usually passes. In some people, however, it does not. It is magnified and long-lasting, upsetting personal relations and overthrowing the ordinary feeling of the flow of existence. The following is an example.

A middle-aged couple, whose grown-up children have left home, take turns in the evening to cook and set the table. On the first night, the woman, Albina, is cooking. She says, "Why don't we use the new tablecloth?". "OK," her husband replies, and changes the cloth. The next night the husband is cooking. He says, "Why don't we use the other knives?". She erupts, "Do you think I am so stupid that I can't even set a table?". Mystified by her vehemence, the husband responds angrily. Soon they are fighting (Meares, 2000: p.53).

She has a past of relational trauma, a family milieu in which, day after day, she could expect belittling and criticism. In this incident, ordinary consciousness is overtaken by an unconscious traumatic memory system (UTMS), triggered by her husband's suggestion which she interprets as criticism. She does not realise she is in the grip of the past. She is unaware of the origin of her vehemence and locates it in the present. Her unconsciousness is not usefully conceived as the outcome of repression, a point which will be more fully explored.

Types of relational trauma

Early studies of the effects of trauma concerned survivors of events such as combat, earthquakes, bushfires and so forth, including, more recently, motor vehicle accidents. Terror was an important aspect of these life-threatening experiences. A realisation began to develop however that sexual and physical abuse, although they might also involve terror, were not in the same category of traumatic disruption. They involve an additional component which adds to their degree of pathogenicity and the complexity of their symptomology; the social context in which these inflictions occur is also part of the trauma. Physical abuse, for example, involves not only pain and fear, but also humiliation. Sexual abuse damages that which is at the core of self, a centre of feeling sometimes called the "tender emotions". To some degree or other, relational traumata are attacks upon humanity.

The sense of "value" at the core of self is a main casualty of relational trauma. "Attacks upon value" have a malign effect, whether or not they are an aspect of physical or sexual abuse. They range in degrees of severity from the apparently well-meaning, as in the case of Albina, to the actively devaluing, and finally to the vicious. In Albina's case, the family environment was intended to be instructional, and to "help" her in not becoming "big-headed". Other developmental contexts involving, for example, derision, ridicule, and systematic devaluation are more destructive. The vicious extreme is clearly abusive. "Slut," "ugly slut," "stupid bitch" are examples of epithets heaped upon the victim.

Even in the least harmful of this range of attacks there is mingled another fundamental relational trauma, separation fear. So small a negative expression as the raised eyebrow of the critical parent may be enough to set off a tremor in the child, a fear that the essential bond with the attachment figure has been lost. More severe breaks may arouse a fear greater than that produced by physical abuse.

Finally, there is a form of relational trauma which occurs very early in life. Increasing evidence suggests that it may be extremely destructive. It arises through repeated disruptions of the sense of union and connection between the infant and caregiver, usually the mother, which is necessary to the baby's sense of existing. In early life, the ordinary interplay between mother and child is a game that Colwyn Trevarthen called a "proto-conversation" (Trevarthen, 1974). It has a subtle rhythm which constitutes the infant's state of being. It depends upon a series of responses from the mother which picture, in the "shape" of the sound of her voice and the features of her face, the baby's immediate experience. When these responses are grossly out of kilter with the baby's personal reality at that moment, they "have an impact on the child rather like that of a loud noise" (Stevenson and Meares, 1992: p.358), like a shock. For an instant, the infant is plunged into non-being. It was further proposed that a caregiving environment characterised by a multitude of such "shocks" could be a forerunner of Borderline Personality Disorder. A series of reports from Giovanni Liotti appear to support this hypothesis (Liotti, 2000).

The therapeutic field

When a victim of relational trauma is encountered, a field dominated by two main forces, positive and negative, is entered. The positive drive is towards well-being and "health"; in essence, towards self. The negative and opposing force is that of unconscious traumatic memory, a form of mental life differing in structural terms from the flow of ordinary, healthy, consciousness. The

UTMS has the effect of constantly influencing, intruding upon, or even overthrowing, the potential towards the establishment of the stream of personal existing that William James called "self". The outcome of this conflict is an ongoing state of existence lacking the main features of a healthy selfhood. It is a depleted, stunted condition, with main features of disintegration and constriction. The subject is plagued with a chronic dysphoria, not, in the usual case, publicly evident. This disconnect between affect and expression can be explained by a disconnectedness between neural systems which usually function together in a coordinated manner but which in the cases of repetitive relational trauma may no longer do so (Meares, 2012).

Treatments have tended to focus on the more salient of the two main effects of repetitive trauma, that is, the "storms" of the kind demonstrated by Albina to a minor degree. Relatively little attention has been paid to the self-deficit, and how it might be rectified. Yet in the case of severe repetitive trauma this must be the primary therapeutic target. This is so not only because of the unsatisfactory kind of existence consequent upon this deficit, but also because the UTMS is not properly treated in isolation from this deficit. Some sense of self is necessary to it. The UTMS needs to be transformed so as to be integrated into the larger consciousness of everyday existing. Janet called this process "mental liquidation" (Janet, 1925). In some cases, the "liquidation" may occur without any apparent or systematic processing of UTMS (Meares, 2005).

The tiers of self

In order to conceive a logically devised system of treatment, there is a need to know something of the structure of self and the UTMS. Self can be conceived in terms of functional "layers" which operate together in a cooperative and coordinated way. It is traditional to speak in terms of three such metaphoric tiers, as Hughlings Jackson did (Jackson, 1958). Their nature is illustrated using the development of memory, which, of course, is part of every form of consciousness (Meares, 2012).

The earliest layer is sensorimotor, made up of procedural memory, concerned with motor repertoires, and the perceptual representation system. The latter is a fast, accurate, and atomised mode of processing, a system of rapid recognition of pieces of sensory information which are, as yet, not connected.

The second level, in operation towards the end of the first year of life, is "semantic", to do with meaning. The world of the infant has now become more integrated. Larger organisations of sensory data are recognised and given a meaning. A familiar cupboard, for example, is known to contain toys.

The third layer of self appears late in development and evolution. This kind of consciousness is reflective. It involves an awareness of "inner" events, indicated by access to autobiographical memory when events from long ago can be re-visioned in the "mind's eye". This developmental stage is reached at about the age of four, when the concept of secrecy is discovered (Meares and Orlay, 1988). The child now knows that he or she lives simultaneously in two worlds, one private and the other public. This double consciousness is also indicated in tests of "false belief" in which the child watches a scene in which he or she knows something that the person being watched does not (Wimmer and Perner, 1983).

The capacity to hold in mind two models of reality is of the utmost significance in the evolution of homo sapiens. It enables us to use symbols, of which the archetype is metaphor. In using metaphor, we make one thing have two meanings. We use symbols all the time, hardly aware of what we are doing. Something of the outer world is however "transferred" to an inner state, in order to give it the "visibility" necessary to communication. Symbols, we might say, are the coins of intimacy. With the achievement of dual consciousness, the hominid becomes a human, able to participate in a new form of relatedness, a to-and-fro patterning in which that which is "inner" is exchanged.

The capacity to symbolise has a consequence more immense than the interpersonal. It enables us to create "culture", the vast system which surrounds us, in which we live, and which, in part, creates us (Meares, 2016).

This "reflective" level of mental life does not emerge automatically, without much help from the environment. Scientists concerned with the development of the consciousness peculiar to human beings, for example, Gerald Edelman and Wolf Singer, agree that this late stage in development and evolution depends upon the use of language (Singer, 2001; Edelman, 2004; Meares, 2016). They do not, however, speculate upon the form of this language or how it is to be used. But it can be suggested that what is required is a conversation which has the effect of coordination. Through such means the third tier, which is that of self, is constructed.

Coordinating the tiers

Jackson was the first to develop a plausible neural model of self (Meares, 1999). He believed that self is a hierarchy of function evolved through increasing coordination between the units of brain function. He pointed out that, of course, there are no "tiers", or layers. These are only words used to describe the working of a complex system which – at all times – is operating as a totality, not at discrete levels.

Jackson proposed that the hierarchy develops not through any new kind of tissue being "tacked on" to the brain, but through the elaboration of existing structures. The coordination leading to the late stages of evolution, he said, is particularly dependent upon the enlargement of the prefrontal cortex. The enhanced capacity for inhibitory control consequent upon this development contributes to the finer differentiation in the processing of sensory data which accompanies the integration characteristic of the higher order consciousness.

Self grows as an increased coordination between brain systems. It is accompanied, at each level, by an enhanced capacity for inhibitory control. This enhancement is paralleled by an increase in voluntary control in higher order function. In the function of memory, for example, the most primitive forms are automatic, whereas autobiographical memories can be brought to mind by an effort of will.

Whereas the coordination of the early levels seems to take place with little help from the social world, this is not so for higher order consciousness. Vygotsky considered that the functions of higher order consciousness arise in the context of an interplay between two people (Vygotsky, 1978). The form of the interplay, he proposed, resembles the form of the function which is emergent. The function of consciousness might be seen, however paradoxical and circular this may seem, as coordination. Self is not only constituted by a process of coordination; it is also a manifestation of coordination. As Jackson put it, citing Ribot, "Le moi est une co-ordination" (Jackson, 1958: p.82). The conversation generative of self involves a patterning in which the expressions of the partners in the interplay coordinate with each other, in the manner of analogic resemblance.

Trauma and unconscious traumatic memory

Jackson found that an insult to the brain–mind system causes a retreat in function down the hierarchy decreed by evolutionary history. He called this process "dissolution". It leads to states of consciousness which are essentially disintegrated. Coordination between brain systems is lost so that the various functions that compose the complex of self become disconnected from each other. For example, the system that deals with the bodily aspect of self, its shape, density, kinaesthetics, and so forth, might become separated from the main organisation, leading to an experience in which the body sense floats away, "watching" the self below.

The fine differentiation between elements of consciousness normal to self is lost. The duality of consciousness dwindles. Fundamental distinctions such as those between self and other, past and present, are compromised. Paradoxically, the patient is both disconnected from the therapist and experientially fused with the therapist. The conversation may become confused by an ambiguous use of the word "you". The past is experienced as if it were the present.

Higher order inhibitory functions are lost leading to the "release phenomena" of Hughlings Jackson. That which can be excluded from consciousness for adaptive purposes is no longer excluded. Emotional expression is unmodulated. In this state, actions are automatic. Voluntary control over memory, attention, motivation, and other main functions of self is diminished. The individual no longer has the capacity to roam around in the "spaces" of the past, as in autobiographical memory, nor in those imagined zones yet to come, of the future; the future barely exists. The sense of time passing which Bergson called "durée", is impaired; Bergson considered durée to be the hallmark of the higher order consciousness peculiar to the human (Bergson, 1913).

This state of consciousness, as Janet frequently pointed out, is constricted, tending to be confined to the shifting stimuli of the present. Attention is difficult to fix. After a series of repetitive "shocks", this constellation of disintegrated psychic material becomes the core of the UTMS. Since the material is pre-reflective, involving lower elements of the hierarchy, it is cut off from reflective memory, the episodic and autobiographical. In this way, it is "unconscious".

The traumatic script – reversals and the expectational field

Further complexity of the UTMS is illustrated by Albina's encounter with her therapist after she and her husband presented to the Westmead Psychotherapy Clinic, referred by an enlightened GP. She was depressed, and he was drinking.

An early meeting – within the first month – with her therapist opens with Albina speaking a jumble of incomplete sentences, disconnected from each other and interspersed with long pauses. This is followed by an account of oscillating moods, "throwing things," and so forth. Finally, she comes to her feelings about therapy, "I said I wasn't coming, I wasn't coming back here anymore, and when I finally realised why I didn't want to come back, one, I'm embarrassed that I have to come, that I need to come, and two, I'm ashamed" (Meares, 2000: p.108).

At this point, the words, "don't be silly" come into the therapist's mind. This is strange because it would be unlike him to say such a thing. He begins to reflect on what has happened in these opening few minutes. He realises that his patient is in the grip of a traumatic script, a primitive encapsulation of the main features of an early damaging relationship. It tells of the main features of the protagonists, the abuser and the victim, and the nature of this relational trauma. Elements of this script are often most evident at the start of a session, when anxiety is high, and the ameliorating effect of the self-system is in partial abeyance. The script is played out, in this case with Albina occupying the victim pole, with the therapist as critic. Where the traumatic script is triggered, the patient may tell a story, apparently unrelated to the immediate therapeutic situation, which intimates a main aspect of what has just been happening. The patient does not usually know that he or she is doing this, but in Albina's case the communication is more direct. She uses the words "embarrassed" and "ashamed"; she has been made to feel embarrassed and ashamed by the demeanour of the therapist. He had listened to her in silence, trying to make out what she was trying to say. However, the silence signified to her that she made no sense, she was stupid, and was being exposed as such.

He now recognises that to have uttered the words "don't be silly" would have potentiated the shame, had he used them, which of course he did not. They would have had the effect of criticism. How then had these words come into his mind? They can be understood as an effect of an "expectational field" (Meares, 2005). The expectational field is presumably the outcome of the activity of the UTMS unmodified by the prefrontal inhibitory systems from which it is now disconnected. Under these circumstances the unfettered amygdala exerts much greater influence than in a state when the individual is conscious of the traumatic memory (Meares, 2005). The negative emotion generated in the amygdaloid system is magnified, affecting the whole body, its postures, expressions and gestures. They indicate the role the individual is playing out in the traumatic script. In Albina's case they included a hanging head, downcast eyes, and a dismal voice. Subliminally, the expectation is conveyed to the therapist that the patient is to be criticised. The expectation crystallises in his mind as subtle kind of coercion, an impetus to behave in a particular way, to become a critic (Meares, 2005). The therapist at this point of realisation does not attempt to convey his "insight" to the patient. Rather, he changes his behaviour. He becomes affirming and validating. Over the next few weeks and months a remarkable improvement takes place. Towards the end of this very successful therapy, the patient, without any questions or probing, observed that although her parents' intentions were well-meaning they always made her feel like an "idiot".

Closely related to the phenomena of the "expectational field" is another, the "reversal" (Meares, 2005). This was displayed, at times, by Albina, during her "oscillations". Sometimes she would become someone unlike her usual self, almost as if she were inhabited by another person. She would become hard, dominating, and critical. Such a shift can be conceived as the outcome of a switch in which the poles of the traumatic script reverse. She becomes the traumatiser and critic. Some patients may present in such a state. It may be relatively persistent, collapsing intermittently into helpless, fearful timidity.

Traumatic attachment and satellites of trauma

Hedged about the central UTMS are a series of habitual relationships which are designed to protect the individual from re-experiencing the trauma, or to restore or maintain some sense of existing. They might be seen as "satellite" scripts. The most important of these is fuelled by the fear of separation and the drive to attachment. These forces become magnified in a state of traumatic consciousness, an effect which can be understood in terms of Jackson's "release phenomena".

The impacts of trauma do not only cause a retreat down the hierarchy of consciousness. They also induce a regression in the forms of relatedness associated with each level of consciousness. The relationship necessary to self is lost, and the earlier forms of relatedness become exaggerated. Intimacy is no longer possible. Separation fears and the attachment drive become much more powerful. These attachments often have a paradoxical or contradictory quality. One of the most common is attachment to the trauma, which is either to a person or the traumatic experience. The former case has the usual background of the abuser being also the carer, the one who could guarantee the child's sense of existing and whose care made the child feel alive, special, and worthwhile. This paradoxical relationship tends to determine a pattern of life in which repeated choices of abusive partners are made.

Attachment to the traumatic experience is often difficult to detect and results in therapeutic impasse. For example, a woman of about 35 always begins a session as if she were in acute psychic pain. She moans and is barely able to speak. This inarticulate state is odd. She is a lawyer involved in high level corporate negotiations. Before her session she chats amiably with the receptionist. The behaviour can be understood as an unconscious replay of developmental experience, an early life spent as an only child on an isolated farm with a remote and affectless mother who barely responded to her child's ordinary expressions of distress, such as crying. The only way the child could gain care was through the almost silent expression of extreme distress. She became attached, one might say addicted, to the traumatic experience itself. It had become associated with the relief of anxiety following restoration of the attachment bond.

Another example of an apparent "false self" driven by attachment needs is accommodative. This system is extremely common and, again, difficult to recognise. It may also lead to therapeutic impasse. The accommodative form of pathological attachment arises from a developmental situation in which the child learns that to be "difficult," to exhibit needs or distress, is likely to upset the mother, so breaking the bond with her. The anxiety produced by the break is so powerful that the child will do anything, even to the extent of sacrificing a personal reality, in order to avoid its recurrence. The child lives only to accommodate to what is required. In therapy, the subject is a "good" patient.

Another important satellite system has the purpose of avoidance, of shielding the subject from repetition of the traumatic impact either through a new infliction of the trauma or by triggering the UTMS. Any potential triggers are prevented from having their effect by manoeuvres of evasion which are usually unconscious and automatic but may be conscious. Neural inhibitory activity blocks renewed traumatic experiencing, a mechanism resembling Freud's repression.

Treatment

Treatment of relational trauma involves two main and interwoven themes of therapeutic activity, one relating to the UTMS and the other to the self-deficit. Space allows consideration only of the latter. The former is discussed elsewhere (Meares, 2000, 2005; Meares et al., 2012; Haliburn, 2017).

The person habitually in the grip of traumatic consciousness relates to the world of others in ways which are inimical to the emergence of self. Pathological attachment, for example, is associated with subtle interpersonal disconnectedness. The patterns of activity induced in the brain by these relationships are alien to the state of self. The result, it has been suggested (Meares, 2012), is relative atrophy of those parts of the brain most associated with higher order consciousness as a consequence of under-use.

Considerable volumetric differences are found between the brains of traumatised people and controls. The outstanding differences, between traumatised and un-traumatised adult brains, is the smaller hippocampi in the former (Meares, 2012). This is not so, however, for children and adolescents (Rinne-Albers et al., 2013). This difference might be explained by different ways of processing sensory data at various developmental levels.

Despite the difficulty of the variety of these findings, a hypothesis can be put forward that the differences in the volumes of various brain areas in traumatised people are the outcome of social construction, the effect of a noxious environment which deprives those areas of stimulation necessary to maturation.

It must not however be supposed that these changes are quite immutable. Particular brain areas can grow, with suitable stimulation. For example, the hippocampi, associated with spatial learning, "shaping," and navigation, became larger in London taxi drivers learning the layout of their city over a four-year period (Woollett and Maguire, 2011). What kind of stimulation is necessary for those who have suffered relational trauma? An answer can be inferred, in a negative way, by studies of people, now called "Borderline", who have been found, in the typical case, to have suffered relational trauma. Their conversational style tends to be "concrete and linear" (Meares, 1977: p.110), suggesting a deficit in right hemispheric function and a domination by the left (Meares, 1977). They speak in the manner of a chronicle (Meares, 1998), an asymbolic catalogue of events.

Neurophysiological studies support the hypothesis that a right hemispheric deficit is characteristic of those who have suffered relational trauma (Meares et al., 2011; Meares, 2012). They also demonstrate, as Hughlings Jackson might have predicted, a failure of coordination, of connectedness, between neural systems which usually work together (Meares et al., 2005).

These data suggest that the regenerative kind of therapeutic conversation should, first of all, have the quality of connecting. This is consistent with the Vygotsky proposal mentioned earlier, that the functions of higher order consciousness appear first as relationships between people. Secondly, the conversation should stimulate right hemisphere activity. It should "fit" the way in which the right hemisphere works.

Since the investigations of Sperry and colleagues of people with "split brains" (Sperry, 1966), it has become well known that the right and left hemispheres process sensory data in different ways and have different functions. The left hemisphere underpins an analytic, linear, and logical mode of thought, whereas the outstanding quality of the right is the capacity for "spatial synthesis" (Levy et al., 1972). It has a "shaping" function, which is made with a non-linear movement of thought.

Both these qualities are at the heart of the proto-conversation which is the beginning of the developmental theme of right hemispheric function which includes symbolic play, and which leads to the capacity for symbolisation. The scenes of this developmental progress give a basis to the principles which guide a therapeutic conversation generative of self (Meares, 2016). In this chapter, the focus is on the proto-conversation. The essential feature of the proto-conversation is a kind of maternal responsiveness which shows the "shape," gives a picture of her baby's experience, at a particular moment. The "shaping" is made by the melodic contours of her voice and by her facial expression. By this re-presentation of the baby's presentation of his or her feeling state, the mother provides an analogue of the baby's sense of existing, an analogue being a thing which has a similar shape or proportion similar to, but is not a copy of, another thing. This analogue is coupled to the baby's expression in a way which gives the infant the sense that mother and child are connected as if two parts of a single system. In the therapeutic context, this analogue of co-created experience has been called a "form of feeling" (Hobson, 1985).

Whereas this representational, or analogic, kind of coupling is momentary, a second kind of coupling is also evident in the proto-conversation. It is serial. Each iteration of presentation by the baby and re-presentation by the mother is followed by another, with which it is continuous. Something of one mini-episode is carried on to the next. In the therapeutic situation, this "chain" of connecting is created by the therapist taking something from the patient's last remark to fashion his or her response (Meares, 2000). Both kinds of connecting response have within them something larger than the original presentation; this amplification may be as simple as a tone of voice. The main components, then, of the proto-conversation are coupling, of which there are two kinds, serial and momentary, amplification, and representation. These are the features of a self-organising system. The emergence of self can be conceived as the outcome of a self-organising process (Meares, 2000).

The analogical theme of the brain–mind development is fragile. It depends upon a particular kind of relationship, which is not always established. The parallel theme of development – the left brain, logical system – is relatively robust. Its development takes place through encounters with the "outer" world. The therapy, then, of relational trauma will have a right hemispheric focus, and will be conducted by means of a language having, for much of the time, a "right hemispheric" quality (Meares, 2016). It will be abbreviated, condensed, and feeling-laden, tending to be ungrammatical in the strict syntactical sense. Sentences, for example, will very often lack a subject (Vygotsky, 1962). Above all, however, the conversation will have the purpose of "connecting". Although complex, flexible, and shifting, it will have the main forms of coupling, amplification, and representation.

Conclusion

A history of relational trauma creates a therapeutic field governed by two main forces, positive and negative. The positive drive is toward selfhood; the negative is a system of unconscious traumatic memories (UTMS). Therapy is initially dominated by the latter force, which tends to create forms of relationships which excite patterns of brain activity which are antagonistic to the development of self. The hypothesis is put forward that when this kind of relating becomes habitual, areas of the brain necessary for the emergence of self become atrophic through disuse. Hobson pioneered an approach to this problem. He called it the Conversational Model. In essence, the main aspect of the treatment of relational trauma is relational. The therapeutic aim is to transform a conversation characteristic of and created by traumatic consciousness into another one, having a different structure, which is conducive to the emergence of self (Hobson, 1971).

References

Bergson H (1913) *Creative Evolution*. New York, NY: Henry Holt.

Edelman G (2004) *Wider than the Sky*. London, UK: Penguin, Allen Lane.

Haliburn J (2017) *An Integrated Approach to Short-term Dynamic Interpersonal Psychotherapy: A Clinician's Guide*. London, UK: Karnac Books.

Hobson RF (1971) Imagination and amplification in psychotherapy. *Journal of Analytical Psychology* 16: 79–105.

Hobson RF (1985) *Forms of Feeling: The Heart of Psychotherapy*. London, UK: Tavistock.

Jackson JH (1958) *Selected Writings of John Hughlings Jackson*. New York, NY: Basic Books.

Janet P (1925) *Psychological Healing*. London, UK: George Allen and Unwin.

Levy J, Trevarthen C and Sperry RW (1972) Perception of bilateral chimeric figures following hemispheric deconnexion. *Brain* 95: 61–78.

Liotti G (2000) Disorganized attachment, models of borderline states, and evolutionary psychotherapy. In: Gilbert P and Bailey K (eds) *Genes on the Couch: Essays in Evolutionary Psychotherapy*. Hove, UK: Psychology Press, pp.232–256.

Meares R (1977) *The Pursuit of Intimacy: An Approach to Psychotherapy*. Melbourne, Australia: Nelson.

Meares R (1998) The self in conversation: On narratives, chronicles and scripts. *Psychoanalytic Dialogues* 8: 875–891.

Meares R (1999) The contribution of Hughlings Jackson to an understanding of dissociation. *American Journal of Psychiatry* 156: 1850–1855.

Meares R (2000) *Intimacy and Alienation: Memory, Trauma and Personal Being*. London, UK: Routledge.

Meares R (2005) *The Metaphor of Play: Origin and Breakdown of Personal Being, Revised and Enlarged Edition*. London, UK: Routledge.

Meares R (2012) *A Dissociation Model of Borderline Personality Disorder*. New York, NY and London, UK: WW Norton and Company.

Meares R (2016) *The Poet's Voice in the Making of Mind*. London, UK and New York, NY: Routledge Taylor & Francis Group.

Meares R, Bendit N, Haliburn J, et al. (2012) *Borderline Personality Disorder and the Conversational Model: A Clinician's Manual*. New York, NY and London, UK: WW Norton and Company.

Meares R, Melkonian D, Gordon E, et al. (2005) Distinct pattern of P3a event-related potential in borderline personality disorder. *Neuroreport* 16: 289–293.

Meares R and Orlay W (1988) On self-boundary: A study of the development of the concept of secrecy. *British Journal of Medical Psychology* 61 (Pt 4): 305–316.

Meares R, Schore A and Melkonian D (2011) Is borderline personality a particularly right hemispheric disorder? A study of P3a using single trial analysis. *Australian and New Zealand Journal Psychiatry* 45: 131–139.

Rinne-Albers MA, van der Wee NJ, Lamers-Winkelman F, et al. (2013) Neuroimaging in children, adolescents and young adults with psychological trauma. *European Child and Adolescent Psychiatry* 22: 745–755.

Mental health impacts

Significant childhood trauma causes such a degree of self-disruption that those experiencing it often have no sense of having functioned well and cannot recall ever having felt healthy or happy. People so affected often struggle to indicate what they "want" because they do not feel entitled to express their preference, and sometimes they cannot even identify what it is. They also find it difficult to experience a sense of safety or feel confident or joyous. Child abuse can also seriously erode an individual's self-esteem, including self-concept and sense of cohesion, and emotional effects can also frequently involve pervasive negative self-attitudes, including guilt, self-blame and shame, and difficulty developing a sense of meaning about themselves, others, and the world.

Sufferers also struggle to manage their internal states and to "regulate" their levels of arousal, emotion, and behaviour, and may be irritable and "moody". They may have difficulty maintaining attention and consciousness, and can appear "spaced out", disconnected, and confused. Forming and maintaining healthy relationships is often a significant problem, with issues around trust, intimacy, and sexuality. Many withdraw and become socially isolated. There is no "one-size-fits-all" approach, but a reduced quality of life is almost universal.

More specifically, in one study, child abuse has been associated with between 26 and 32 per cent of adolescent and adult psychiatric disorders (Green et al., 2010). Of adults reporting child physical abuse and neglect, 76 per cent experience at least one psychiatric disorder in their lifetime and nearly 50 per cent have been diagnosed with three or more psychiatric disorders (Borger et al., 2005). Women sexually abused as children are also two to three times more likely to suffer a psychiatric or substance abuse disorder, and the risk increases with the severity of abuse (Kendler et al., 2000). Childhood trauma is in fact the single most significant predictor that a person will present to a mental health system; the more severe and prolonged the trauma, the more severe are the psychological and physical health consequences (Kezelman and Stavropoulos, 2012).

Mental health diagnoses commonly applied to survivors of child abuse and other childhood trauma vary widely and include PTSD, Borderline Personality Disorder, Depression (Widom et al., 2007) or other Affective Disorders, Anxiety Disorders or Psychosis (Shevlin et al., 2007) including Schizophrenia and Bipolar Disorder, also Dissociative Disorders (Dorahy et al., 2016) and Somatic Symptom Disorder, previously known as Somatoform Disorder (Spitzer et al., 2008). Though not all childhood trauma leads to Psychosis, and not all Psychosis is trauma-related, trauma is also a well-documented potential risk factor for psychosis (Schäfer and Fisher, 2011).

Other challenges include multiple coexisting conditions such as Substance Abuse, Eating Disorders, self-harming behaviours, and suicidality (Cutajar et al., 2010). It is important to recognise here that any diagnosis or comorbid diagnosis may be a manifestation of what is in fact the major condition, C-PTSD, or may be related to a coping mechanism used to assist in the wake of abuse (for example, Substance Abuse).

Singer W (2001) Consciousness and the binding problem. *Annals of the New York Academy of Sciences* 929: 123–146.

Sperry R (1966) Brain bisection and mechanisms of consciousness. In: Eccles JC (ed) *Brain and Conscious Experience*. New York, NY: Springer Verlag, pp.298–313.

Stevenson J and Meares R (1992) An outcome study of psychotherapy for patients with borderline personality disorder. *American Journal of Psychiatry* 149: 358–362.

Trevarthen C (1974) Conversations with a two-month old. *New Scientist* 62: 230–235.

Vygotsky LS (1962) *Thought and Language*. Cambridge, MA: MIT Press.

Vygotsky LS (1978) *Mind in Society: The Development of Higher Psychological Processes*. Cambridge, MA: Harvard University Press.

Wimmer H and Perner J (1983) Beliefs about beliefs: Representation and constraining function of wrong beliefs in young children's understanding of deception. *Cognition* 13(1): 103–128.

Woollett K and Maguire EA (2011) Acquiring "the knowledge" of London's layout drives structural brain changes. *Current Biology* 21: 2109–2114.

3 Childhood trauma – the long-term impact and the human cost

Cathy Kezelman

> Over the past two decades, vast amounts of knowledge have accumulated about what we call "Complex Trauma", a psychiatric condition that officially does not exist, but which possibly constitutes the most common set of psychological problems to drive human beings into psychiatric care.
>
> Bessel van der Kolk, 2009, p.455

Introduction

Trauma results from an event or series of events or circumstances which harm or threaten to harm a person, physically and/or emotionally. In so doing, trauma overwhelms or threatens to overwhelm an individual's capacity to cope. When interpersonal trauma occurs in childhood, particularly in the early years, it can be especially damaging. When unresolved, it can have long-lasting impacts on mental and physical health, relationships, and daily functioning. Child abuse and other childhood trauma not only affects individuals but also their families, communities, and society more broadly.

"Child abuse and neglect" or "child maltreatment" refer to any non-accidental behaviour of parents, caregivers, other adults or older adolescents, outside the norms of conduct, which have a significant risk of physical or emotional harm to a child or young person. "Child maltreatment" includes sexual, emotional, and physical abuse, neglect, and exposure to family violence (Australian Institute of Family Studies, 2015). When caregivers have their own unresolved childhood trauma histories they can also unwittingly transmit trauma intergenerationally to their children via "disrupted attachment" relationships, which might involve any of the above categories. Other forms of childhood trauma include but are not limited to medical trauma, bullying and cyber-bullying, socio-economic disadvantage, social isolation, racism, oppression, community violence including civil unrest, war, and terrorism. Child maltreatment can be intentional or unintentional, and includes acts of omission or "neglect", and/or of commission or "abuse".

For most people, the word "trauma" connotes single incidents and events. "Single-incident trauma" relates to an unexpected and "out of the blue" event such as a natural disaster, accident, terrorist attack or single episode of assault, abuse or witnessing of such an event, and is typically associated with the development of Posttraumatic Stress Disorder (PTSD). The abuse of children, on the other hand, is of a different nature, most often varied, repetitive, cumulative, and perpetrated by one human being on another. The common element is the powerlessness of the child, due to age and dependency, to prevent or minimise it. "Complex Trauma" is the term frequently used to describe the effects of repeated abuse in childhood or in adulthood, and the varied potential sequelae have been described in the concept of a Complex Post-Traumatic Stress Disorder (C-PTSD) (Herman,1992). This category clusters together a range of effects on mood, memory, consciousness, relationships, and world view that may all occur in the wake of repeated traumas, and by so doing gives meaning to the difficulties and helps clinicians avoid making multiple discrete diagnoses, a situation encouraged by the classification systems currently in use.

In the Australian context it is also worth noting that although many Indigenous children grow up in safe environments, many do not. Large numbers of Aboriginal and Torres Strait Islander people have experienced the trauma of colonisation, displacement, forced removal, institutionalisation, racism, and collective and intergenerational violence and abuse, and are at risk of repeated victimisation (Atkinson, 2013). Other groups are also at higher risk of trauma, and they include refugees and culturally and linguistically diverse minorities, older Australians, people with disabilities, and people who are lesbian, gay, bisexual, transgender, queer, and intersex.

Prevalence

Statistics in this area are always difficult to interpret because different definitions of abuse and maltreatment are used, different age ranges are used, and different techniques are used to gather data. Some reviews for example have concluded that child physical abuse has been experienced by between 10–31 per cent of men and 6–40 per cent of women, and sexual abuse by 3–29 per cent of men and 7–36 per cent of women, widely varying figures (Springer et al., 2003). The pivotal US study, the Adverse Childhood Experiences Study (or ACE Study), carefully explored with retrospective surveys the association between childhood trauma and adult health in more than 17,000 predominantly white, middle class Americans (Felitti et al., 1998). In addition to emotional, physical, and sexual abuse, the original study included five types of household dysfunction: mother treated violently; living with an alcohol or drug user; living with a family member who is chronically depressed, mentally ill, institutionalised, or suicidal; having a household member incarcerated; or not being raised by both biological parents (Felitti and Anda, 2010). In the second wave of the study, physical and emotional neglect were added. Each category is given a score of one, regardless of the amount of trauma involved, and as there are 10 categories, the maximum score is 10.

The study concluded that ACEs are significantly more common than recognised or acknowledged, and they also have a powerful effect on adult health, decades later. Two-thirds of study participants reported at least one ACE category, one in six reported four or more, and one in nine reported five or more (Felitti and Anda, 2010). Considering the 10 chosen categories of childhood maltreatment, these US figures also showed that 28 per cent of respondents reported physical abuse, 27 per cent parental substance use, 23 per cent separation or divorce, 22 per cent sexual abuse (28 per cent for women), 17 per cent household mental illness, 15 per cent emotional neglect, 13 per cent mother treated violently, 11 per cent overt emotional abuse, 10 per cent physical neglect, and 6 per cent an incarcerated household member (Felitti and Anda, 2010).

A 2007 Australian University-initiated study of more than 21,000 older Australians – another retrospective survey – found that more than 13 per cent of those surveyed reported having been either physically or sexually abused in childhood, or both (Draper et al., 2008); it is important to record that this study did not include those who experienced emotional abuse, neglect, or family violence. That said these prevalence figures are lower than those of other studies. Possible influencing factors include the use of postal questionnaires which may be seen as somewhat impersonal. The surveys were also directed to people 60 years and over – people who might be less likely to identify that what happened to them was abuse in comparison with a younger cohort.

The relative prevalence of maltreatment subtypes via official child protection records are completed differently, contemporaneously, and only after official concerns about child care are lodged and investigated. Nationally in 2016–17, emotional abuse was the most common primary type of abuse or neglect that was substantiated for children (48 per cent). This was followed by neglect (24 per cent), physical abuse (16 per cent), and sexual abuse (12 per cent); the categories do not follow those in the ACE Study, and the numbers do not total more than 100 per cent as substantiations in Australia are categorised into one of the four types, although in reality there is frequently overlap (Australian Institute of Health and Welfare, 2018). Overall, in Australia, aggregated prevalence data across all categories of childhood trauma estimates that conservatively one in four adults – approximately five million people – have experienced significant childhood trauma in diverse settings, including within the home, family, neighbourhood, and within institutions (Kezelman et al., 2015).

Extensive research has also established that by far the majority of those people presenting to public mental health services have experienced sexual, physical, or psychological trauma (Cusack et al., 2006), with two out of three patients presenting to emergency, inpatient, or outpatient mental health services suffering the effects of Complex Trauma related to childhood physical or sexual abuse (Read et al., 2005). If emotional abuse, chronic neglect, and the impacts of growing up with substance abuse and family violence are included, the number affected increases substantially.

A vignette – "Helen"

Helen was a 65-year-old single health professional with tertiary qualifications and skills, who lived with her beloved cat. She had been in a long-term relationship until 20 years ago, when she left due to domestic violence, including sexual exploitation. Thereafter she stole narcotics from her workplace, of which she has no memory, and as a result, lost her job, and she retired five years ago. She had two long-standing friendships but was estranged from her family.

Helen had been treated by several psychiatrists for Depression since her late 20s, with Electro-convulsive Therapy and a range of medications, many of which she still took. Helen had also been amnestic for large periods of her childhood, and as an adult has struggled with chronic low mood, self-hatred, flashbacks and nightmares, loss of lengthy periods of time, and episodes of self-harm and suicidality.

Helen disclosed her history of trauma to a psychologist when she was hospitalised for Depression only two years ago. She divulged that although she was unable to remember large periods of her childhood, she knew that she had not only been sexually abused from the age of eight by her father, but that he had also involved other groups of men. Her mother was cold toward her and had offered her no protection.

On interview, Helen presented as polite, childlike, and deferential. Wide-eyed, often startled, she sometimes "jumped" out of her chair. Generally slow in her movements, however, she often appeared to be "zoned out" or in a trance-like state, and she gave short simple answers to questions, preferring not to talk about herself.

Her most recent psychiatrist provisionally diagnosed a Dissociative Disorder, which was confirmed by the knowledge that Helen had been seriously abused. She was appropriately referred for psychotherapy.

Physical health and psychosocial impact

Child abuse survivors often have a problematic relationship to their body. A person who has been sexually abused can view their body as alien, treacherous, contaminated, and/or detached from their self, and this can place them at risk of suicide. Overwhelming childhood experiences also compromise other systems of the body including but not limited to the hormonal, endocrine, and immune systems (Karr-Morse, 2012). Survivors experience approximately twice the incidence of Fibromyalgia, Chronic Fatigue, Chronic Pain syndromes, and "medically unexplained symptoms", as well as disorders of the digestive, circulatory, endocrine, and immune systems, for example, Irritable Bowel Syndrome (Seng et al., 2006).

Several studies, including the ACE study, have demonstrated a direct relationship between the number of categories of ACEs and the risk for a range of negative health and wellbeing outcomes across the life course. When people had an ACE score of four or more, the odds ratio, or measure of the strength of an association between an exposure and a physical health outcome, was 1.6 times for Diabetes, 1.8 for any Cancer, 2.2 for Ischaemic Health Disease, 2.4 for Stroke, and 3.9 for Chronic Obstructive Pulmonary Disease; the link between abuse, smoking, and Lung Disease appears to be particularly important to note. The odds ratios for Skeletal Fractures, Hepatitis, and poor self-rated health were 1.6, 2.3, and 2.2, respectively (Felitti et al., 1998). ACEs are also related to premature mortality: the risk of death before the age of 50, for those with an ACE score of only two or more, is 57 per cent higher for men and 80 per cent higher for women (Kelly-Irving et al., 2013).

Abuse and other traumas in childhood are also strongly associated with significant social impacts, including educational and vocational. An Irish longitudinal study on ageing, involving a nationally representative survey of people aged 50 and over, showed that male victims of child sexual abuse are almost three times more likely to be out of the labour force due to sickness and disability, have significantly lower incomes, and are more likely to live alone (Barrett and Kamiya, 2014). People who have experienced abuse and violence in childhood are also often at risk of further re-victimisation and re-traumatisation later in life and are more likely to be a victim or perpetrator of violence, both within and outside of relationships.

Adaptations to abuse

The physiological responses of "fight", "flight", and "freeze" to the perception of extreme threat help protect the child from being overwhelmed and maximise their chances of survival. The freeze response is common because young children are disempowered around adults and less able to fight or flee. In the absence of effective coping skills, the best option for a child to psychologically survive in the short term is often to dissociate or shut off the experience from his or her consciousness. Inevitably though, the dissociation fails and those who have been abused suffer from a range of emotional difficulties.

In the longer term, many of the negative health outcomes related to child abuse are associated with the adoption of health "risk" behaviours, most of which are "adaptations" to help modulate these emotions, these adaptations in fact being maladaptive coping strategies, and include smoking, overeating, alcohol and drug misuse, physical inactivity, high risk sexual behaviours, self-harm (including cutting and burning), chronic suicidal ideation, overwork, and extreme sports. The risk of each behaviour occurring increases as the number of ACEs increases. To illustrate, males with an ACE score of six or more are 46 times more likely than those with a score of zero to be intravenous drug users (Felitti, 2003). Additionally, risk-taking behaviour not only negatively impacts health, but also contributes to social problems such as criminal convictions and gaol sentences, vulnerability to abusive, violent and unhealthy relationships, and economic problems such as gambling debt. Other coping strategies used by both children and adults who have experienced child abuse and other childhood traumas include denial, minimisation, pleasing and appeasing, and rationalisation.

The cost of suicide

Though it follows that those who have been abused suffer with a range of psychological, psychiatric, and physical disorders, and are more likely to attempt and in fact complete suicide, the literature shows that the relationship is complex, and that child abuse is one of several associated factors (Beautrais, 2000). People with childhood trauma histories do however find it difficult to cope with stress, manage negative emotions, and maintain feelings of hope and optimism. A meta-analysis showed a strong association between child sexual and physical abuse and neglect and attempted suicide in young adults (Gilbert et al., 2009). One particular study completed in New Zealand demonstrated that 11–21 per cent of young adults or adolescents who had suffered severe physical abuse or penetrative sexual abuse reported suicide attempts, in comparison with 1–3 per cent of controls (Fergusson et al., 2008).

Research has further established a powerful graded relationship between ACEs more broadly and the risk of attempted suicide throughout the lifespan, a relationship probably partially mediated by substance use and emotional dysregulation. Notably, the risk of suicide attempt is increased two to five-fold by any single ACE, no matter what category, and an ACE score of seven or more increases the risk of suicide attempts 30-fold among adults and 51-fold for children and adolescents (Dube et al., 2001). Furthermore, 64 per cent of all suicide attempts in adults can be attributed to ACEs, and 80 per cent among children and adolescents (Dube et al., 2001), or approximately two-thirds of all suicide attempts.

A 2010 study of 21 countries also showed that childhood adversity measured over nine categories increased the risk of suicidal thoughts and attempts with an odds ratio ranging from 1.2 to 5.7; the greater the number of adverse childhood events, the greater the risk (Bruffaerts et al., 2010). For those who had attempted suicide, nearly a third (29.3 per cent) reported physical abuse, about one in four (24.8 per cent) family violence, and one in six (14.5 per cent) sexual abuse. People who have experienced sexual and/or physical abuse also had more persistent suicidal behaviour and an earlier onset (Bruffaerts et al., 2010). Large population-based studies of suicide attempts have also shown a strong association with other traumas, for example, parental mental health and substance abuse issues, parental suicide, and socio-economic disadvantage (Fergusson et al., 2000; Molnar et al., 2001).

Several rigorous studies report significant links between child sexual abuse and suicidality more specifically (Fergusson et al., 2000; Molnar et al., 2001). A study of 2,759 Australian medically identified victims of child sexual abuse found significantly higher rates of suicide in the child sexual abuse group compared with the general population, with females over 40 times more at risk of suicide, and males over 14 times, with females at 88 times higher risk of death by accidental fatal overdose, and men 38 times (Cutajar et al., 2010). Another Australian study into those who had suffered child sexual abuse found that 32 per cent had attempted suicide, and 43 per cent had considered it, and that the suicide rate in sexually abused children was 10.7–13.0 times that of the Australian national rate (Plunkett et al., 2001).

The Australian Youth Development Index showed that Aboriginal and Torres Strait Islander men between 19 and 25 had the highest rate of suicide in the world (Youth Action and Policy Association, 2016). The standardised death rate for Aboriginal and Torres Strait Islander persons was 23.8 deaths per 100,000 persons, compared with 11.4 deaths per 100,000 for non-Indigenous persons (Australian Bureau of Statistics, 2016). Suicide deaths also accounted for a greater proportion of all Aboriginal and Torres Strait Islander deaths (5.5 per cent) compared with deaths of non-Indigenous Australians (1.7 per cent) (Australian Bureau of Statistics, 2016). The disproportionately high rate of Indigenous suicide is significantly associated with the prevalence of inter-generational individual and collective trauma experienced by Aboriginal and Torres Strait Islander peoples (Dudgeon et al., 2017).

A vignette – "Rowena"

Rowena was admitted at the age of 44 to the high dependency unit of an acute mental health facility. She had tried to kill herself with both prescription and "over the counter" medication, and she was still actively suicidal on the ward. She had been hearing and seeing things for several weeks, and she felt like someone was trying to kill her. Rowena had also been drinking heavily and smoking marijuana. Prior to her suicide attempt she hadn't been able to eat or sleep, and she was admitted in a very agitated state.

In background, Rowena gave a history of being an unwanted child. One of her earliest memories was of her mother trying to drown her. Her father had "a short fuse", and when he drank, which was often, he became violent. She watched her mother and brother being physically and verbally abused by him, and she was often hiding her own bruises at school. Her sister who had an intellectual disability was largely ignored. Her mother left the family on a few occasions as she could no longer cope, but she always returned. Rowena got thrown out of home when she was only 15 for fighting back. Thereafter she started smoking marijuana frequently, and she was admitted for the first time to a psychiatric ward when she was only 17, after "losing the plot" she said. Rowena fell in and out of relationships which made her feel even worse about herself, and hospital admissions had the same effect. The psychiatrists she said just kept giving her medications which "zonked" her out. No one, she added, sat down and talked to her.

The most recent admission occurred after Rowena finally left her last partner after a three-year "on and off" relationship. He was a heavy drinker who lost his temper whenever Rowena "spoke out of turn". He had also controlled everything, her money, who she could see, what she could do, and he always told her that if she ever tried to leave him that he would come after her. But the doctors just "didn't get it", she said. She tried to explain about him and why she took the overdose, but, again, no one listened. After five days, Rowena was discharged, as she was thought to be no longer suicidal. Outpatient follow-up was organised, but Rowena felt that they only wanted to see if she would take her medication and stop using marijuana and alcohol. She also thought that the medical and nursing staff had primarily diagnosed her with Schizophrenia because she was paranoid and heard things, but she thought she suffered from "stress" and struggled to trust people because of all the things that had happened to her. She told the staff that she had no intention of following up because no one seemed interested in her or her story.

The public health impact of childhood trauma

Most people treated by public mental health, substance abuse services and the human services sector have trauma histories (Jennings, 2004). National and international research has established that childhood trauma is a major public health issue, with high prevalence and substantial individual and community health, welfare, and economic repercussions (Kezelman and Stavropoulos, 2012).

It is evident then that an adequate response to the issue of childhood trauma requires a public health approach (Magruder et al., 2016).

A 40-year longitudinal prospective study on a Dunedin birth cohort of more than 1,000 people looking at childhood risk predictors and adult economic outcomes supports this position. It found that nearly 80 per cent of the adult economic burden of that birth cohort could be attributed to 22 per cent of the subjects who often came from low socio-economic backgrounds, struggled with self-control, were maltreated, and received low scores on IQ tests (Caspi et al., 2016). They also used a disproportionate amount of costly services across health, criminal justice, and social welfare systems. The study established the strongest effect sizes documented to date, measuring the connection between an at-risk childhood and costly adult outcomes.

Unresolved childhood trauma also substantially erodes national productivity and wellbeing, including through educational failure, low workforce participation, and premature death (Segal, 2015). In Australia, childhood trauma has been shown to have substantial long-term economic consequences (Reeve and van Gool, 2013). Another economic study estimated that if the impact of childhood trauma on adults in Australia was adequately addressed, the budgetary positions of federal, state, and territory governments could be improved by a minimum of $9.1 billion annually, and by as much as $24 billion annually. These figures represent the combined effect of higher government expenditure and foregone tax revenue (Kezelman et al., 2015).

It is also important to note that research into recovery from such trauma shows promising results. A synthesis of the work of researchers, academics, and clinicians in the trauma field suggests that it is possible for even profound early trauma to be resolved, and the negative impacts on the next generation consequently interrupted (Siegel, 2003). World Mental Health Surveys from 21 countries conducted by the World Health Organisation have indicated that eradicating adverse experiences in childhood would lead to a 22.9 per cent reduction in Affective Disorders, a 31.0 per cent decrease in Anxiety Disorders, a 41.6 per cent drop in Behaviour Disorders, a 27.5 per cent decline in Substance Disorders, and a 29.8 per cent fall overall in the disorders studied (Kessler et al., 2010). Another study suggested that 12 per cent of binge drinking, 14 per cent of poor diet, 23 per cent of smoking, 42 per cent of violence perpetration, 38 per cent of unintended teenage pregnancy, and 59 per cent of heroin and "crack" cocaine use, could all be attributed to maltreatment before the age of 18 (Bellis et al., 2014). It is also known that the way in which a community responds to an individual's trauma influences that individual's trauma experience and its impact. Communities that foster understanding and encourage self-determination facilitate recovery, whereas those which avoid or misunderstand the impact of trauma can re-traumatise individuals and interfere with their recovery process (Substance Abuse and Mental Health Services Administration, 2014).

The above studies demonstrate that childhood trauma has a very wide array of long-term effects, and that effective and efficient interventions can reduce both the personal and the economic burden. But despite these findings, child abuse and other such traumas are not considered by governments or policy makers to be major public or preventative health issues. Services remain largely inadequate, inaccessible, unaffordable, and poorly matched to need (Kezelman and Stavropoulos, 2012), with, historically, an endemic failure to invest comprehensively into the trauma-informed services necessary to facilitate recovery across the lifespan (Mental Health Coordinating Council, 2013). Although several programs have recognised the need for trauma-informed practice and embedded the requisite changes, the absence of larger policy directives to drive systemic change means that any such changes are sporadic.

An effective public health response to trauma will therefore require comprehensive political engagement and leadership (Mental Health Coordinating Council, 2013). It will also require a prioritisation of services, organisations, and professions which acknowledge trauma across diverse sectors and integration of evidence-based policy with vision and vigour. Initial US evaluation of trauma-informed practice suggests that it is cost-effective (Domino et al., 2005), reducing the risk of inadvertent harm, improving client outcomes, and fostering staff safety, wellbeing, and community connectedness (Mental Health Coordinating Council, 2013).

The reality is that the cost of child abuse and other childhood trauma, including suicide, is vast. An informed, coordinated public health approach integrated across systems and governments is needed if these escalating costs, both human and economic, are to be mitigated.

References

Atkinson J (2013) *Trauma-informed Services and Trauma-specific Care for Indigenous Australian Children. Resource Sheet no. 21.* Produced for the Closing the Gap Clearinghouse. Canberra, Australia: Australian Institute of Health and Welfare and Melbourne, Australia: Australian Institute of Family Studies.

Australian Bureau of Statistics (2016) *Intentional Self-harm in Aboriginal and Torres Strait Islander People.* Canberra, Australia: Australian Bureau of Statistics.

Australian Institute of Family Studies (2015) *What is Child Abuse and Neglect? Child Family Community Australia Resource Sheet.* Canberra, Australia: Australian Government.

Australian Institute of Health and Welfare (2018) *Child Protection Australia 2016–17.* Child welfare series no. 68. Cat. no. CWS 63. Canberra, Australia: Australian Institute of Health and Welfare.

Barrett A and Kamiya Y (2014) Childhood sexual abuse and later-life economic consequences. *Journal of Behavioral and Experimental Economics* 53: 10–16.

Beautrais AL (2000) Risk factors for suicide and attempted suicide among young people. *Australian and New Zealand Journal of Psychiatry* 34(3): 420–436.

Bellis MA, Hughes K, Leckenby N, et al. (2014) National household survey of adverse childhood experiences and their relationship with resilience to health-harming behaviours in England. *BMC Medicine* 12: 72.

Borger S, Cox B and Amundson G (2005) PTSD and other mental health problems in adults who report histories of severe physical abuse and neglect. In: Corales T (ed) *Trends in Posttraumatic Stress Disorder Research.* Hauppage, NY: Nova Science Publishers, pp.249–261.

Bruffaerts R, Demyttenaere K, Borges G, et al. (2010) Childhood adversities as risk factors for onset and persistence of suicidal behaviour. *British Journal of Psychiatry* 197(1): 20–27.

Caspi A, Houts RM, Belsky DW, et al. (2016) Childhood forecasting of a small segment of the population with large economic burden. *Nature Human Behaviour* 1: 005.

Courtois CA and Ford JD (eds) (2009) *Treating Complex Traumatic Stress Disorders: An Evidence-based Guide.* New York, NY: The Guilford Press.

Cusack KJ, Grubaugh AL, Knapp RG, et al. (2006) Unrecognized trauma and PTSD among public mental health consumers with chronic and severe mental illness. *Community Mental Health Journal* 42(5): 487–500.

Cutajar M, Mullen P, Ogloff J, et al. (2010) Suicide and fatal drug overdose in child sexual abuse victims: a historical cohort study. *Medical Journal of Australia* 192(4): 184–187.

Domino ME, Morrissey JP, Chung S, et al. (2005) Service use and costs for women with co-occurring mental and substance use disorders and a history of violence. *Psychiatric Services Journal* 56: 1223–1232.

Dorahy MJ, Middleton W, Seagar L, et al. (2016) Child abuse and neglect in complex dissociative disorder, abuse-related chronic PTSD, and mixed psychiatric samples. *Journal of Trauma and Dissociation* 17(2): 223–236.

Draper RB, Pfaff J, Pirkis J, et al. (2008) Long-term effects of childhood abuse on the quality of life and health of older people: Results from the depression and early prevention of suicide in General Practice project. *Journal of the American Geriatrics Society* 56(2): 262–271.

Dube SR, Anda RF, Felitti FJ, et al. (2001) Childhood abuse, household dysfunction, and the risk of attempted suicide throughout the lifespan: Findings from the Adverse Childhood Experiences Study. *Journal of the American Medical Association* 286: 3089–3095.

Dudgeon P, Calma T and Holland C (2017) The contexts and causes of suicide of Indigenous people in Australia. *Journal of Indigenous Wellbeing* 2(2): 6–15.

Felitti VJ (2003) Origins of addiction: evidence from a study of stressful childhood experiences. [Article in German] *Praxis der Kinderpsychologie und Kinderpsychiatrie* 52(8): 547–559.

Felitti VJ, Anda RF, Nordenberg D, et al. (1998) The relationship of adult health status to childhood abuse and household dysfunction. *American Journal of Preventive Medicine* 14(4): 245–258.

Felitti V and Anda R (2010) The relationship of adverse childhood experiences to adult medical disease, psychiatric disorders and sexual behaviour: Implications for healthcare. In: Lanius RA, Vermetten E and Pain C (eds) *The Impact of Early Life Trauma on Health and Disease: The Hidden Epidemic*. Cambridge, UK: Cambridge University Press, pp.77–87.

Fergusson DM, Woodward LJ and Horwood LJ (2000) Risk factors and life processes associated with the onset of suicidal behaviour during adolescence and early childhood. *Psychological Medicine* 30(1): 13–39.

Fergusson DM, Boden JM and Horwood LJ (2008) Exposure to childhood sexual and physical abuse and adjustment in early adulthood. *Child Abuse and Neglect* 32: 607–619.

Gilbert R, Spatz Widom C, Browne K, et al. (2009) Burden and consequences of child maltreatment in high-income countries. *Lancet* 373: 68–81.

Green JG, McLaughlin KA, Berglund PA, et al. (2010) Childhood adversities and adult psychiatric disorders in the National Comorbidity Survey Replication I: Associations with first onset of DSM-IV disorders. *Archives of General Psychiatry* 67(2): 113–123.

Herman J (1992) *Trauma and Recovery*. New York, NY: Basic Books.

Jennings A (2004) *Models for Developing Trauma-informed Behavioral Health Systems and Trauma-specific Services*. Rockville, MD: United States Department of Health and Human Services.

Karr-Morse R (2012) *Scared Sick: The Role of Childhood Trauma in Adult Disease*. New York, NY: Basic Books.

Kelly-Irving M, Lepage B, Dedieu M, et al. (2013) Adverse childhood experiences and premature all-cause mortality. *European Journal of Epidemiology* 28(9): 721–734.

Kendler KS, Bulik C, Silberg J, et al. (2000) Childhood sexual abuse and adult psychiatric and substance abuse disorders in women: An epidemiological and cotwin control analysis. *Archives of General Psychiatry* 57(10): 953–959.

Kessler RC, McLaughlin KA, Green JG, et al. (2010) Childhood adversities and adult psychopathology in the WHO World Mental Health Surveys. *The British Journal of Psychiatry* 197(5): 378–385.

Kezelman CA and Stavropoulos PA (2012) *Practice Guidelines for Treatment of Complex Trauma and Trauma Informed Care and Service Delivery*. Sydney, Australia: Blue Knot Foundation (formerly, Adults Surviving Child Abuse).

Kezelman C, Hossack N, Stavropoulos P, et al. (2015) *The Cost of Unresolved Childhood Trauma and Abuse in Adults in Australia*. Sydney, Australia: Adults Surviving Child Abuse and Pegasus Economics.

Magruder KM, Kassam-Adams N, Thoresen S, et al. (2016) Prevention and public health approaches to trauma and traumatic stress: A rationale and a call to action. *European Journal of Psychotraumatology* 18(7): 29715.

Mental Health Coordinating Council (2013) *Trauma-informed Care and Practice: Towards a Cultural Shift in Policy Reform Across Mental Health and Human Services in Australia, A*

National Strategic Direction. Position Paper and Recommendations of the National Trauma-Informed Care and Practice Advisory Working Group. Sydney, Australia: Adults Surviving Child Abuse (ASCA).

Molnar BE, Berkman LF and Buka SL (2001) Psychopathology, child sexual abuse and other childhood adversities: Relative links to subsequent suicidal behaviour in the US. *Psychological Medicine* 31(6): 965–977.

Plunkett A, O'Toole B, Swanston H, et al. (2001) Suicide risk following child sexual abuse. *Ambulatory Pediatrics* 1(5): 262–266.

Read J, Os JV, Morrison AP, et al. (2005) Childhood trauma, psychosis and schizophrenia: A literature review with theoretical and clinical implications. *Acta Psychiatrica Scandinavica* 112(5): 330–350.

Reeve R and van Gool K (2013) Modelling the relationship between child abuse and long-term health care costs and wellbeing: Results from an Australian community-based survey. *Economic Record* 89(286): 300–318.

Schäfer I and Fisher HL (2011) Childhood trauma and psychosis – what is the evidence? *Dialogues in Clinical Neuroscience* 13(3):360–365.

Segal L (2015) Economic issues in the community response to child maltreatment. In: Matthews B and Bross DC (eds) *Mandatory Reporting Laws and the Identification of Severe Child Abuse and Neglect. Child Maltreatment 4.* Dordrecht, the Netherlands: Springer Science and Business, pp.193–216.

Seng JS, Clark MK, McCarthy AM, et al. (2006) PTSD and physical co-morbidity among women: Results from service use data. *Journal of Traumatic Stress* 19: 45–56.

Shevlin M, Dorahy MJ and Adamson G (2007) Trauma and psychosis: An analysis of the National Comorbidity Survey. *American Journal of Psychiatry* 164: 166–169.

Siegel DJ (2003) An interpersonal neurobiology of psychotherapy: The developing mind and the resolution of trauma. In: Solomon MT and Siegel DJ (eds) *Healing Trauma: Attachment, Mind, Body and Brain.* New York, NY: Norton, pp.1–56.

Spitzer C, Barnow S, Gau K, et al. (2008) Childhood maltreatment in patients with somatisation disorder. *Australian New Zealand Journal of Psychiatry* 42(4): 335–341.

Springer KW, Sheridan J, Kuo D, et al. (2003) The long-term health outcomes of child abuse: An overview and call to action. *Journal of General Internal Medicine* 18 (10): 864–870.

Substance Abuse and Mental Health Services Administration [SAMHSA] (2014) *Trauma-informed Care in Behavioral Health Services.* Treatment Improvement Protocol (TIP) Series, No. 57. Rockville, MD: SAMHSA.

Van der Kolk BA (2009) Afterword. In: Courtois CA and Ford JD (eds) *Treating Complex Traumatic Stress Disorders: An Evidence-based Guide.* New York, NY: The Guilford Press, pp.

Widom CS, DuMont K and Czaja SJ (2007) A prospective investigation of major depressive disorder and comorbidity in abused and neglected children grown up. *Archives of General Psychiatry* 64(1): 49–56.

Youth Action and Policy Association, NSW (2016) *Australian Youth Development Index: A Jurisdictional Overview of Youth Development. 2016 Report.* An electronic publication. Wooloomooloo, NSW: Youth Action.

4 The relationship between child maltreatment, inequalities and later health outcomes

Jackie Amos and Leonie Segal

Introduction

Childhood maltreatment is a major public health, human rights, ethical, legal and social problem, and a significant adversity faced by children and their families (Norman et al., 2012). The impact on an infant, child or adolescent depends on the characteristics of the maltreatment and the context in which it occurs. Age of onset, severity, chronicity, exposure to multiple forms of maltreatment, and relationship to the perpetrator are some of the pertinent characteristics of maltreatment. The availability of practical and emotional support, socioeconomic status, poverty, welfare dependency, long-term parental unemployment, discord in the parenting relationship, paucity of familial and other social supports, poor educational opportunities, criminality, living in a violent neighbourhood, dispossession and war are examples of important contextual factors. The layering of adversity and exposure to multiple types of maltreatment compound negative consequences.

This chapter explores the relationship between familial maltreatment in childhood, general health, mental health and socioeconomic outcomes in adulthood. It is argued, drawing on theory and epidemiological evidence, that child maltreatment is a primary determinant of the observed relationship between socioeconomic status and health: higher socioeconomic status being associated with better health, and lower socioeconomic status with poorer health. If this is the case, effectively addressing child maltreatment offers an opportunity to improve the health, social and economic outcomes of the most vulnerable in society, and to redress health and social inequalities (Segal and Dalziel, 2011).

The relationship between child maltreatment, health and mental health

The variety of poor outcomes that have been consistently linked with childhood maltreatment are extraordinary, but most important and consistent is the serious threat that early life trauma poses to the developing nervous system (Teicher and Samson, 2016), and to the immune and stress modulation systems (Danese and Baldwin, 2017).

The direct suffering experienced in childhood by those exposed to abuse and neglect is, in itself, a major concern. Failure of adequate nurturing or protection and direct violation results in a range of negative outcomes including emotional and behavioural dysregulation, aggressive outbursts, severe anxiety, changes in mood and motivation, exaggerated compliance, indiscriminate affection, developmental delay, poor physical health, poor school attendance and performance, difficulty in establishing peer relationships and risk of premature death (Cook et al., 2017). Though designed to increase safety, child removal can also exacerbate the difficulties of a child.

Mental health difficulties in adulthood with good evidence for potential causality include Depression and Anxiety, Substance Use Disorders, Posttraumatic Stress Disorder (PTSD) (Gilbert et al., 2009), Obsessive-Compulsive symptoms (Mathews et al., 2008), Personality Disorders (Battle et al., 2004), Sleep Disorders (Kajeepeta et al., 2015), Eating Disorders (Gilbert et al., 2009; Molendijk et al., 2017), mental health problems in the perinatal period (Choi and Sikkema, 2016), as well as self-harm, suicidal ideation and dissociation (Gilbert et al., 2009). Associations between childhood maltreatment and Bipolar Disorder (Marangoni et al., 2016) and Schizophrenia (Matheson et al., 2013) have also been reported. Interpersonal relationships too are affected, with increases in interpersonal sensitivity, hostility, anger, low self-esteem, and rates of re-victimisation (Lalor and McElvaney, 2010).

Physical health difficulties in adolescence and adulthood associated with histories of sexual abuse include functional somatic disorders (Afari et al., 2014), now officially referred to as Somatic Symptom Disorders in DSM-5 (American Psychiatric Association, 2013); Obesity (Danese and Tan, 2014); Sexually Transmitted Infections (Norman et al., 2012); gynaecological conditions; Chronic Pain (Irish et al., 2010); gastrointestinal, neurological, musculoskeletal, cardiovascular, respiratory, and metabolic disorders, including Type Two Diabetes (Wegman and Stetler, 2009); and seizures (Paras et al., 2009).

Socioeconomic outcomes of great concern include homelessness (Sundin and Baguley, 2015), increased adolescent and adult criminal behaviour (Gilbert et al., 2009; Braga et al., 2017), sexual victimisation (Lalor and McElvaney, 2010), high-risk sexual behaviours, poor educational outcomes and employment (Gilbert et al., 2009), negative perceptions of health care services and reduced quality of life (Weber et al., 2016).

The seriousness and the scale of the problem of child maltreatment becomes clearer when the relationship to adult outcomes is more thoroughly understood. In 1998, Felitti and others published the initial findings of the Adverse Childhood Experiences study (ACE study) (Felitti et al., 1998). This landmark research challenged the commonly held opinion at the time that poor physical and mental health in adulthood could not be explained by exposure to early life adversities (Nemeroff, 2016). The ACE study was the first to establish, empirically, the existence of strong correlations between exposure to adverse childhood experiences and poor health outcomes in adulthood, with the experiences including emotional, physical and sexual abuse, neglect, as well as not being raised by both biological parents, being exposed to domestic violence, living with household members who had substance abuse problems, were suicidal or mentally ill, and had ever been imprisoned. These results captured the imagination of the research community. The authors of this chapter identified more than 100 systematic reviews and meta-analyses published between 2000 and 2017 devoted to the outcomes in adulthood of exposure to child maltreatment. There is now a considerable body of research that provides a consistent message: childhood maltreatment is associated with poorer outcomes in adulthood (Wegman and Stetler, 2009; McCrory et al., 2012; Norman et al., 2012; Nemeroff, 2016; Afifi et al., 2016; Weber et al., 2016). The literature on the sequelae of child maltreatment is so vast that only one example is described in detail, namely, the links between sexual abuse and poor perinatal mental health.

Perinatal mental health and sexual abuse

Traditionally, Depression and Anxiety were thought to be uncommon during pregnancy, however, quantitative research has revealed a strong association between childhood maltreatment, Depression, Anxiety disorders and PTSD, both during pregnancy and childbirth, and after childbirth (Choi and Sikkema, 2016). Sexual abuse, particularly more invasive abuse, increases the risk of both Depression and Anxiety during pregnancy (Choi and Sikkema, 2016). Clinically, there are a range of connections between pregnancy in a woman with a history of sexual abuse and triggers for posttraumatic distress. For example, a woman with a history of invasive sexual abuse could react to the actual presence of another human being inside her body, she could have concerns about the sort of world that her infant is being born into, harm befalling her child, as well as her own capacity to keep her child safe.

Qualitative research, which privileges the voices of survivors, offers further insights into the subjective experiences of women during pregnancy and in childbirth. One systematic review relating to the experiences of childbirth in survivors of sexual abuse examined 10 reports spanning 25 years (LoGiudice, 2016). This review identified that childbirth itself can be extremely distressing for women with histories of sexual abuse and noted that a lack of perceived control, routine aspects of childbirth such as vaginal examination, pushing in the second stage of labour, having an epidural anaesthetic, or seeing others touch the vulnerable infant may all trigger severe anxiety, flashbacks, and dissociative experiences for women with these histories.

Difficulties in the postnatal period can also affect the quality of the new mother's relationship with her infant. Another systematic review, examining observational studies of mother–infant dyads, confirmed the association between early abuse and difficulties in the emerging relationship between mother and infant (Vaillancourt et al., 2017). Overall, studies identify that mothers with histories of childhood maltreatment struggle to be sensitive to the needs of their infants. As the infant becomes a toddler, the dyad can become inverted, with the toddler attempting to provide care for the mother, who can alternate between being overprotective, to prevent the abuse of her child, and being oblivious to the dangers that particular individuals, such as potential romantic partners, might pose. Children can also become prematurely self-reliant, parentified and hostile, while also being brittle, anxious and extremely vulnerable at other times (Amos et al., 2011).

The importance of research and making connections between child maltreatment and sequelae

Associations and correlations are only considered causal if nine criteria, set down by Sir Bradford Hill, are met (Anda et al., 2006). These criteria include plausibility, a strong and specific correlation between two variables, in this case childhood maltreatment and later health difficulties; consistency of evidence across multiple studies; evidence that the insult occurs before the outcome; a dose–response relationship; a well described biological mechanism to explain the association; experimental evidence to support the mechanisms; and that the findings do not contradict existing knowledge of a disease. The evidence relating maltreatment in childhood and subsequent poor health meets all of these criteria, supporting a causal association.

First, research consistently reveals a strong correlation between child maltreatment and a wide range of mental and physical health conditions. The ACE studies clearly demonstrate a graded, dose-response relationship between early adversity and difficulties in adult life (Anda et al., 2006). For example, exposure to one adverse experience increased the risk of Depression 1.5 times, whereas exposure to four or more adverse experiences increased the risk 3.6 times. The risk of severe Obesity was increased 1.3 times with a single exposure and 1.9 times with four or more. The risk of using injectable illicit drugs was increased 2.3 times with one adverse experience and 11.1 times with four or more.

Paralleling the evidence regarding the strength of the observed association between exposure to childhood maltreatment and poor outcomes in childhood, adolescence, and adulthood is the surge of interest and research into the biological mechanisms underpinning these associations, such as the effects on the brain, the immune and endocrine systems, and memory. There is an emerging consensus that, at a basic biological level, infants, children, and adolescents adapt to endangering early environments by "permanently embodying environmental information in their structure and function" (Grassi-Oliveira et al., 2008: p.62). To give some sense of the explanatory power of the biological research, the relationship between perinatal Depression, Anxiety, and PTSD is used as an example of how a series of interlocking mechanisms initiated in infancy could give rise to maternal Depression and Anxiety in the perinatal period.

Thinking about a mother, maltreated as an infant, and drawing on the work of Danese and Baldwin (2017), it is likely that the psychological distress and pain caused by experiences of maltreatment provoke an immune response, just as bacterial or viral infections do. The difference is that, when the immune system responds to an acute infection, this response is attenuated once the infection subsides. Where the threat continues, as frequently occurs in child maltreatment, the immune system becomes chronically hyper-reactive.

This chronic hyper-reactivity has been shown to affect the functioning of the hypothalamic–pituitary axis, leading to persistently high levels of cortisol, which in turn, is toxic to the developing brain, causing cell death in areas that are sensitive to its effects, for example, the hippocampus (Teicher and Samson, 2016). The hippocampus is involved in the encoding and retrieval of autobiographical memory, as well as the placing of memories in context (Teicher and Samson, 2016); a fact that is important in understanding the link between immune dysregulation and mental health difficulties. Adults suffering from Depression, Anxiety, and PTSD have consistently been observed to have reduced hippocampal volume which has been linked with immune dysfunction (Teicher and Samson, 2016), findings that point to a shared neurobiological substrate in infancy and adulthood. Disturbances in autobiographical memory and in the contextualisation of memory are hallmarks of PTSD and contribute to the context-dependent intrusion of memory in situations reminiscent of the original context within which the maltreatment was experienced, linking immune hyper-reactivity in infancy with core symptoms of PTSD in adulthood (Elbert et al., 2015).

In her research, LoGiudice (2016) clearly demonstrates how the loss of bodily control experienced by a birthing woman, who is subject to invasive genital procedures by medical and nursing staff, and the feeling of the infant moving down the birth canal, acts as a contextual trigger for memories of invasive sexual abuse. This is an example of how disturbances in memory systems, of which the hippocampus is a part, can affect what might otherwise be considered routine health care. Depending on the timing of the abuse, or the relative levels of dissociation of these memories from the rest of the personality (Van der Hart et al., 2006), the woman may not be aware that her distress is related to her past traumatic experiences (as well as the inevitable discomfort of birthing), leaving her vulnerable to misattributing her distress to the infant's entry into the world. This potentially sets the scene for a difficult relationship between mother and infant, thus continuing the cycles of disrupted relationships, neglect, and abuse (Amos et al., 2011).

More than 10 years ago, Anda and colleagues, citing the increasing convergence between the findings in neuroscience and epidemiology, proposed that research findings of a relationship between childhood maltreatment and later health outcomes met the Bradford Hill criteria for causality (Anda et al., 2006). Since then, in addition to the research referred to in the preceding paragraphs, biological research in the areas of functional neuro-imaging, affective neurobiology and the psychological sciences have yielded increasingly comprehensive explanations of the impact of childhood maltreatment. The argument that the associations are causal continues to strengthen.

Child maltreatment as a determinant of the socioeconomic gradient in health

Social determinants of health are defined by the World Health Organization as

> the conditions in which people are born, grow, live, work and age. These circumstances are shaped by the distribution of money, power and resources at global, national and local levels. The social determinants of health are mostly responsible for health inequities – the unfair and avoidable differences in health status seen within and between countries.
>
> (World Health Organization, 2011)

This definition incorporates the proposition that social determinants are largely responsible for the observed socioeconomic gradient in health.

The World Health Organization established a Commission on Social Determinants of Health in 2005, publishing a major report in 2008 (World Health Organization, 2008), covering matters such as early childhood education, employment, participatory communities, income and social welfare protection, universal health care, fair taxation, gender equity, and sharing of political power. This work extends the scope of traditional public health and is focused on the social conditions in which people live as well as public health infrastructure (water, housing, health care, sewerage, and related areas), underpinned by income, status, and power imbalances. There is particular focus on national and global policies and the distribution of income, wealth, and power. Early childhood is identified here as a priority for action. Though economic circumstances are undoubtedly related to health (as both cause and consequence), it can be argued that it is the early nurturing environment, or failure thereof, as typified by child abuse and neglect, that is pivotal in either exacerbating or potentially disrupting disadvantage.

Child maltreatment is therefore postulated as a fundamental cause of the documented relationship between socioeconomic status and health, and poorer social and economic outcomes (Segal et al., 2011). This proposition rests on two core arguments: first, that child maltreatment has large direct and indirect effects on health (mental and physical), and second, that child maltreatment also impacts on the social determinants of health. As described earlier, the evidence that child maltreatment impacts on physical and mental health is extensive and incontrovertible. Research, including the numerous ACE studies (Centers for Disease Control and Prevention, 2016), report that, for almost every condition looked at, child maltreatment poses additional risk (Gilbert et al., 2009; Fryers and Brugha, 2013; Centers for Disease Control and Prevention, 2016). Increasingly well-defined mechanisms support this relationship as causal (Shonkoff et al., 2009; Amos et al., 2015). The impact of child maltreatment on the likelihood of mental disorders is extreme, with risk ratios from 100 to more than 1000 per cent (for example, four to 12 times the risk for attempted suicide) (Dube et al., 2001) and for physical health generally in the 25 to 50 per cent excess risk range (Norman et al., 2012; Gilbert et al., 2015). The adoption of harmful life-style behaviours such as early use of tobacco, illicit drugs, and alcohol, disordered eating (including Anorexia Nervosa and Morbid Obesity) and risky sexual behaviour further exacerbate the effects on health (Felitti et al., 1998).

Child maltreatment also impacts on what are known as "the social determinants of health" such as education, employment, welfare dependency, income, and housing. The primary mechanism is through the toxic effects of child maltreatment and early life trauma on brain development, which in turn influences behaviour, affect regulation, and sometimes intellectual capacity. Children might exhibit poor impulse control, have difficulty in focus and planning, and a reduced capacity to form and maintain successful peer relationships, so that many victims of child maltreatment have difficulty engaging with school, observed in lower school attendance, high rates of increased suspensions and expulsions, and poor academic performance (Productivity Commission, 2017). These outcomes will be worse for children of parents who through their own trauma histories are unable to offer a supportive learning environment at home. Child maltreatment can also disturb relational understandings, profoundly affecting sense of self and capacity for agency (Amos et al., 2015), potentially increasing risk of justice involvement and welfare dependency.

Furthermore, the initial vulnerability attracts additional adversities. A compromised education, when combined with problematic behaviours, poorer mental and physical health, possible drug and alcohol use from an early age (as a form of self-medication to deal with the distress), further exacerbates likely harms. These compounding adversities inevitably impact on other key social determinants, such as the ability to secure and maintain employment, or the ability to navigate the social welfare system, with deleterious effects on the ability to earn an income and to afford and sustain secure housing. Relationship breakdown, which has its own negative effects on the family system, can further aggravate the social difficulties.

To illustrate the strength of the impact of child maltreatment on the socioeconomic gradient, it is helpful to look at child protection data. In Australia, child protection rates, the number of children per 1000 in notifications and substantiations, in the lowest socioeconomic decile are 10 to 20 times the rates for children in the top decile (increased by 1,000 to 2,000 per cent) (Hirte, 2006; O'Donnell et al., 2010). The relationship is non-linear, with differences exaggerated in the bottom and top deciles. There is no evidence to suggest this is primarily a surveillance bias issue, especially in the context of decades of mandatory reporting.

The authors of this chapter argue that child abuse and neglect is "the cause of the causes": that child abuse and neglect is the cause of the profound and intractable disadvantage evident in the well documented socioeconomic gradient of health. As outlined above, child maltreatment has both direct impacts on health and well-being but also inevitably attracts additional adversity, compounding the risk of poor health, social and economic outcomes. Furthermore, as child maltreatment is implicated in intergenerational transmission (Segal and Dalziel, 2011; Amos et al., 2011, 2015; Amos, 2017; Vaillancourt et al., 2017), it is a source of entrenched disadvantage across generations, locking in socioeconomic disparities.

Policy implications

The problem of child maltreatment has profound policy implications with respect to existing health, social, and economic inequalities. That families and their histories of trauma be given paramount importance is the message intended in this chapter. Supporting families in healing from past trauma, as well as helping currently stressed and distressed parent–child relationships, must be given priority.

This model of illness and health, and the pivotal role of the family environment is captured in Figure 4.1, which is taken from an earlier description of the argument published elsewhere (Segal et al., 2011). The immediate and more distant consequences of the early family environment are shown as the central cause–consequence pathway, responsible for setting up a destructive and entrapping cycle, or a virtuous and life-enhancing cycle. The community, state, and national level social and health policy environment is shown to be relevant, but on the periphery, in the sense that policies are either working "hard" to overcome early disadvantage, or for those who are already advantaged, likely extend their potential even further. These policies are unlikely to reduce disparities. The model in effect argues that the best path to reducing general health and social disparities is via the family – ensuring a nurturing early family environment.

The need to consider and enhance protective factors must also be emphasised, so that maltreated children can be set on a more favourable trajectory that will maximise their potential, rather than on a destructive trajectory that will undermine their life chances. The resilience of human beings must also be recognised. Many children faced with multiple adversities (Guy et al., 2016) can go on to live successful, fulfilled, and long lives, although this is not the typical experience of children with a serious history of child maltreatment.

Conclusion

Child maltreatment is a significant public health issue, likely affecting more than 25 per cent of Australians (Segal, 2015). Its impact on mental and physical health leading to a wide range of social and economic outcomes is considerable and can be experienced from infancy across the entire life course. The biological and psychosocial mechanisms that underpin this impact are becoming increasingly well understood, and causality is being increasingly inferred. This knowledge, combined with new understandings of the pathways into maltreatment and how to disrupt them, makes the prevention of child maltreatment and its associated negative consequences a realistic possibility (Amos, 2017). Investing in

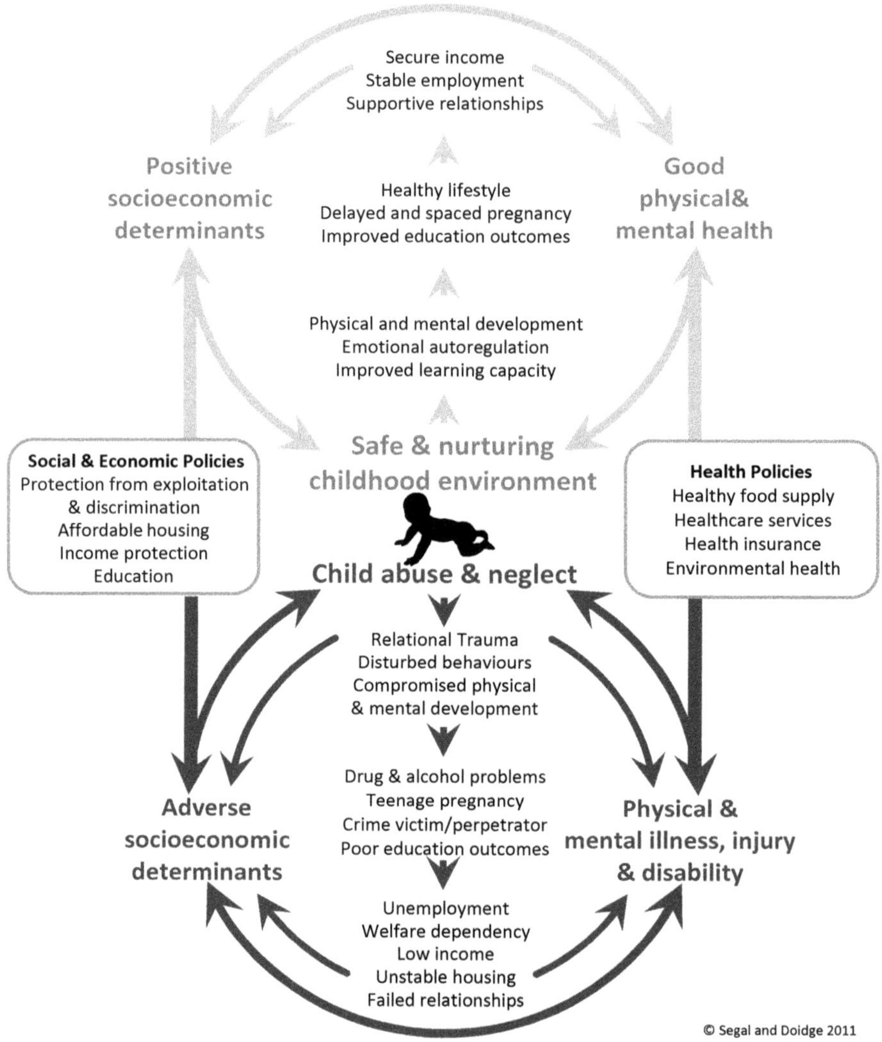

Figure 4.1. Direct and indirect mechanisms through which the childhood environment drives health and wellbeing. The CHOICES model: Changing Health Outcomes by Improving Childhood Environments. Reproduced from Segal et al. (2011).

well-designed, adequately resourced, and targeted programs and services to address child maltreatment will certainly help not only alleviate current distress for children and parents, but also avert the cascade of downstream consequences, including intergenerational transmission.

Society has acknowledged the need to prioritise health, social and economic inequalities, and to address child maltreatment, so that all children can grow up in a safe and nurturing environment. However, that these issues are intimately related is rarely considered. The cost of child maltreatment in terms of the suffering of children, adults, and families, its impact on government, and on the fabric of society, is immense. Putting in place an adequate service response that involves at its core mental health workers with adequate levels of training in the treatment of trauma, to work in collaboration with other services, for example, early childhood education and family support services, is critical. This conclusion is consistent with other research that finds there is a need for a considerable expansion of high quality infant, child, adolescent, and family mental health services (Segal et al., 2018). The entire human services sector needs to work together with vulnerable families in a more trauma-informed way. As has been outlined earlier, child maltreatment perpetuates a vicious cycle of negative consequences that attract additional adversities and transfers disadvantage across generations. In fact, child maltreatment might just be the most pivotal and potentially modifiable variable, offering the best opportunity to intervene and indeed reverse the socioeconomic gradient in health. There can be no better place to focus the community effort with the prospect of the greatest possible returns on investment.

In contrast to the conventional social determinants argument, which emphasises the distribution/redistribution of income, wealth, and power, a focus on the family environment and the quality of family relationships offers a pathway through which real change is possible.

References

Afari N, Ahumada SM, Wright LJ, et al. (2014) Psychological trauma and functional somatic syndromes. *Psychosomatic Medicine* 76(1): 2–11.

Afifi TO, MacMillan L, Boyle M, et al. (2016) Child abuse and physical health in adulthood. *Health Reports* 27(3): 10–18.

American Psychiatric Association (2013) *Diagnostic and Statistical Manual of Mental Disorders, Fifth Edition*. Arlington, VA: American Psychiatric Publishing.

Amos JA (2017) *When wounds from infancy collide: The mother child relationship as trauma, trigger, and treatment*. PhD Thesis. Adelaide, Australia: University of South Austalia.

Amos J, Furber G and Segal L (2011) Understanding maltreating mothers: A synthesis of relational trauma, attachment disorganization, structural dissociation of the personality, and experiential avoidance. *Journal of Trauma and Dissociation* 12(5): 1–16.

Amos J, Segal L and Cantor C (2015) Entrapped mother, entrapped child: Agonic mode, hierarchy and appeasement in intergenerational abuse and neglect. *Journal of Child and Family Studies* 24(5): 1442–1450.

Anda RF, Felitti VJ, Bremner DG, et al. (2006) The enduring effects of abuse and related adverse experiences in childhood: A convergence of evidence from neurobiology and epidemiology. *European Archives of Psychiatry and Clinical Neuroscience* 256 (3): 174–186.

Battle CL, Shea TM, Johnson DM, et al. (2004) Childhood maltreatment associated with adult personality disorders: Findings from the collaborative longitudinal personality disorders study. *Journal of Personality Disorders* 18(2): 193–211.

Braga T, Concalves LC, Basto-Pereira M, et al. (2017) Unraveling the link between maltreatment and juvenile antisocial behavior: A meta-analysis of prospective longitudinal studies. *Aggression and Violent Behavior* 33: 37–50.

Centers for Disease Control and Prevention (2016) *Adverse Childhood Experiences (ACEs)*. Available at: cdc.gov/violenceprevention/acestudy.

Choi KW and Sikkema KJ (2016) Childhood maltreatment and perinatal mood and anxiety disorders: A systematic review. *Trauma, Violence and Abuse* 17(5): 427–453.

Cook A, Spinazzola J, Ford J, et al. (2017). Complex Trauma in children and adolescents. *Psychiatric Annals* 35(5): 390–398.

Danese A and Tan M (2014) Childhood maltreatment and obesity: Systematic review and meta-analysis. *Molecular Psychiatry* 19: 544–554.

Danese A and Baldwin JR (2017) Hidden wounds? Inflammatory links between childhood trauma and psychopathology. *Annual Review of Psychology* 68: 517–544.

Dube SR, Anda RF, Felitti VJ, et al. (2001) Childhood abuse, household dysfunction, and the risk of attempted suicide throughout the life span: Findings from the Adverse Childhood Experiences Study. *Journal of the American Medical Association* 286: 3089–3096.

Elbert T, Schauer M and Neuner F (2015) Narrative Exposure Therapy (NET): Reorganizing memories of traumatic stress, fear, and violence. In: Schnyder U and Cloitre M (eds) *Evidence Based Treatments for Trauma-related Psychological Disorders*. Basel, Switzerland: Springer International Publishing, pp.229–254.

Felitti VJ, Anda RF, Nordenberg D, et al. (1998) Relationship of childhood abuse and household dysfunction to many of the leading causes of death in adults: The Adverse Childhood Experiences (ACE) Study. *American Journal of Preventive Medicine* 14(4): 245–258.

Fryers T and Brugha T (2013) Childhood determinants of adult psychiatric disorder. *Clinical Practice and Epidemiology in Mental Health* 9: 1–50.

Gilbert R, Spatz Widom C, Browne K, et al. (2009) Child Maltreatment Series 1: Burden and consequences of child maltreatment in high-income countries. *The Lancet* 373: 68–81.

Gilbert LK, Breiding MJ, Merrick MT, et al. (2015) Childhood adversity and adult chronic disease: An update from ten states and the District of Columbia, 2010. *American Journal of Preventative Medicine* 48(3): 345–349.

Grassi-Oliveira R, Ashy M and Stein LM (2008) Psychobiology of childhood maltreatment: Effects of allostatic load? *Revista Brasileira de Psiquiatria* 30(1): 60–68.

Guy S, Furber G, Leach M, et al. (2016) How many children in Australia are at risk of adult mental illness? *Australian and New Zealand Journal of Psychiatry* 50(12): 1146–1160.

Hirte C (2006) *Contact with the South Australian Child Protection System: A Statistical Analysis of Longitudinal Child Protection Data*. Adelaide, Australia: Government of South Australia, Department for Families and Communities.

Irish L, Kobayashi I and Delahanty DL (2010) Long-term physical health consequences of childhood sexual abuse: A meta-analytic review. *Journal of Pediatric Psychology* 35(5): 450–461.

Kajeepeta S, Gelaye B, Jackson CL, et al. (2015) Adverse childhood experiences are associated with adult sleep disorders: A systematic review. *Sleep Medicine* 16: 320–330.

Lalor K and McElvaney R (2010) Child sexual abuse, links to later sexual exploitation/high risk sexual behavior and prevention/treatment programs. *Trauma, Violence and Abuse* 11(4): 159–177.

LoGiudice JA (2016) A systematic literature review of the childbearing cycle as experienced by survivors of sexual abuse. *Nursing for Women's Health* 20(6): 582–594.

McCrory E, De Broto SA and Viding E (2012) The link between child abuse and psycho-pathology: A review of neurobiological and genetic research. *Journal of the Royal Society of Medicine* 105(4): 151–156.

Marangoni C, Hernandez M and Faedda G (2016) The role of environmental exposures as risk factors for bipolar disorder: A systematic review of longitudinal studies. *Journal of Affective Disorders* 193: 165–174.

Matheson SL, Shepard AM, Pinchbeck RM, et al. (2013) Childhood adversity in schizophrenia: A systematic analysis. *Psychological Medicine* 43(2): 225–238.

Mathews CA, Kaur N and Stein MB (2008) Childhood trauma and obsessive-compulsive symptoms. *Depression and Anxiety* 25: 742–751.

Molendijk ML, Hoek HW, Brewerton TD, et al. (2017) Childhood maltreatment and eating disorder pathology: A systematic review and dose-response meta-analysis. *Psychological Medicine* 47(8): 1402–1416.

Nemeroff CB (2016) Paradise lost: The neurobiological and clinical consequences of child abuse and neglect. *Neuron* 89(5): 892–909.

Norman RE, Byambaa M, De R, et al. (2012) The long-term health consequences of child physical abuse, emotional abuse, and neglect: A systematic review and meta-analysis. *Plos Medicine* 9(11): e1001349.

O'Donnell M, Nassar N, Leonard H, et al. (2010) Characteristics of non-Aboriginal and Aboriginal children and families with substantiated child maltreatment: A population-based study. *International Journal of Epidemiology* 39: 921–928.

Paras ML, Murad MH, Chen LP, et al. (2009) Sexual abuse and lifetime diagnosis of somatic disorders. A systematic review and meta-analysis. *Journal of the American Medical Association* 302(5): 550–561.

Productivity Commission (2017) *Report on Government Services*. Canberra, Australia: Australian Government.

Segal L (2015) Economic issues in the community response to child maltreatment. In: Mathews B and Bross D (eds) *Mandatory Reporting Laws and the Identification of Severe Child Abuse and Neglect. Child Maltreatment, Volume 4 (Contemporary Issues in Research and Policy)*. New York, NY: Springer, pp.193–216.

Segal L and Dalziel K (2011) Investing to protect our children: Using economics to derive an evidence-based strategy. *Child Abuse Review* 20(4): 274–289.

Segal L, Doidge J and Amos J (2011) Determining the determinants: Is child abuse and neglect the underlying cause of the socio-economic gradient in health? In: Laverty M and Callaghan L (eds) *Determining the Future: A Fair Go and Health for All*. Melbourne, Australia: Connor Court Publishing, pp.159–176.

Segal L, Guy S, Leach M, et al. (2018) A needs-based workforce model to deliver tertiary-level community mental health care for distressed infants, children and adolescents in South Australia: A mixed methods study. *Lancet Public Health* 3: e296–303.

Shonkoff J, Boyce W and McEwen B (2009) Neuroscience, molecular biology, and the childhood roots of health disparities: Building a new framework for health promotion and disease prevention. *Journal of the American Medical Association* 301: 2252–2259.

Sundin EV and Baguley T (2015) Prevalence of childhood abuse among people who are homeless in western countries: A systematic review and meta-analysis. *Social Psychiatry and Psychiatric Epidemiology* 50(2): 183–194.

Teicher MH and Samson JA (2016) Annual Research Review: Enduring neurobiological effects of childhood abuse and neglect. *Journal of Child Psychology and Psychiatry* 57(3): 241–266.

Vaillancourt K, Pawlby S and Fearon RMP (2017) History of childhood abuse and mother–infant interaction: A systematic review of observational studies. *Infant Mental Health Journal* 38(2): 226–248.

Van der Hart O, Nijenhuis ERS and Steele K (2006) *The Haunted Self: Structural Dissociation of the Personality and the Treatment of Chronic Traumatization*. New York, NY: Norton.

Weber S, Jud A and Landolt MA (2016) Quality of life in maltreated children and adult survivors of child maltreatment: A systematic review. *Quality of Life Research* 25(2): 237–255.

Wegman H and Stetler C (2009) Meta-analytic review of the effects of childhood abuse on medical outcomes in adulthood. *Psychosomatic Medicine* 71(8): 805–812.

World Health Organization (2008) *Closing the Gap in a Generation: Health Equity Through Action on the Social Determinants of Health. Commission on Social Determinants of Health, Final Report*. Geneva, Switzerland: World Health Organization.

World Health Organization (2011) *Gender Equity and Human Rights*. Available at: who.int/gender-equity-rights/understanding/sdh-definition/en.

5 Adult trauma and Posttraumatic Stress Disorder – contemporary concepts

Alexander C McFarlane

Historical background

Posttraumatic Stress Disorder (PTSD) is now so much a part of modern nomenclature and broader society that it is difficult to comprehend just how far psychiatry has advanced in this area over the last four decades. Prior to the inclusion of PTSD in the Third Edition of the *Diagnostic and Statistical Manual of Mental Disorders*, the DSM-III, in 1980 (American Psychiatric Association, 1980), there was no diagnostic category that captured the concept that adult exposure to extreme stress could lead to a prolonged psychological injury. The new more scientific approach to classification introduced in the DSM-III represented a remarkable renaissance in both academic and clinical psychiatry. Rigorous observational phenomenology came to replace the theoretical hypotheses of psychoanalysis, involving infantile sexuality, fantasy and unconscious conflict as the cause of most adult psychopathology, and the concept of neurosis was removed from diagnostic systems. This change allowed for a reformulation of the enduring effects of traumatic stress and its relevance to psychopathology.

It is important to realise that the concept of PTSD has a long history, dating back at least to Oppenheim's definition of Traumatic Neurosis in 1889, where it was asserted that psychological trauma brought about actual organic changes (Oppenheim, 1889). World War I and World War II led to this disorder being discarded for political and nationalistic reasons, rather than over questions of validity (Shephard, 2003). In World War I, in particular, the acknowledgment of psychological disability was seen to undermine the fighting spirit. At that time, the combination of suggestibility and the process of diagnosis were seen to be the cause of illness, not exposure to the enduring horrors of war. The effects of stress were also seen to be acute and short-lived, so that soldiers could be managed by brief interventions that could be followed by a return to the front. Long-term disability was similarly seen to be a response to the possibility of compensation by the authorities, so that it was also thought that there should be no pension payments. The realities of war, however, prevented this philosophy from being enforced. In the wake of World War II, the focus on the acute effects of stress led to the introduction of the category of "Transient Situational Disturbance" in the DSM-II.

It should also be noted that a significant amount of research was conducted in the 1960s and 1970s about the effects of a broad range of life stressors and their contribution to adult psychiatric disorders. This body of work provided part of the foundation for the re-emergence of interest in catastrophic events, such as disasters, bereavement and sexual assaults perpetrated upon both children and adults. It was this work, along with a renewed understanding of the devastating long-term effects of war seen in veterans returning from Vietnam, that led to the creation of the diagnostic category of PTSD.

Current conceptualisations of Posttraumatic Stress Disorder

Classification issues

The initial criteria for PTSD required the direct experience of an event that was "outside the range of usual human experience", regular re-experiencing of the event, and persistent symptoms of avoidance and arousal (American Psychiatric Association, 1980); a three-factor model. Those involved in the development of the original diagnosis were focused on stressors like war, torture, rape, and natural disasters, and categorised PTSD as a type of Anxiety Disorder. The traumatic stressor, occurring externally, was thought to be the most important factor. Symptomatically, those suffering with PTSD may suffer from a broad range of difficulties including memories and nightmares of the trauma, hypervigilance, withdrawal, irritability, insomnia, aggression and self-harm, substance abuse, depression and anxiety, a number of physical problems, and have a higher risk of developing significant cognitive dysfunction (Yehuda et al., 2015).

The diagnosis of PTSD has always been somewhat controversial, and the criteria used in different versions of the DSM system, the major classification system in use, have changed substantially since the condition was first included (North et al., 2016). Over this period, for example, the number of potential symptoms has increased from 12 to 20. A range of significant variations were introduced more recently with the publication of the Fifth Edition of the system, the DSM-5 (American Psychiatric Association, 2013). First, the condition was moved out of the Anxiety Disorders category into a newly created section called "Trauma and Stressor-Related Disorders". This move reflected both the relevant aetiology and the understanding that symptoms other than anxiety may be predominant. In particular, the significance of negative alterations in cognitions and mood were introduced as a subset of criteria in the new manual. These focus on overly and often distorted negative thoughts and assumptions about oneself and the world, a loss of interest in activities, estrangement from others, exaggerated blame of the self or others, and an inability to recall key features of the trauma. As such, PTSD is now seen as a four, rather than a three, factor model.

A "Dissociative Subtype" of PTSD has also been added into the DSM-5. This specifier is used when there are high levels of depersonalisation or derealisation in response to trauma-related stimuli. The new subtype is associated with greater symptom severity and is based upon symptom clustering studies via latent class analysis, brain imaging studies, and varying treatment responses for this group (Lanius et al., 2012). A pre-school type of PTSD has also been added, in recognition of the possibility that such a serious condition can present in children of this age group.

The changes involving negative thoughts have been driven by the increasing dominance of Cognitive Behavioural theorists in the trauma field. However, the narrowness of this approach has been challenged by numerous senior clinicians and academics (Hoge et al., 2016). Importantly, the cognitive approach does not address the breadth of affective responses that may occur at the time of the traumatic exposure, such as horror. Trauma may also lead to a broader range of subsequent problems with affect dysregulation including irritability, guilt, anger, and shame.

Fear, sensitisation, and kindling

In contrast with earlier views in which PTSD was seen as a disorder of memory, PTSD is now conceptualised primarily as a fear-based disorder. This view emphasises the importance of the fear response at the time of the traumatic exposure, which leads to a secondary cascade of conditioned reactivity and responses to environmental triggers. Research data repeatedly demonstrate abnormalities in fear conditioning and extinction learning (Yehuda et al., 2015), and this is particularly thought to involve impaired regulation of the amygdala by the prefrontal cortex (Rauch et al., 2006).

Importantly, there is a growing body of research that highlights that it is the cumulative burden of trauma exposure that increases the risk of PTSD developing (Brewin et al., 2000), and that the delayed onset of PTSD is common (Bryant et al., 2015), suggesting that traumatic exposure may progressively lead to a disruption of an individual's interpretation of and adaptation to the environment. This has not previously been well understood because of the relative lack of long-term follow-up studies of trauma-exposed populations; often researchers will follow a population in the acute aftermath of an event in the months that follow and in so doing miss the morbidity that can emerge even 20 years later (McFarlane et al., 2017). One large multi-site study with extended follow-up demonstrated that there are five potential pathways after a traumatic event (Bryant et al., 2015). Whereas 73 per cent were resilient and 6 per cent recovered, 4 per cent remained chronically ill, 8 per cent got worse and then improved, while 10 per cent worsened and did not improve. The two groups that deteriorated involved 18 per cent of those studied, substantially more than had been previously anticipated, and was more common than those who had elevated levels of acute symptoms. These findings highlight the progression of the disorder through a subsyndromal phase that is underpinned by sensitisation and kindling to environmental stimuli (Bryant et al., 2015).

These models suggest that trauma can sensitise neural circuitry. The term "kindling" refers to electrophysiological changes that occur in the brain as a result of repeated exposures to a subthreshold stimulus such that there is a permanent decrease in the threshold for excitability; the word kindling originally meant to "set fire to". It seems likely that some who have been exposed to trauma may not experience obvious psychological symptoms in the immediate aftermath, but when exposed to stressors reactivate previously conditioned trauma responses. The sensitisation model suggests that individuals may respond excessively to subsequent and potentially less stressful events, and that these effects will be compounding. Memories of traumatic events, originally contained, may become increasingly dominant and drive increasing hyperarousal when repeatedly triggered by traumatic reminders, such that sensitised neurobiological systems are unable to return to their homeostatic baseline (McFarlane, 2010).

This more recent work highlights the importance of focusing on emerging symptoms for preventive intervention before a more complete PTSD diagnosis is manifest. In clinical practice, these subsyndromal symptoms are often minimised and their predictive significance underestimated.

The importance of traumatic memory

Early perspectives regarding PTSD as a disorder of memory concentrated on the re-experiencing of memory in various ways, including reflexive recurrent involuntary memories, nightmares, and dissociative reactions or flashbacks that involved a sense of reliving the event by transposition in time and place. The importance of memory in PTSD occurred as a consequence of the contribution of early theorists, including Horowitz, who focused on the importance of imagery in the disorder (Horowitz, 1986). More contemporary observations have highlighted that a striking aspect of traumatic memories is their relative lack of verbal representations and their somatosensory quality (Brewin, 2001). The impact on the sufferer is that the present is often experienced very acutely through the prism of the past. Current experience in some situations ceases to be primary, and the past trauma comes to sit between the present environment and the individual's experience; there is a sense of being disembodied in the present as traumatic triggers repeatedly draw the individual back to the traumatic re-enactment. In contrast to more day-to-day memories that utilise explicit memory systems, traumatic memories are held primarily in implicit memory systems that are not as verbally accessible, and they are also more perceptual types of memory that are less associatively linked (Brewin, 2001). This occurs as a result of stress disrupting hippocampally-dependent memories, the hippocampus being the structure that consolidates information from short-term to long-term memory. This model has proposed a dual representation theory where there is a separate memory system underlying the vivid experiencing of the intrusive memories versus the ordinary autobiographical memories of trauma (Brewin et al., 1996). This has considerable implications for therapy as it is not possible to talk about material that is essentially inaccessible to memory.

Freud raised the relevance of traumatic memory to mental illness through his study of Hysteria with Breuer over 100 years ago (Breuer and Freud, 1895/1955). He advocated the exploration of the factual detail of the memory and the associated emotion; the key to improvement in therapy was to develop the expression of the emotion in language, in the context of the traumatic memory. The irony is that Freud's original conceptualisation has largely been adapted by the Cognitive Behaviourists in a range of constructs without acknowledgement of the original authors.

Psychobiological underpinnings

The final dimension of the original formulation of PTSD, not generally considered in contemporary versions, is Kardiner's formulation that it was a type of "physioneurosis", with soldiers suffering from a range of intense physical reactions to combat (Yehuda et al., 2015). Current diagnostic criteria largely ignore this domain and the significance of those somatic manifestations of distress that are frequently the presenting symptoms of patients, classically gastrointestinal and digestive disturbances. There is in fact now substantial evidence that PTSD is associated with inflammatory responses at a physiological level, which in turn can contribute to these non-specific physical symptoms of PTSD (Michopoulos and Jovanovic, 2015). A range of physical illnesses are also more common in individuals with PTSD, including Cancer, Autoimmune Disease, Cardiovascular Disease, as well as various pain conditions including chronic back and headache (O'Donovan et al., 2015). There is also sufficient evidence to suggest that the extent of the physical morbidities in PTSD lead to premature ageing and a decreased life expectancy on average of four years (Lohr et al., 2015).

These physical accompaniments of PTSD highlight the neurobiological underpinnings of the effects of traumatic stress and that their role in PTSD needs to be a primary focus of discussions about prevention and treatment. The evidence suggests that these disruptions in homeostasis are linked with the up-regulation of activation systems and compensatory up-regulation of inhibitory systems. The concept of allostasis has been used to characterise the increased physiological "wear and tear" arising from these shifts in physiological regulation that are a central part of PTSD (Michopoulos and Jovanovic, 2015). This area is not necessarily addressed in treatment because most therapies for PTSD are psychologically based, and most of these with cognitive and behavioural foci. A recent growth in the literature highlighting the extensive physical comorbidities of PTSD is however forcing a reconsideration of the importance of these bodily-based dimensions and, therefore, the need for new therapeutic approaches.

Prevalence of trauma and PTSD

One recent survey has shown that rates of trauma exposure and PTSD were higher in Australia than would have been expected in contrast to countries such as Italy and Spain (Dückers et al., 2016). These higher rates of accidents and violence have largely gone unnoticed in the wider community and are of concern given their potential consequences to mental health. Within Australia, there have been two National Mental Health and Wellbeing Surveys conducted, in 1997 and 2007 (Creamer et al., 2001; Slade et al., 2009). An intriguing finding from the 2007 study was that PTSD was the most common psychiatric disorder in the Australian community, at 4.4 per cent of the population, using ICD-10 criteria (the alternate classification system, the World Health Organization's International Classification of Diseases) – a higher prevalence than the 4.1 per cent rate of Major Depressive illness (Slade et al., 2009). It was also noteworthy that the rates had risen considerably from the 12-month prevalence estimate of 3.3 per cent in the 1997 survey. One explanation for this change in prevalence was the difference in the way that traumatic events were recorded in the two studies, as well as how these events were linked to the symptoms of PTSD. It is also increasingly recognised that the concept of a subthreshold form of PTSD needs to be recognised as it almost as prevalent as full PTSD (Stein et al., 1997), and as it causes significant dysfunction, with no significant differences found in degree of impairment in comparison with full PTSD (Zlotnick et al., 2002).

Data further highlight the cost of interpersonal trauma in relation to PTSD, in contrast to impersonal trauma (Forbes et al., 2012). Violence has a substantially greater impact on mental health than both accidents and disasters, which indicates the need for prevention in this area to be made a critical priority.

Those who suffer sexual abuse and rape, domestic violence, robbery, home invasion, and other types of violence may all develop severe PTSD, and at significant levels. Rape, for example, may produce rates of PTSD approximately 10 times that immediately following a natural disaster (Forbes et al., 2012). In Australia, for reasons primarily relating to intergenerational trauma, the situation for Indigenous Australians is substantially amplified; the lifetime prevalence of PTSD in one remote Indigenous community for example was recorded at 55 per cent (Nadew, 2012).

There has also been a recent focus through a "Beyond Blue" initiative (Beyond Blue is a major Australian mental health support and advocacy body) on the rates of PTSD in the emergency services sector (Beyond Blue, 2018). There are more than 500,000 paid and volunteer workers in this sector (Varker et al., 2018), and they are repeatedly exposed to vicarious, or secondary, trauma, which can result from being directly involved in distressing scenes of severe injuries and/or death, or from listening repeatedly to the trauma of others. With the newer understanding of cumulative burden and the effects of sensitisation and kindling, it is clear that emergency services workers are particularly at risk over the course of their careers. This is an important challenge because the diagnostic criteria for PTSD require the nomination of a specific traumatic event, although the inclusion of the category of indirect exposure to aversive details, such as first responders collecting body parts, has been included in the DSM-5 (American Psychiatric Association, 2013), which will assist with diagnosis and treatment. The Beyond Blue initiative involves a large study of the effects of trauma across a wide range of workers and will be followed up with a series of practical strategies to improve the mental health of those involved. The study is currently underway.

The Royal Commission into Institutional Responses to Child Sexual Abuse has also brought into sharp focus the significant adult consequences of childhood abuse (Royal Commission into Institutional Responses to Child Sexual Abuse, 2017). This is also in part due to the cumulative effects of trauma exposure, but particularly focuses on the detrimental consequences of sexual abuse. The long-term effects of these traumas are particularly mediated by the development of childhood Anxiety and Depressive disorders. With possible further exposure to trauma in adulthood, this burden of childhood abuse is a significant risk factor, highlighting the public health impact of trauma on child development, and the imperative for this to be addressed as a national priority in order to create resilient adult populations.

Military and veterans' mental health

The last 15 years has been a period of significant upheaval in the provision of health care to military personnel and veterans in Australia. Firstly, the Commonwealth Department of Veterans' Affairs has divested itself of Veterans' Affairs hospitals. These facilities previously provided an important network and coalition of health care providers, as well as opportunities for training in trauma-related mental health care. This change in service provision has coincided with a period of high operational tempo, with the Australian Defence Force (ADF) having been deployed continuously since 1999, first into East Timor and subsequently from 2001 into Afghanistan and Iraq.

A series of major studies has been carried out into the long-term health consequences of these deployments, and the entire ADF was surveyed to produce the 2010 ADF Mental Health Prevalence and Wellbeing Survey. This latter survey utilised the same methodology as the National Mental Health and Wellbeing Survey and was able to compare the ADF with the broader civilian community. The ADF experienced a 12-month prevalence of 22 per cent of any mental health disorder, with a higher rate of Affective Disorder (9.5 per cent versus 5.9 per cent) and a lower rate of Alcohol Abuse (5.2 per cent versus 8.3 per cent) than the civilian population (McFarlane et al., 2011). PTSD itself was present in 8.3 per cent of the military population in comparison with 5.2 per cent of a matched civilian cohort (McFarlane et al., 2011). An important finding of this study was that the rates of disorder were similar within the deployed and non-deployed populations. Several protective factors were identified in the deployed group, including a lower life-time history of trauma exposure, for example childhood interpersonal trauma, the existence of more stable relationships, and the holding of a higher rank.

An important issue for the ADF were the higher rates of PTSD than the civilian population, particularly in the younger age groups that represent a particularly vulnerable population if they are to transition to civilian life. These rates occur despite personnel being healthier on enlistment than the general population, because of recruitment standards, and highlight the importance of ongoing awareness of the delayed consequences of the Middle East Area of Operations deployments in ex-serving personnel, and the need to monitor for subsyndromal symptoms.

A further important body of work has been the ongoing study of the Vietnam veterans' cohort which has found that the rates of PTSD have continued to increase over the decades since the war ended. In one longitudinal follow-up study, although approximately 20 per cent were seen to suffer with PTSD in the 1990s, that number increased to 28 per cent in the 2000s (O'Toole et al., 2009). The costs of combat exposure in the Vietnam veterans were further demonstrated in a study showing the impact of a veteran's PTSD on the mental health of their children (Commonwealth of Australia, 2014).

Other trauma groups

Australia has continued to contribute to the broad body of research in the traumatic stress field above and beyond its own population. The multi-site study previously mentioned was carried out in teaching hospitals across Australia and involved more than 1000 patients admitted after a motor vehicle accident, assault, or a fall (Bryant et al., 2015). In addition to the work on delayed onset PTSD, this study further demonstrated the importance of PTSD in predicting the physical morbidity and quality of life in this population. For example, PTSD played an important role in the long-term outcome in terms of chronic pain and physical disability in these injury survivors (Liedl et al., 2010). Given its longitudinal nature, this study additionally illustrated the role of PTSD in disrupting the social support available to these individuals. Though levels of social support are often seen to be causally related to PTSD, this study highlighted that the emotional withdrawal, numbing, and the irritability of PTSD sufferers has a major disruptive effect on the quality of their ongoing social environments and that poor social support may be more the consequence of PTSD, rather than the cause. Importantly, the incidence of PTSD was not impacted upon by whether an individual was receiving compensation. However, the stress of the compensation process was shown to significantly compound the impairments and distress of the individuals. This further illustrates that compensation systems need to be subject to scrutiny because an excessively vigilant attitude on the part of the insurers can lead to adverse outcomes of those rightfully being compensated for their injuries.

The Black Saturday Bushfires of 2009 – Australia's worst bushfire disaster with 173 deaths, and more than 2000 houses destroyed – and the devastating downstream effects on Victorian communities demonstrates the ongoing challenges our country faces from fire, flood, and storm (Bryant et al., 2014). Despite often extensive planning, significant rates of morbidity still emerge in the aftermath when studied (Bryant et al., 2010). This is despite the existence of an awareness in the community of the potential for treatment via various mental health services. A critical strategy in dealing with disaster-affected populations is to use these events as an opportunity to strengthen and improve rural and remote mental health services in the aftermath. Traumatic events in the form of motor vehicle and agricultural accidents are common in these communities. Hence, the need for services does not suddenly dissipate in the aftermath of the disaster; rather, these events should be used to upskill the mental health workforce and to ensure adequate ongoing support for these communities.

Trauma and its role in other psychiatric disorders

PTSD is a restrictive lens that does not address the broader consequences of traumatic events in the Australian community. For example, Major Depressive Disorder occurs 12 months after accidents in 16 per cent of the population, Generalised Anxiety Disorder in 11 per cent, in contrast to PTSD in only 10 per cent (Bryant et al., 2010). This highlights that traumatic stress is an important aetiological factor in Affective and Anxiety Disorders, as well as in PTSD. Equally, Obsessive-Compulsive Disorder can also occur in the aftermath of traumatic events, with checking rituals focusing on safety and ruminations about inactions being impacted upon by these traumas (Grabe et al., 2008).

A broad literature also indicates that trauma exposure is a risk factor for the onset of Psychotic Disorders, and also predicts the probability of illness chronicity (Spauwen et al., 2006). This relationship is further complicated by the fact that individuals with Psychotic Disorders are a population at risk of interpersonal violence due to their social disadvantage and substance abuse. The impact of traumatic experiences that occur as a consequence of the psychotic illness should not be under-estimated. As a result, services for the severely mentally ill need to have an equal focus on the relevance of traumatic stress compared with the obviously trauma-affected populations.

The evidence of the role of trauma exposure and PTSD in the use of substances continues to grow. The drug crystal methamphetamine, or "ice", is particularly worthy of mention because of its increasing usage (McKetin et al., 2014) and because of the multiple ways that it may be associated with PTSD. One study has demonstrated that individuals with PTSD are more likely to have used crystal methamphetamine than those without PTSD, that those with PTSD are more likely to have used the drug for longer, and that they preferentially use the drug to manage avoidance and hyperarousal symptoms, but not the re-experiencing symptoms (Smith et al., 2010). One suggestion is that substance use has a feed forward effect on levels of consumption in those who are becoming symptomatic. However, it is not straightforward to infer causality as there are multiple other explanations, for example, those using substances being at risk of violence and PTSD. In any case, the use of substances like crystal methamphetamine may lead to more interpersonal violence, social disruption, and psychiatric difficulty. Substance abuse programs need to focus not only on substances but also on the effects of traumatic stress and the prevention of further episodes of violence and their unwanted consequences.

The need for neuroscience-informed treatment

Neuroscience has made substantial strides in the last three decades in elucidating the underlying psychobiological mechanisms of PTSD. Paradoxically, this has not led to improvements in treatment based on these novel neurobiological findings. Pharmacological treatments, for example, have had minimal advances in the last decade. The relative lack of innovation is highlighted when the 2013 Treatment Guidelines produced by the Australian Centre for Posttraumatic Mental Health (Australian Centre for Posttraumatic Mental Health, 2013) are compared with those first developed by the International Society of Stress Studies in 2000 (Foa et al., 2000), where few differences are seen. Ensuring evidence-based care is provided is a critical aim in improving treatment outcomes. Equally, improving the uptake of treatment, where as few as 40 per cent in the general population receive any care (Slade et al., 2009), should be made a priority. However, even with evidence-based care, in some populations where there has been cumulative trauma exposure, such as the military, after courses of treatment with Cognitive Processing Therapy or Prolonged Exposure therapy, 66 per cent of patients continue to meet the criteria for PTSD (Steenkamp et al., 2015). Similarly, substantial residual impairments are apparent in 80 per cent of participants in trials of psychotropic medication (Hoskins et al., 2015). Hence, despite the expanding repertoire of evidence-based care, substantial morbidity continues, and new strategies are required to improve treatment outcomes.

One approach that has promise is the use of "personalised medicine" that targets interventions according to the type and stage of a patient's presentation (Phillips et al., 2015). Some research has been done in Depression, but there is currently little to guide optimal treatment in PTSD. For example, higher levels of C-reactive protein, an inflammatory marker associated with PTSD, have been shown to predict treatment response to Bupropion (an antidepressant) when a Selective Serotonin Reuptake Inhibitor (SSRI) (another antidepressant) is added in Depression, whereas an SSRI alone is superior when inflammation is absent (Jha et al., 2017). Similar trials using augmentation strategies targeting inflammation in PTSD have not been carried out but are an important priority (Michopoulos and Jovanovic, 2015). To date, the issue of neurobiological profiling and treatment resistance have rarely been considered in the PTSD literature.

The absence of integration of neuroscience knowledge into clinical practice and planning care is in fact striking (Yehuda et al., 2015). If neuroscience is going to contribute to improved standards of care this will require structural strategies, such as providing items in the Australian Government's medical remuneration system, the Medical Benefits Schedule. For example, event-related potentials (measurable brain responses to specific stimuli) that examine information processing in PTSD could be utilised. Optimally, this type of work would initially be undertaken in specialist research clinics, involving agreed suites of phenomenological assessments and batteries of neuropsychological and neurobiological tests. Such a national strategy would allow the development of predictive algorithms to optimise the most appropriate choice of care. Equally, this strategy could assist in improving the treatment outcomes from those who are currently treatment resistant.

Systems of care

One of the most notable issues involving the care of adult trauma victims in Australia is the fragmentation that has occurred secondary to uncoordinated funding streams at multiple levels of government. For example, there are different funding streams for accident victims, victims of crime, and for veterans. Another challenge involving the fragmentation of services occurs within state government jurisdictions as different departments – health, emergency services, criminal justice, and child protection – also take uncoordinated approaches, with little focus on improving treatment outcomes (McFarlane and Bryant, 2017). This is above and beyond any other care that may be delivered by the private health sector.

The situation has been exacerbated for veterans with the privatisation of the Repatriation Hospitals and their devolution to the state health systems; their national coordinating role has been significantly lost. The state-based mental health services are often primarily focused on the treatment of Psychotic Disorders and invest little in the consequences of traumatic stress despite the evidence of its major impact. Also, state governments are increasingly trying to limit their liability for psychological injuries from motor vehicle accident and workers' compensation accidents, including for emergency services personnel (McFarlane and Bryant, 2017). These restrictive practices have a significantly detrimental impact in that they often harbour significant stigma and prejudice against the victims of traumatic stress. The absence of an integrated "whole of government" approach to the treatment of traumatic stress is an ongoing challenge.

The superficial coverage of PTSD in some clinical psychology training programs and in the training of psychiatrists also means that the next generation of mental health staff are not being well prepared for challenging practice. There are also increasingly fewer opportunities for clinical placements in services specifically designed to provide expert care for trauma sufferers.

The limited advocacy for services for PTSD is also in conspicuous contrast to the advocacy provided by organisations like Beyond Blue which focus primarily on Depression, despite there being a roughly equivalent burden of disease between the conditions managed.

This situation regarding the treatment of trauma occurs despite Australia being a leader internationally in the research field as well as in the development of evidence-based treatment guidelines by Phoenix Australia (Phoenix

Australia, 2013). This institution has provided an important focal point for professional development and for fostering areas of clinical and research excellence.

Challenges for the future

The improvement of care for victims of traumatic stress is not simply about improving the interventions offered in the settings of consultations. Broader questions involve systems of care, funding streams, and the range of therapies available. Both federal and state government input, co-operation, and funding are necessary to develop a national strategy for managing the effects of traumatic stress in the Australian community, and the establishment of a network of academic centres of clinical excellence across the nation is paramount. These centres would also serve as a prime resource for disasters and terrorism.

It is also important to note that health professionals carry collective experience and wisdom about the challenges that the system presents to patients. It is critical that a broad range of individuals and professional groups provide an advocacy role to improve the standards of care for those who have suffered trauma. Real change in the area of traumatic stress will only transpire when this occurs.

References

American Psychiatric Association (1980) *Diagnostic and Statistical Manual of Mental Disorders, Third Edition.* Washington, DC: American Psychiatric Publishing.

American Psychiatric Association (2013) *Diagnostic and Statistical Manual of Mental Disorders, Fifth Edition.* Arlington, VA: American Psychiatric Publishing.

Australian Centre for Posttraumatic Mental Health (2013) *Australian Guidelines for the Treatment of Acute Stress Disorder and Posttraumatic Stress Disorder.* Melbourne, Victoria: Australian Centre for Posttraumatic Mental Health.

Beyond Blue (2018) *National Mental Health and Wellbeing Study of Police and Emergency Services.* Available at: beyondblue.org.au/about-us/about-our-work/workplace-mental-health/pes-program/national-mental-health-and-wellbeing-study-of-police-and-emergency-services.

Breuer J and Freud S (1895/1955) Studies on hysteria. In: Strachey J (ed and trans) *The Standard Edition of the Complete Psychological Works of Sigmund Freud, Volume II.* London, UK: Hogarth Press.

Brewin CR (2001) A cognitive neuroscience account of posttraumatic stress disorder and its treatment. *Behaviour Research and Therapy* 39(4): 373–393.

Brewin CR, Dalgleish T and Joseph S (1996) A dual representation theory of posttraumatic stress disorder. *Psychological Review* 103(4): 670–686.

Brewin CR, Andrews B and Valentine DJ (2000) Meta-analysis of risk factors for posttraumatic stress disorder in trauma-exposed adults. *Journal of Consulting and Clinical Psychology* 68(5): 748.

Bryant RA, O'Donnell ML, Creamer M, et al. (2010) The psychiatric sequelae of traumatic injury. *American Journal of Psychiatry* 167(3): 312–320.

Bryant RA, Waters E, Gibbs L, et al. (2014) Psychological outcomes following the Victorian Black Saturday bushfires. *Australian and New Zealand Journal of Psychiatry* 48 (7): 634–643.

Bryant RA, Nickerson A, Creamer M, et al. (2015) Trajectory of post-traumatic stress following traumatic injury: 6-year follow-up. *The British Journal of Psychiatry* 206(5): 417–423.

Commonwealth of Australia (2014) *Vietnam Veterans Health Study. Volume 1, Introduction and Summary of the Studies of Vietnam Veterans Families*. Canberra, Australia: Department of Veterans' Affairs.

Creamer M, Burgess P and McFarlane AC (2001) Post-traumatic stress disorder: Findings from the Australian National Survey of Mental Health and Well-being. *Psychological Medicine* 31(7): 1237–1247.

Dückers ML, Alisic E and Brewin CR (2016) A vulnerability paradox in the cross-national prevalence of post-traumatic stress disorder. *The British Journal of Psychiatry* 209(4): 300–305.

Foa EB, Keane TM, Friedman MJ, et al. (2000) *Effective Treatments for PTSD: Practice Guidelines from the International Society for Traumatic Stress Studies, First Edition*. New York, NY: Guilford Press.

Forbes D, Fletcher S, Parslow R, et al. (2012) Trauma at the hands of another: Longitudinal study of differences in the posttraumatic stress disorder symptom profile following interpersonal compared with non-interpersonal trauma. *The Journal of Clinical Psychiatry* 73(3): 372–376.

Grabe HJ, Ruhrmann S, Spitzer C, et al. (2008) Obsessive-compulsive disorder and posttraumatic stress disorder. *Psychopathology* 41(2): 129–134.

Hoge CW, Yehuda R, Castro CA, et al. (2016) Unintended consequences of changing the definition of posttraumatic stress disorder in DSM-5: Critique and call for action. *JAMA Psychiatry* 73(7): 750–752.

Horowitz MJ (1986) *Stress Response Syndromes*. Northvale, NJ: J Aronson.

Hoskins M, Pearce J, Bethell A, et al. (2015) Pharmacotherapy for post-traumatic stress disorder: Systematic review and meta-analysis. *The British Journal of Psychiatry* 206(2): 93–100.

Jha MK, Minhajuddin A, Gadad BS, et al. (2017) Can C-reactive protein inform antidepressant medication selection in depressed outpatients? Findings from the CO-MED trial. *Psychoneuroendocrinology* 78: 105–113.

Lanius RA, Brand B, Vermetten E, et al. (2012) The dissociative subtype of posttraumatic stress disorder: Rationale, clinical and neurobiological evidence, and implications. *Depression and Anxiety* 29: 701–708.

Liedl A, O'Donnell M, Creamer M, et al. (2010) Support for the mutual maintenance of pain and posttraumatic stress disorder symptoms. *Psychological Medicine* 40(7): 1215–1223.

Lohr JB, Palmer BW, Eidt CA, et al. (2015) Is post-traumatic stress disorder associated with premature senescence? A review of the literature. *The American Journal of Geriatric Psychiatry* 23(7): 709–725.

McFarlane AC (2010) The long-term costs of traumatic stress: Intertwined physical and psychological consequences. *World Psychiatry* 9(1): 3–10.

McFarlane AC, Hodson S, Van Hooff M, et al. (2011) *Mental Health in the Australian Defence Force: 2010 ADF Mental Health Prevalence and Wellbeing Study, Full Report*. Canberra, Australia: Department of Defence.

McFarlane AC and Bryant RA (2017) PTSD: The need to use emerging knowledge to improve systems of care and clinical practice in Australia. *Australasian Psychiatry* 25(4): 329–332.

McFarlane AC, Lawrence-Wood E, Van Hooff M, et al. (2017) The need to take a staging approach to the biological mechanisms of PTSD and its treatment. *Current Psychiatry Reports* 19(2): 10.

McKetin R, Lubman DI, Najman JM, et al. (2014) Does methamphetamine use increase violent behaviour? Evidence from a prospective longitudinal study. *Addiction* 109(5): 798–806.

Michopoulos V and Jovanovic T (2015) Chronic inflammation: A new therapeutic target for post-traumatic stress disorder? *The Lancet Psychiatry* 2(11): 954–955.

Nadew GT (2012) Exposure to traumatic events, prevalence of posttraumatic stress disorder and alcohol abuse in Aboriginal communities. *Rural Remote Health* 12(4): 1667.

North CS, Suris AM, Smith RP, et al. (2016) The evolution of PTSD criteria across editions of the DSM. *Annals of Clinical Psychiatry* 28(3): 197–208.

O'Donovan A, Cohen BE, Seal KH, et al. (2015) Elevated risk for autoimmune disorders in Iraq and Afghanistan veterans with posttraumatic stress disorder. *Biological Psychiatry* 77(4): 365–374.

Oppenheim H (1889) *Die Traumatischen Neurosen*. Berlin, Germany: Hirschwald.

O'Toole BI, Catts SV, Outram S, et al. (2009) The physical and mental health of Australian Vietnam veterans three decades after the war and its relation to military service, combat, and post-traumatic stress disorder. *American Journal of Epidemiology* 170 (3): 318–330.

Phillips ML, Chase HW, Sheline Y, et al. (2015) Identifying predictors, moderators, and mediators of antidepressant response in major depressive disorder: Neuroimaging approaches. *American Journal of Psychiatry* 172(2): 124–138.

Phoenix Australia – Centre for Posttraumatic Mental Health (2013) *Australian Guidelines for the Treatment of Acute Stress Disorder and Posttraumatic Stress Disorder*. Melbourne, Australia: Phoenix Australia.

Rauch SL, Shin LM and Phelps EA (2006) Neurocircuitry models of posttraumatic stress disorder and extinction: Human neuroimaging research – past, present and future. *Biological Psychiatry* 60: 376–382.

Royal Commission into Institutional Responses to Child Sexual Abuse (2017) *Royal Commission into Institutional Responses to Child Sexual Abuse, Final Report*. Sydney, Australia: Commonwealth of Australia.

Shephard B (2003) *A War of Nerves: Soldiers and Psychiatrists in the Twentieth Century*. Cambridge, MA: Harvard University Press.

Slade T, Johnston A, Teeson M et al. (2009) *The Mental Health of Australians 2: Report on the 2007 National Survey of Mental Health and Wellbeing*. Canberra, Australia: Department of Health and Ageing.

Smith RC, Blumenthal H, Badour C, et al. (2010) An investigation of relations between crystal methamphetamine use and posttraumatic stress disorder. *Addictive Behaviors* 35 (6): 625–627.

Spauwen J , Krabbendam L, Lieb R, et al. (2006) Impact of psychological trauma on the development of psychotic symptoms: Relationship with psychosis proneness. *The British Journal of Psychiatry* 188(6): 527–533.

Steenkamp MM, Litz BT, Hoge CW, et al. (2015) Psychotherapy for military-related PTSD: A review of randomized clinical trials. *Journal of the American Medical Association* 314(5): 489–500.

Stein MB, Walker JR, Hazen AL, et al. (1997) Full and partial posttraumatic stress disorder: Findings from a community survey. *American Journal of Psychiatry* 154: 1114–1119.

Varker T, Metcalf O, Forbes D, et al. (2018) Research into Australian emergency services personnel mental health and wellbeing: An evidence map. *Australian and New Zealand Journal of Psychiatry* 52(2): 129–148.

Yehuda R, Hoge CW, McFarlane AC, et al. (2015) Post-traumatic stress disorder. *Nature Reviews Disease Primers* 1: 15057-1–15057-22.

Zlotnick C, Franklin CL and Zimmerman M (2002) Does "subthreshold" posttraumatic stress disorder have any clinical relevance? *Comprehensive Psychiatry* 43(6): 413–419.

6 Complex Post-Traumatic Stress Disorder, Developmental Trauma Disorder, Borderline Personality Disorder, and the Dissociative Disorders

Mary-Anne Kate and Martin J Dorahy

Introduction

Trauma-informed care is critical for all individuals who have experienced traumatic events, but the value is increased where exposure to trauma is "complex". This generally refers to situations in which trauma has occurred early in childhood, when it has occurred repeatedly, when it has occurred over prolonged periods of time, and when it is primarily interpersonal in nature. Under these circumstances, the individual is more likely to meet criteria for a trauma-related disorder. These conditions frequently present with a wide array of psychiatric and somatic symptoms; difficulties with affect regulation, identity, relationships with others; and a vulnerability to self-harm or victimisation (Herman, 1992). This chapter discusses mental disorders that are characterised by exposure to this type of trauma: Complex Post-Traumatic Stress Disorder (C-PTSD), Developmental Trauma Disorder (DTD), Borderline Personality Disorder (BPD), and the Dissociative Disorders (DDs). These disorders collectively make up a considerable number of those in hospital inpatient and outpatient programs, and those requiring acute care. The psychological impact of exposure to traumatic stress, especially when interpersonal in nature, creates not only a prolonged emotional burden for those affected and those connected with them, but there are also substantial medical, financial, and social costs. It is important to identify and accurately diagnose individuals with these disorders, as evidence-based treatments are available and effective.

Prevalence of trauma-related disorders in Australia

C-PTSD is now recognised as an official diagnosis in the International Classification of Diseases (ICD-11) (more below). General awareness of C-PTSD is lower than it is for Posttraumatic Stress Disorder (PTSD). With studies in the early stages, and considerable overlap with PTSD, statistics are complicated. Recent international epidemiological studies have however found that 0.6 per cent of the general population currently meet criteria for C-PTSD, that 2.6 per cent will meet criteria for C-PTSD during their lifetime, and that around one quarter to one half of individuals meeting criteria for PTSD will also meet criteria for C-PTSD (Wolf et al., 2015; Ben-Ezra et al., 2018). An earlier study of adults reporting childhood physical abuse, sexual abuse, or both, found that half met criteria for C-PTSD, and that women who had been both physically and sexually abused were 14.5 times more likely to develop C-PTSD than women who had suffered physical or sexual abuse only (Roth et al., 1997). The presence of C-PTSD is further intimated by Australian research showing rates of PTSD of 40–55 per cent in populations where a greater exposure to Complex Trauma has been documented – Indigenous Australians living in remote communities, sex workers, women fleeing domestic violence, and in children who have been sexually abused; these rates of PTSD are at least four times higher than those found in populations exposed to adult trauma, including those serving in the military, police force, and emergency services (Kate and Jamieson, 2017). More work is required, but it appears likely that as C-PTSD garners more interest as an official diagnostic entity it will be seen to be a very common mental disorder.

DTD is not yet an official diagnosis, and the prevalence is not known. The number of substantiated cases of child abuse and neglect, and the high proportion of individuals self-reporting adverse experiences in childhood indicate that it is likely that DTD is widespread (Van der Kolk, 2005).

It is estimated that approximately 1.6 per cent of all Australians meet the criteria for BPD, with prevalence rates increasing to 6 per cent in primary care settings. 10 per cent of outpatient populations and 20 per cent of inpatients receiving psychiatric care have a diagnosis of BPD (National Health and Medical Research Council, 2012).

The prevalence of the DDs in Australia is currently unknown, but international studies indicate that DDs may be much more common than typically believed. A general population study in New York State found a rate of 8.6 per cent, however this study did not conduct a full diagnostic assessment on all participants (Johnson et al., 2006). General population studies in Canada and Turkey using structured clinical interviews found the rate of DDs to be 13 per cent and 18 per cent, respectively (Kate and Middleton, 2018). The higher rate of DDs in Canada and Turkey is largely attributable to the higher prevalence of Dissociative Amnesia (7.5 per cent) than was evident in the American study (1.8 per cent), which is most likely the result of the American pre-screening process not effectively detecting Dissociative Amnesia. Rates of Dissociative Identity Disorder (DID) were broadly similar in all three studies, ranging from 1 to 3 per cent, which suggest it may be as common as BPD (Kate and Middleton, 2018). Other international studies have found that 1 per cent to 5 per cent of patients in general inpatient psychiatric units, in adolescent inpatient units, and in programs that treat Substance Abuse, Eating Disorders, and Obsessive-Compulsive Disorder, meet DSM diagnostic criteria for DID (International Society for the Study of Trauma and Dissociation, 2011). These findings are likely to be contested given scepticism surrounding the DDs, and further epidemiological studies using structured clinical interviews with all participants would be instructive to determine replicability.

Although studies of prevalence of trauma-related disorders are scarce in Australia, and issues like comorbidity with other disorders impact on accurate assessment, from the available data it seems likely that a substantial number of Australians will meet the diagnostic criteria for at least one of these trauma-related disorders in their lifetime, and that the area merits substantial attention.

Diagnostic categories

Complex Post-Traumatic Stress Disorder

For much of the twentieth century it was believed that exposure to traumatic events did not cause mental illness, and the role of trauma was essentially overlooked until the impact of external events was recognised when PTSD was introduced into the Diagnostic and Statistical Manual of Mental Disorders (DSM-III) in 1980 (Muir, 2007). C-PTSD found its way into the psychiatric lexicon through the astute clinical observations of Judith Herman, who recognised that the DSM diagnosis of PTSD did not capture the range and complexity of symptoms and characterological features of those describing exposure to multiple, chronic, and deliberate traumatic events (Herman, 1992).

The features of C-PTSD as outlined by Herman were operationalised under the moniker of Disorders of Extreme Stress Not Otherwise Specified (DESNOS) for the DSM-IV field trials, and included six psychobiological domains of dysregulation that captured the essence of the proposed symptom and characterological markers of C-PTSD (Van der Kolk et al., 2005). These were alterations in: 1) affect and impulses; 2) attention and consciousness, including amnesia and depersonalisation; 3) self-perception; 4) relations with others; 5) somatic symptoms; and, 6) systems of meaning (for example, hopelessness). Evidence supports the inclusion of C-PTSD as a unique diagnostic entity (Cloitre et al., 2013; Hyland et al., 2016) and also challenges it (Wolf et al., 2015). Individuals with DESNOS or C-PTSD can easily be mistaken for having a Mood, Anxiety, Personality, and/or Psychotic Disorder due to their complex presentation.

A vignette – the relevance of inquiring about trauma

A man arrived for treatment with very low mood, and anxiety about leaving his house. He reported hearing voices that commented on his behaviour, and they often informed him that he wasn't safe. His concerns for his safety could have been construed as paranoia, had his history of being bundled into a car while walking down the street and tortured for several days not been asked about. He had times when he would "tune-out", become confused or very agitated, and he could be volatile in relationships. He attempted to manage his internal experience by self-harming and with substance use, and the chronic nature of his problems, along with his efforts at managing them, led to him becoming quite socially isolated, fearing other people. His history revealed multiple incidences of child abuse by several of his mother's boyfriends, victimisation and perpetration as part of an adolescent gang, and multiple assaults, including the episode where he was held for several days.

DESNOS was omitted from the DSM-5 with the expansion of the diagnostic criteria of PTSD to explicitly capture alterations in self-perception related to emotions like shame and guilt, and because of the creation of the Dissociative Subtype of PTSD, which captures depersonalisation and derealisation in addition to the usual discriminating symptoms of PTSD (Friedman, 2013). Between 12–30 per cent of individuals with PTSD meet criteria for the new Dissociative Subtype, and this group has a greater exposure to childhood abuse and neglect than those who do not meet the criteria (Lanius et al., 2012); these individuals are more likely to fit the symptom profile of C-PTSD.

Although it is not recognised in the DSM-5, C-PTSD was introduced in the new edition of the ICD (ICD-11), and particularly apply to posttraumatic responses to exceedingly threatening or horrific events of an extreme, prolonged, or repetitive nature from which escape is difficult or impossible. Examples include repeated childhood sexual or physical abuse, prolonged domestic violence, torture, slavery, and genocide campaigns. The individual must meet the diagnostic requirements for PTSD as well as experiencing at least one symptom from each of the following domains: emotional dysregulation (for example, reactivity, outbursts, frequent dissociative episodes), negative self-perception (for example, shame, worthlessness), and relationship disturbance (for example, difficulties maintaining relationships) (World Health Organization, 2017). The presence of the core PTSD symptoms immediately distinguishes the C-PTSD criteria in the ICD-11 from DESNOS where these symptoms were not diagnostically required. The inclusion of C-PTSD in the ICD-11 provides international recognition of the significant impact of chronic interpersonal trauma on mental health.

Developmental Trauma Disorder

Emerging from studies of C-PTSD came a focus on the types of chronic, relational trauma which gave rise to the pervasive symptoms of C-PTSD that cut across multiple domains of body-mind functioning (Van der Kolk, 2014). These traumas were often of deliberate intent, beginning in childhood, and repeated often over lengthy periods, having major implications for neurobiological, psychosocial, and relational development. Numerous studies have shown the developmental impact of early relational trauma on brain maturation, which underpins other developmental processes (Teicher and Samson, 2016).

In an attempt to obtain adequate recognition of the mental health consequences of repetitive early-life trauma and adequate treatment for those living with its consequences, calls were made for the introduction of "Developmental

Trauma Disorder" (DTD) into the DSM-5 (Van der Kolk, 2005). Maltreated children are not served well by the current diagnostic system as many do not meet the criteria for PTSD, which also prevents a diagnosis of C-PTSD in the ICD-11. DTD was designed to, "capture the reality of the clinical presentations of children and adolescents exposed to chronic interpersonal trauma, and thereby guide clinicians to develop and utilize effective interventions, and for researchers to study the neurobiology and transmission of chronic interpersonal violence" (Van der Kolk, 2014: p.359). Like DESNOS, DTD was developed to encapsulate under the one category a number of clinical disorders that seem to be outcomes of traumatic stress. This removes the comorbidity issue: rather than having a vast array of symptoms (for example, anxiety, affect dysregulation, dissociation), and a number of discrete comorbid problems (for example, PTSD, Depression, Somatic Disorder), a unifying diagnosis allows sense to be made of an otherwise complex presentation. DTD was however not included in the DSM-5, but studies are currently underway to explore the validity of the construct in more depth. These studies have adopted the formulation that prolonged or multiple traumas occurring over the course of at least a year and which started in childhood or adolescence lead to major dysregulations in affective and physiological functioning, attentional and behavioural functioning, and self and relational functioning, as well as producing no less than one symptom from at least two of the PTSD clusters (Van der Kolk, 2014).

The symptom profiles of DTD and ICD-11's C-PTSD have considerable overlap but differ with regard to the aetiological stressor. DTD restricts trauma exposure to a sustained period during childhood or adolescence (Van der Kolk, 2005), whereas C-PTSD also covers exposure to repetitive or persistent trauma in adulthood. C-PTSD's requirement that the trauma is experienced as extremely threatening or horrific may prevent a diagnosis in some individuals who meet the proposed DTD criteria. Hence, even with the inclusion of C-PTSD, there are still many maltreated traumatised children and adults whose experiences and symptomology do not enable them to be classified in the current diagnostic systems of the DSM-5 or the ICD-11. As a result, some may be diagnosed with BPD (see below), which shares similar antecedents and symptoms, but is often diagnosed without giving due regard for the impact of a traumatic upbringing.

Borderline Personality Disorder

The term "borderline" originally referred to mental illnesses characterised by both psychosis and neurosis, without clearly meeting the criteria for either (Stern, 1938). The disorder was further defined in the 1960s when it came to be viewed as a distinct entity from psychosis and neurosis, and was formalised in 1980 with its inclusion in the third edition of the DSM, although it was not until 1992 that the diagnosis of "Emotionally Unstable Personality Disorder, Borderline Type" was added to ICD-10 (Hooley et al., 2012). BPD is characterised by a pervasive pattern of marked impulsivity and instability of interpersonal relationships, self-image, and affects, along with a fear of abandonment, and externalised affect regulatory strategies (for example, self-harm, substance abuse). The majority of people with BPD have histories of childhood trauma, including physical and sexual abuse, neglect, hostile conflict, and early parental loss (American Psychiatric Association, 2013). Children with documented early abuse or neglect are 7.7 times more likely to develop BPD than their peers without these adverse experiences (Johnson et al., 1999). Research also indicates that BPD is linked to less overt forms of maltreatment and neglect, such as absent parents, being degraded or ignored by caregivers, parental discord, and attachment disturbances (Hooley et al., 2012). This is important to recognise, as those who have experienced these early adversities may not understand these experiences are the basis of their difficulties.

Because of the high prevalence of developmental trauma, leading trauma experts suggest BPD be conceptualised as a posttraumatic syndrome (Herman et al., 1989). However, genetic factors may be equally as influential as environmental factors, with each contributing around half the variance in features of BPD such as affective instability, identity problems, negative relationships, and self-harm (Distel et al., 2010).

A vignette – a man with Borderline Personality Disorder

A man in his mid-20s described relationship volatility, confusion, and instability about his identity, with difficulty holding stable images of himself and others: he would see people asynchronously as having both endearing and displeasing features. He struggled to talk about his feelings as they felt too intense, and as a result he would try to distance himself from his feelings by hurting himself, or by verbally abusing others. Early in treatment, he often expressed the idea that the therapy was not going anywhere, but he found it challenging to discuss the problem with his therapist. Rather, he would get into cycles where he thought that one or the other was at fault, and the relationship between them often looked like it would end. Both would often leave sessions confused, despondent, and negatively self-evaluating. The pain, confusion, negativity, anger, and desire evoked from his early chaotic family relationships was repeated in therapy, playing out in actions. Reflections and words to describe his internal experience, which would allow containment and understanding of what he was experiencing, were not an available part of his psychological armamentarium at that stage of the therapy.

The diagnosis of BPD has been criticised for its lack of specificity, with the same constellation of symptoms being manifest across a range of possible disorders, leading some theorists and clinicians to believe that BPD describes largely unrelated patterns of symptomology occurring in challenging patients who do not fit traditional diagnostic categories. However, the majority of clinicians agree that BPD is a distinct entity with a phenomenological core, although they fail to reach agreement as to whether this core encompasses a single unifying pattern, no core symptom, or a complex of symptoms (Meares et al.,

2011). For example, Clarkin and others suggest there are three core factors: identity problems and interpersonal difficulties, affect difficulties and self-harm, and impulsivity (Clarkin et al., 1993), whereas Meares suggests that the core symptom is a painful sense of "personal incoherence", a term that encompasses psychic pain, personality fragmentation and dissociation (Meares et al., 2011). The overlap between BPD and dissociation is not surprising given BPD and the DDs share some similar features and are often comorbid, and both have a high correlation with early traumatic experience.

Dissociative Disorders

As doctors were beginning to systematically study the psychology of mental health problems in earnest at the end of the nineteenth century, dissociation was at the forefront of their investigations and explanations (Ellenberger, 1970). They were attempting to understand the psychological mechanisms that allowed people to present with conversion and somatic symptoms, report episodes of amnesia, appear as seemingly different people without necessarily having awareness of different aspects of themselves, and who were distressed one moment and calm the next (Ellenberger, 1970; Van der Hart and Dorahy, 2009). This work coincided with investigations around hypnosis, automatic writing, and possession, which viewed dissociation as a key explanatory mechanism. Advocates for the central role of dissociation in the understanding of disorders that would now fall under the Somatoform, Dissociative and Personality Disorders, included Jean-Martin Charcot, Pierre Janet, and a young Sigmund Freud. In the USA, Morton Prince founded the *Journal of Abnormal Psychology* in 1906, and used it as an avenue for his writings and ideas about dissociation and what are now called the DDs (Prince, 1906).

Dissociation is currently characterised by a disruption and discontinuity in the normal integration of consciousness, memory, identity, emotion, perception, body representation, motor control, and behaviour (American Psychiatric Association, 2013), and has often been conceptualised and studied as a reactive response to trauma. At the turn of the twentieth century, dissociation was understood as reflecting a division of the personality, which gave rise to autobiographical and traumatic amnesia, and somatoform symptoms captured by the diagnosis of "Hysteria". Hysteria continued to be used as a diagnosis until 1980, when it was finally abandoned by the American Psychiatric Association. Studies of dissociation proliferated in the 1970s, and the DDs entered into psychiatric nomenclature in the DSM-III in 1980 (Van der Hart and Dorahy, 2009).

The DDs contain three specific diagnoses. Depersonalisation/Derealisation Disorder is characterised by persistent or recurrent experiences of unreality or detachment from one's mind, self, or body, and/or experiences of unreality or detachment from one's surroundings. Dissociative Amnesia is characterised by an inability to recall autobiographical information that may be localised to an event or period of time, to a specific aspect of an event, or generalised to identity and life history. A more severe subtype of amnesia, fugue, involves purposeful travel or bewildered wandering with loss of identity. Dissociative Identity Disorder, or DID, previously known as Multiple Personality Disorder, is defined by the presence of two or more distinct personality states alongside recurrent episodes of amnesia. The most common disordered manifestation of dissociative symptoms seen in clinical settings falls under the category, "Other Specified Dissociative Disorder", which is a subclinical form of DID. Here the person experiences intrusive emotions, thoughts, actions, speech, and impulses from personality states that are less marked than in DID, or they have dissociative identities but little amnesia (American Psychiatric Association, 2013; Kate and Middleton, 2018).

Clinically, DDs can be hard to detect. For example, a person with DID might present with other concerns (for example, depressive symptoms, identity instability, somatic complaints), and may be quite fearful or ashamed about disclosing losing time, "coming to" in unfamiliar places, hearing voices that seem unfamiliar, being told they engage in behaviours that are foreign to, or uncharacteristic of, them, and feeling like they engage in actions outside their control. The DDs represent some of the most controversial disorders in the DSM, with DID arguably being the most contentious. Proponents of DID argue that exposure to chronic childhood trauma, especially by an attachment figure or trusted other, creates dissociative separations in the mind which attempt to partition away the psychobiological correlates of such abuses (Dorahy et al., 2014; Şar et al., 2017). Opponents of DID argue the disorder is created by a complex mix of factors including sleep difficulties, suggestions from a therapist, fantasy proneness, and media protrayals of such presentations, where reports of abuse in childhood become exaggerated or confabulated (Lynn et al., 2012). The term "False Memory Syndrome", which is not a medically recognised condition, was coined to describe individuals who reported elaborate memories of sexual abuse that had lain dormant for years before resurfacing. These "recovered memories" were widely regarded as being false, despite long-standing evidence that traumatic memories can be lost and then recovered (Van der Kolk, 2014). Furthermore, the hypothesis that dissociation renders individuals prone to fantasy and subsequently leads to false memories of trauma lacks robust empirical support (Staniloiu and Markowitsch, 2014).

Comorbidity

The similar symptom profiles across C-PTSD, DTD, BPD, and the DDs point to the traumatic etiology of these disorders. Comorbidity between these disorders is common, and some patients may meet the diagnostic criteria for all four. For instance, the criteria for PTSD is met by the overwhelming majority of patients with DID (Middleton and Butler, 1998) and around 40 per cent of individuals with BPD (Lawn and McMahon, 2015). Nearly two-thirds of individuals with BPD meet criteria for a DD (Sar, 2011), and dissociative symptoms are central to the diagnostic criteria for C-PTSD and PTSD (for example, flashbacks, numbing), with some capturing the features of the Dissociative Subtype of

PTSD in the DSM-5. As well as being interrelated, C-PTSD, BPD and DID all have high rates of comorbid Depression, Anxiety Disorders, Substance Abuse, Eating Disorders, and suicidal ideation (International Society for the Study of Trauma and Dissociation, 2011; American Psychiatric Association, 2013; Lawn and McMahon, 2015). If an individual presents with a myriad of symptoms that cut across multiple domains, it is indicative of a trauma history. Yet, this may be overlooked where treatment centres on psychiatric diagnoses made with a purely symptom focus. If the underlying trauma-related disorder is not recognised, interventions to address the presenting disorder may be ineffective.

Complex Trauma and mental health services

Complex Trauma and its effects are often unrecognised or misdiagnosed, even amongst individuals who present to multiple services over a long period of time (Bateman et al., 2013). Despite their prevalence, the DDs are generally considered "fringe" diagnoses, potentially indicating that the vast majority of people living with DDs are undiagnosed. Statistically, Australians with complex and early trauma are less likely to be users of mental health services, with usage being nearly twice as high for those who experienced traumas such as natural disasters and car accidents than those experiencing interpersonal trauma, and four times higher for those experiencing trauma as an adult than those who experienced trauma before the age of 16 (Australian Bureau of Statistics, 2008). The data suggest that although a subset of individuals with both identified and unidentified histories of Complex Trauma may be high users of mental health care, many individuals with early and interpersonal trauma do not access mental health care. Survivors of Complex Trauma are faced with societal, community, and familial pressures to remain silent, as well as the individual's own drive to minimise negative feelings such as shame, guilt, and fear. Survivors often have a legitimate fear of being accused of fantasising, lying, seeking attention, or seeking revenge, and this is particularly true of survivors of childhood abuse (Phoenix Australia – Centre for Posttraumatic Mental Health, 2013). In Australia, the situation has slowly improved over the last 30 years as a result of increased awareness, advocacy and support, the conviction of high-profile members of the community including politicians and celebrities, and national attention garnered by the Royal Commission into Institutional Responses to Child Sexual Abuse. Yet more needs to be done to improve access to trauma-informed mental health care for at-risk populations.

Focusing on symptomology and missing the trauma

The complexity of the presenting symptoms in C-PTSD, DTD, BPD, and the DDs, and their pervasiveness, especially those associated with dysregulated affect, sense of self, and relationship functioning, can mean a traumatic origin might be overlooked, especially by those not working in specialty trauma services or who are not familiar with the trauma literature and the type of therapeutic responses required. This is more likely to be the case in both generic hospital and acute mental health wards, but it may also occur in many outpatient settings. Trauma-informed education in inpatient settings and in primary care is particularly important. Having specific, directed, succinct, and well-formed assessment questions that examine both adult and childhood trauma, as well as the breadth of psychobiosocial outcomes associated with chronic interpersonal trauma, are likely to heighten trauma-informed practice during assessment. DDs in particular often go undetected as major generic psychiatric diagnostic instruments do not incorporate questions that detect dissociation and the DDs, and clinicians may be unfamiliar with screening and diagnostic tools for identifying DDs, including the Structured Clinical Interviews for DSM Dissociative Disorders (Dorahy et al., 2014). The introduction of the Dissociative Subtype of PTSD provides the opportunity for greater awareness of dissociation amongst clinicians who may otherwise overlook dissociative symptomology. The majority of people with a DD remain undiagnosed, and therefore do not get interventions that have been shown to relieve their symptoms (Brand et al., 2013).

Not treating symptoms separate from the trauma, and communicating the link between symptom development and traumatic experiences, taking into account psychological, physiological, and social development, is likely to increase trauma-informed care options for those presenting with the collection of symptomatic, characterological, and affect regulatory difficulties that characterised the trauma-related disorders. For example, if the complex nature of the trauma is missed in an individual with PTSD, it is possible that exposure therapy could be given as the standard treatment, which can lead to re-traumatisation in a person with Complex Trauma (Van der Kolk, 2000).

Prejudice and scepticism preventing appropriate diagnosis and treatment

An official diagnosis of BPD often has the effect of impeding, rather than facilitating, effective treatment, as individuals with such a diagnosis are often stigmatised as being manipulative, demanding, and attention-seeking. A survey of Australians with the disorder found significant discrimination when attempting to get their needs met within both public and private health services (Lawn and McMahon, 2015). Dismissive and contemptuous interactions are not uncommon, and mirror the rejection, abuse, and neglect that was characteristic of their early lives, which is re-traumatising (Meares and Stevenson, 2000), and may trigger further self-destructive behaviour that reinforces the negative stereotype. Individuals diagnosed with BPD have historically been seen as unresponsive to treatment (Bateman et al., 2013), yet tailored therapeutic interventions such as the Conversational Model can be highly effective (Stevenson et al., 2005). As a result of the negative repercussions for many individuals receiving a BPD diagnosis, clinicians are often reluctant to diagnose the disorder, yet this is counterproductive if evidence-supported treatments for the disorder are not implemented. Clinically, individuals with BPD can provide treatment challenges for therapists in part because the therapeutic relationship is often tenuous, tumultuous, under attack, and moving through difficult cycles of rupture and repair.

Though people with BPD face the problem of being identified, judged, and dismissed, the diagnosis of those with DDs is often missed, or, if made, ignored. Scepticism about recovered memories and dissociation has existed for over a century. Although DDs have been in the DSM for nearly four decades, discussions regarding the validity of DID and other DDs have been more divisive and emotive than discussions involving almost any other mental disorder (Middleton, 2004). Despite compelling scientific evidence supporting the validity of DDs and recovered memory (Dalenberg et al., 2012), disbelief surrounding DDs by clinicians, and health and social care services more generally, presents a serious barrier to both diagnosis and treatment. The International Society for the Study of Trauma and Dissociation produced guidelines for identifying and treating DID, with therapy based on the three phase approach of establishing safety, stabilisation, and symptom reduction; confronting, working through, and integrating traumatic memories; and identity integration and rehabilitation (2011). This method is efficacious, with patients showing significant reductions in dissociation and harmful behaviours (Brand et al., 2013). If the dissociation and trauma go unrecognised and untreated, other therapeutic interventions are likely to be ineffective and may be harmful.

Conclusion

Trauma-informed care hinges on an accurate diagnosis, and an understanding that is reflective of the traumatic origins of the presenting symptoms. Yet a diagnosis of BPD or a DD currently has the potential to both secure and prevent effective engagement and treatment. If attempts to address the pervasive stigma and disbelief experienced by those with these disorders are not successful, then this group of vulnerable individuals are unlikely to receive the tailored therapeutic interventions required for symptom reduction or any marked improvement in quality of life. The introduction in the DSM in 1980 of PTSD, BPD, and DDs was momentous as it provided the foundation for acknowledging the role of trauma in poor mental health. Recent moves to introduce a Dissociative Subtype of PTSD into the DSM-5, and C-PTSD into the ICD-11, demonstrate incremental progress in recognising the significant impact of developmental and repeated trauma on mental health. Now emphasis needs to be focused on providing care for people with C-PTSD, DTD, BPD, and the DDs that is validating, sensitive and informed by the impact of major traumatic rupture on systems for attaching, relating, thinking, feeling, and behaving.

References

American Psychiatric Association (2013) *Diagnostic and Statistical Manual of Mental Disorders, Fifth Edition*. Arlington, VA: American Psychiatric Publishing.

Australian Bureau of Statistics (2008) *2007 Australian National Survey of Mental Health and Wellbeing: Summary of Results*. Canberra, Australia: Australian Bureau of Statistics.

Bateman J, Henderson C and Kezelman C (2013) *Trauma-Informed Care and Practice: Towards a Cultural Shift in Policy Reform Across Mental Health and Human Services in Australia, A National Strategic Direction, Position Paper and Recommendations of the National Trauma-informed Care and Practice Advisory Working Group*. Report. Sydney, Australia: Mental Health Coordinating Council.

Ben-Ezra M, Karatzias T, Hyland P, et al. (2018) Posttraumatic stress disorder (PTSD) and complex PTSD (CPTSD) as per ICD-11 proposals: A population study in Israel. *Depression and Anxiety* 35: 264–274.

Brand BL, McNary SW, Myrick AC, et al. (2013) Supplemental material for a longitudinal naturalistic study of patients with dissociative disorders treated by community clinicians. *Psychological Trauma: Theory, Research, Practice, and Policy* 5(4): 301–308.

Clarkin JF, Hull JW and Hurt SW (1993) Factor structure of borderline personality disorder criteria. *Journal of Personality Disorders* 7: 137–143.

Cloitre M, Garvert DW, Brewin CR, et al. (2013) Evidence for proposed ICD-11 PTSD and Complex PTSD: A latent profile analysis. *European Journal of Psychotraumatology* 4 ArtID: 20706.

Dalenberg CJ, Brand BL, Gleaves DH, et al. (2012) Evaluation of the evidence for the trauma and fantasy models of dissociation. *Psychological Bulletin* 138(3): 550–588.

Distel MA, Willemsen G, Ligthart L, et al. (2010) Genetic covariance structure of the four main features of borderline personality disorder. *Journal of Personality Disorders* 24: 427–444.

Dorahy MJ, Brand BL, Şar V, et al. (2014) Dissociative identity disorder: An empirical overview. *Australian and New Zealand Journal of Psychiatry* 48(5): 402–417.

Ellenberger HF (1970) *The Discovery of the Unconscious*. New York, NY: Basic Books.

Friedman MJ (2013) Finalizing PTSD in DSM-5: Getting here from there and where to go next. *Journal of Traumatic Stress* 26: 548–556.

Herman JL (1992) *Trauma and Recovery*. New York, NY: Basic Books.

Herman JL, Perry JC and Van der Kolk B (1989) Childhood trauma in borderline personality disorder. *American Journal of Psychiatry* 146: 490–495.

Hooley JM, Cole SH and Gironde S (2012) Borderline Personality Disorder. In: Widiger TA (ed) *The Oxford Handbook of Personality Disorders*. Oxford, UK: Oxford University Press.

Hyland P, Shevlin M, Elklit A, et al. (2016) An assessment of the construct validity of the ICD-11 proposal for Complex Posttraumatic Stress Disorder. *Psychological Trauma: Theory, Research, Practice, and Policy* 9(1): 1–9.

International Society for the Study of Trauma and Dissociation (2011) Guidelines for treating Dissociative Identity Disorder in adults, third revision: Summary version. *Journal of Trauma and Dissociation* 12: 188–212.

Johnson JG, Cohen P, Brown J, et al. (1999). Childhood maltreatment increases risk for personality disorders during early adulthood. *Archives of General Psychiatry* 56: 600–606.

Johnson JG, Cohen P, Kasen S, et al. (2006) Dissociative disorders among adults in the community, impaired functioning, and axis I and II comorbidity. *Journal of Psychiatric Research* 40: 131–140.

Kate M-A and Jamieson GA (2017) A soldier and a sex worker walk into a therapist's office – who's more likely to have PTSD? *The Conversation* 28 March. Available at: theconversation.com.

Kate M-A and Middleton W (2018) Dissociative disorders and somatic symptom-related disorders. In: Kring AM, Johnson SL, Kyrios M, et al. (eds) *Abnormal Psychology, First Edition*. Brisbane, Australia: Wiley, pp.279–318.

Lanius RA, Brand B, Vermetten E, et al. (2012) The dissociative subtype of posttraumatic stress disorder: Rationale, clinical and neurobiological evidence, and implications. *Depression and Anxiety* 29(8): 701–708.

Lawn S and McMahon J (2015) Experiences of care by Australians with a diagnosis of borderline personality disorder. *Journal of Psychiatric Mental Health Nursing* 22(7): 510–521.

Lynn SJ, Lilienfeld SO, Merckelbach H, et al. (2012) Dissociation and Dissociative Disorders: Challenging conventional wisdom. *Current Directions in Psychological Science* 21: 48–53.

Meares R and Stevenson J (2000) Borderline personality disorder. *Australian and New Zealand Journal of Psychiatry* 34(5): 869–871.

Meares R, Gerull F, Stevenson J, et al. (2011) Is self disturbance the core of Borderline Personality Disorder? An outcome study of borderline personality factors. *Australian and New Zealand Journal of Psychiatry* 45: 214–222.

Middleton W (2004) Dissociative disorders: A personal "work in progress". *Australasian Psychiatry* 12(3): 245–252.

Middleton W and Butler J (1998) Dissociative identity disorder: An Australian series. *Australian and New Zealand Journal of Psychiatry* 32: 794–804.

Muir K (2007) The predisposition theory, human rights and Australian psychiatric casualties of war. *Australian Journal of Human Rights* 13(1): 195–218.

National Health and Medical Research Council (NHMRC) (2012) *Clinical Practice Guideline for the Management of Borderline Personality Disorder*. Melbourne, Australia: National Health and Medical Research Council.

Phoenix Australia – Centre for Posttraumatic Mental Health (2013) *Australian Guidelines for the Treatment of Acute Stress Disorder and Posttraumatic Stress Disorder*. Melbourne, Australia: Phoenix Australia.

Prince M (1906) Hysteria from the point of view of dissociated personality. *The Journal of Abnormal Psychology* 1(4): 170–187.

Roth S, Newman E, Pelcovitz D, et al. (1997) Complex PTSD in victims exposed to sexual and physical abuse: Results from the DSM-IV field trial for posttraumatic stress disorder. *Journal of Traumatic Stress* 10: 539–555.

Şar V (2011) Developmental trauma, Complex PTSD, and the current proposal of DSM-5. *European Journal of Psychotraumatology* 2(1): 5622. doi:10.3402/ejpt.v2i0.5622.

Şar V, Dorahy MJ and Krüger C (2017) Revisiting the etiological aspects of dissociative identity disorder: A biopsychosocial perspective. *Psychology Research and Behavior Management* 10: 137–146.

Staniloiu A and Markowitsch HJ (2014) Dissociative amnesia. *The Lancet Psychiatry* 1: 226–241.

Stern A (1938) Psychoanalytic investigation of and therapy in the borderline group of neuroses. *Psychoanalytical Quarterly* 7: 467–489.

Stevenson J, Meares R and D'Angelo R (2005) Five-year outcome of outpatient psychotherapy with borderline patients. *Psychological Medicine* 35: 79–87.

Teicher MH and Samson JS (2016) Annual research review: Enduring neurobiological effects of childhood abuse and neglect. *Journal of Child Psychology and Psychiatry* 57: 241–266.

Wolf EJ, Miller M, Kilpatrick D, et al. (2015) ICD–11 Complex PTSD in US national and veteran samples: Prevalence and structural associations with PTSD. *Clinical Psychological Science* 3(2): 215–229.

World Health Organization (2017) *ICD-11 Beta Draft*. Geneva, Switzerland: World Health Organization. Available at: apps.who.int/classifications/icd11.

Van der Hart O and Dorahy MJ (2009) History of the concept of dissociation. In: Dell PF and O'Neil JA (eds) *Dissociation and the Dissociative Disorders: DSM-V and Beyond*. Hoboken, NJ: Taylor & Francis, pp.3–26.

Van der Kolk BA (2000) Posttraumatic stress disorder and the nature of trauma. *Dialogues in Clinical Neuroscience* 2: 7–22.

Van der Kolk BA (2005) Developmental trauma disorder. *Psychiatric Annals* 35(5): 401–408.

Van der Kolk BA (2014). *The Body Keeps the Score: Brain, Mind, and Body in the Healing of Trauma*. New York, NY: Viking.

Van der Kolk BA, Roth S, Pelcovitz D, et al. (2005) Disorders of extreme stress: The empirical foundations of a complex adaptation to trauma. *Journal of Traumatic Stress* 18: 389–399.

Part II

Specific populations

7 Trauma-informed care in infancy

Louise Newman

Introduction

The first three years of life are increasingly seen as a foundational period in terms of both neurological and psychological development. During this time, brain development is at its most rapid, with the establishment of neural pathways forming the basis of self-experience, regulation of emotions and interpersonal understanding (Schore, 2000). Abuse or neglect during this particularly sensitive stage can have devastating effects. The Australian Institute of Health and Welfare report (2017) found 45,714 substantiated cases of child abuse in the 12-month period 2015–16, with 61,723 children under care and protection orders. Children under one year of age were the most likely to be in receipt of child protection services at 37.6 cases per 1000 children. Aboriginal and Torres Strait Islander children were seven times more likely to have received child protection services than other children. Importantly, the impacts of child trauma are related to the age of the child, the relationships between the child and the perpetrator, the duration of abuse and the response to any disclosures made; abuse and trauma are more likely to have significant developmental impacts during infancy and early childhood when the child is most dependent on the attachment figure. However, sophisticated early therapeutic interventions targeting the parent–infant dyad are being developed to guide early intervention and may significantly improve outcomes.

Development in infancy

The related fields of infant mental health and developmental psychopathology have expanded considerably over the last 30 years. Progress in the neurosciences and neurobiology have contributed to the evolution of more integrated models of development and to the knowledge base of the origins of mental disorder (Schore, 2009). Infancy is a significant period for the establishment of resilience but is also a period of neuro-vulnerability. As these models are applied to the understanding of adult mental health problems, it is becoming increasingly clear that adversity during crucial early developmental periods is related to a wide range of mental health conditions (Newman et al., 2016).

Compared with many other species, the human infant is born with a relatively under-developed brain. The brain undergoes rapid growth and development in response to environmental input, moving from approximately 20 per cent of the weight of the average adult brain at birth to around 60 per cent by 12 months (Cozolino, 2002). The infant brain has however more nerve cells and connections than the adult and these connections are gradually shaped into pathways or neural networks with an overall loss of neurones, a process known as "pruning". Experiences in infancy – the actual sensory input the brain receives – have a direct effect on emerging connections, architecture, pathways, and overall functioning. These experiences are primarily affective and occur almost solely within the context of caregiving and attachment relationships and are significantly influenced by the quality of care and the caregiver's emotional interactions and sensitivity within the relationship; this is known as the experience-dependent nature of early brain development (Cozolino, 2002). This early care provided literally shapes brain structure and function, particularly in the limbic and prefrontal areas, regions that are particularly crucial with respect to emotion and attachment, and the quality of care has major implications for later psychological organisation and health (Hart, 2008).

Initially, the infant is in a state of total dependency on the caregiver figure to help them regulate their internal states and to maintain arousal within manageable levels (Strathearn, 2007). Infants are however born with the capacity to communicate emotional experience and other internal physiological states from birth, and they seek social connectedness and communication from birth. They also look for comfort and use others to help manage their feelings and internal states, an innate capacity for emotional regulation and self-organisation that drives attachment behaviour and the rapid growth in social understanding that occurs over the first two years of life. Such early experiences in relationships and the ability of the caregiver to engage emotionally with the infant form the basis of healthy self-development, including the capacity to regulate stress and emotional states, and the development of learning and memory systems.

The other crucial component of early infant development related to later psychological functioning is the emergence of representations of self, other, and relationships. The infant, through the relationship with the caregiver, begins, in the language of Bowlby's attachment theory, to develop internal working models of relationships (Bowlby, 1969). The quality of these early interactions and relationships shapes the infant's emerging understanding of human interaction. These models or representations are essentially affective and cognitive schema by which the infant develops a psychological understanding of human interaction, their own inner world, and the inner world of the other. This is crucial in the development of empathic understanding and the broader concept of theory of mind. In healthy relationships, the caregiver has a good capacity to understand and process the social and emotional communication of the infant. This not only provides an external regulatory function, it also allows the caregiver to understand and validate the infant's emotional experience (Stern, 1985).

This process of understanding and processing communications involves the ability to focus very carefully on the infant's states, adapting or "fine tuning" their overall interaction according to the signals that the infant communicates, responding to them in a way that contains anxiety. These processes of a caregiver being able to "read" and respond to the emotional communications of the infant are the essential building blocks of early relationships, and reflect the caregiver's own early experience, their ideas and feelings about parenting and the infant, and their current mood and stress levels. Caregivers with histories of abuse and trauma may have particular difficulties in having empathic and sensitive interactions with their infant and experience a range of anxieties when they attempt to parent.

It is also important to note that the infant is not born with a fully functioning hypothalamic–pituitary–adrenal axis or stress regulating system and is dependent on the caregiver to act as a regulator of overall stress levels in a physiological sense. The study of infants in adverse social environments and poorer quality relationships including inconsistent care, neglect, and maltreatment has focused on infant difficulties in stress regulation and the impact of high levels of stress-related hormones such as cortisol on infant neurodevelopment and developmental outcome (Gunnar and Quevedo, 2007). High levels of stress in infancy are most commonly related to disturbances in early emotional interaction and care. Infants are particularly sensitive to perturbations in early relationships and stress may have long-term impacts on core functions of stress, endocrine, and immune systems (Danese and Lewis, 2017). Studies also show that high degrees of early stress and effects on stress-related hormones impact brain development, particularly emergent capacities to regulate emotions (De Bellis, 2001).

Relational trauma and its effects

Traumatic experiences in infancy may have major developmental implications and consequences for neurological and psychological development, and the establishment of vulnerability for later psychopathology (Teicher, 2003). Definitions of trauma in infancy are varied, but the concept of trauma in infancy is primarily a relational one (Schore, 2010) and effects range from more subtle disturbances in the quality of early emotional interactions with caregivers to more severe maltreatment and abuse. Research into severe abuse and neglect have focused on populations exposed to major care disturbance such as the Romanian and Bulgarian orphans (Zeanah et al., 2009). These studies have found that this level of abuse has significant effects on brain development and growth, psychological functioning, and the ability to relate to others. In the face of severe stress, the infant uses mechanisms of self-protection such as withdrawal and dissociation, which become characteristic patterns in the face of trauma (Perry et al., 1995) and which may have lifelong legacies.

The more common traumas experienced in infancy are not as severe but relate to disturbances in early caregiving relationships with implications for interpersonal functioning and social cognition, and, importantly, for the ability to understand self and others in terms of mental states, known as reflective functioning (Fonagy et al., 2013). Relational trauma may occur in several circumstances, for example parental neglect or depression. The effect is greater when the parent is simultaneously both the provider of a needed sense of security and a source of confusion and terror. These experiences have been described as producing a state of inescapable fear and anxiety which is unable to be resolved. In attachment theory this is the situation that leads to the development of a disorganised attachment style, where the infant is confused about the safety and availability of the caregiver, and the functioning of the social world (Schore, 2009).

From a psychological perspective, infants who experience relational trauma are frequently exposed to distortions in the caregiver's understanding of the infant. Infants are born into a pre-existing network of relationships and meanings which are shaped by the caregiver's own early history, and particularly any unresolved attachment-related trauma that they may have experienced. Caregivers with this type of trauma background are frequently those who present with a range of complex issues from anxiety about the capacity to care, to avoidance of interaction with the infant, to extreme cases where the parents themselves have experienced significant maltreatment and neglect and the unresolved traumatic attachment issues can be re-enacted with the infant (Fraiberg, 1975). These parents are likely to have deficits in their own capacity for psychological understanding, or reflective functioning, and this will significantly impact their capacity to parent in an emotional and psychological sense, the model for the intergenerational transmission of trauma (Fonagy et al., 2013).

In these situations, the parent may be fundamentally conflicted and confused about their capacity to establish a relationship with the infant, and may have difficulties with ambivalence, anger, and hostility. Parents may also experience envy and an unconscious need to devalue their infant's experience. In these high-risk scenarios there is always a need to evaluate risk to the infant and the parent's capacity for therapeutic engagement in terms of developing a more sensitive understanding of their infant. Particularly in scenarios where mothers are diagnosed with Borderline Personality Disorder (BPD), there may be fundamental conflicts around the capacity to nurture and the ability to tolerate dependency. Such parents are more likely to experience unprocessed traumatic memories which can be triggered by the very presence of their infant. In other words, the caregiver re-experiences their own unresolved negative feelings related to poor early experiences of care and may variously experience the infant as anxiety-provoking, persecutory, and even hostile. Under these conditions, there is a risk of re-enactment involving child abuse (Newman and Stevenson, 2005). Clearly, these issues represent opportunities for prevention if they can be identified early.

The effects of early emotional trauma and disruptions during critical early developmental periods are potentially long-term. The evidence suggests that there are continuities between early relational trauma and attachment disorganisation and a range of interpersonal and psychological functioning deficits (Lyons-Ruth and Jacobvitz, 2016). Specifically, infants who develop attachment disorganisation in the context of fearful and confusing early relationships are more likely to exhibit high levels of anxiety, poor modulation of feelings and behaviour, difficulties in interpersonal functioning and understanding, and persistent maladaptive defence mechanisms such as dissociation.

Trauma-related diagnoses can certainly be used in infancy and early childhood but are obviously imprecise and tend to refer to distortions of basic regulatory processes. For example, infants can show acute stress responses including withdrawal, dissociation, and non-organic failure to thrive. Posttraumatic Stress Disorder is certainly recognised in early childhood and children will enact in play specific traumatic scenarios even in the absence of the necessary linguistic skills required to describe the trauma verbally, and they may also show a range of non-specific fears and difficulties in anxiety regulation. It is recognised that in pre-school children, patterns of disrupted behaviours and distorted attachment behaviours are also seen, including the symptoms and behaviours recognised in the diagnosis of Reactive Attachment Disorder. This is described as a disorder of relatedness in which the child is either withdrawn and inhibited, or overfamiliar. These patterns are seen to be the consequence of early care disturbances (Zeanah et al., 2016). It is important to note that even when diagnostic classifications are appropriate it is still vital to examine developmental pathways rather than assume that precisely refined neurobiological and neurochemical disease is present.

Some of the changes may also represent early pathways to the development of personality dysfunction. This includes aspects of BPD, a complex developmental outcome with dysregulation on both neurological and psychological levels which is frequently associated with a history of early trauma and abuse (Cattane et al., 2017), and often transmitted intergenerationally.

Approaches to trauma-focused intervention in infancy

Early intervention is based on the need to support the early parenting relationship, the quality of emotional interactions, and to re-establish the parental capacity to reflect on the inner world of the infant. There are many diverse approaches to early parenting interventions; however, the majority of these do not specify or target the high-risk intergenerational issues that are frequently seen in clinical practice. Parent-focused psychoeducational approaches and generic behaviour management approaches appear to have limited use in these groups, although they may be very appropriate for community-based samples. For intergenerational trauma and other significant issues, relationship and attachment-based approaches are currently undergoing research evaluation, with some evidence relating to their effectiveness in high-risk situations accumulating (Newman et al., 2015). When working with extremely high-risk parents, such as those with BPD, unstructured psychodynamic and psychoanalytic approaches previously utilised have had to be replaced with more structured approaches that also avoid more anxiety-provoking interactions (Newman and Stevenson, 2005).

A vignette – "Anna" and "Lilly"

Anna is a 35-year-old single woman with a three-month old daughter, Lilly. Anna has had a previous child removed from her care due to concerns about neglect and exposure of the infant to domestic violence and drug use. Anna has a history of opiate dependence over 14 years with several brief abstinences. Anna has also had several exploitative partners and describes a pattern of intense relationships driven by a need to find a caring partner whilst simultaneously failing to recognise the risk factors in the men she liaises with. In addition, Anna has long-term feelings of depression and guilt over the loss of her previous child, and says she is motivated to keep Lilly in her care and make up for her previous mistakes. She stopped using drugs during her pregnancy. She has no relationship with the father of the infant, and she has distanced herself from a drug-abusing social group.

Anna's background is one of significant early neglect and exposure to drug using and alcoholic parents. Her father was violent towards her mother, and left the home when Anna was only three. Anna's mother was involved in a series of violent relationships, and Anna describes sexual abuse from the ages of five to 15 years at the hands of several different men. She left home, and became homeless, in her early twenties, and managed feelings of depression with drug abuse. She has a long history of self-harming, and she recalls feeling that being a mother with her first child was her main hope of reworking her life and having a positive identity. The reality for Anna was that she found it difficult to tolerate her infant's emotional states and dependency and she became withdrawn and neglectful. Anna made a suicide attempt after which her baby was placed in care.

Anna however not only enrolled in a substance use program during her second pregnancy, she was better motivated to understand how to parent and to reflect on the complex issues she faced as a woman whose own early experiences disrupted her capacities to deal with strong emotions. As a result, she was referred to a parent–infant therapist, "Carla", whom she started seeing weekly with Lilly. Carla spoke to both Anna and Lilly in a very calm and soothing manner. Over a few weeks, Carla begun to understand how difficult Anna's early life had been, and how hard she was now trying to look after Lilly, and she reflected this to Anna.

As Anna began to trust Carla, she admitted to her that in the middle of the night when Lilly was hard to settle that she felt jealous of the care that Lilly was receiving. She said she found Lilly very needy, just like the last child she had lost. She also thought that Lilly hated her, and she said she sometimes felt the same way toward her. She asked Carla, "How can I care for Lilly when no-one cared about me?". She also worried about losing Lilly. Carla gently speculated with Anna about the background to these feelings, and Anna gradually came to understand that her own history was directly impacting on her day-to-day care of Lilly, particularly the repeated failures of her own mother to protect her. As the work progressed, Carla helped Anna to wonder about what Lilly might be feeling, in a range of mood states, and Anna developed a better and a more "here-and-now" understanding of Lilly's feelings. She also learnt to re-interpret Lilly's distress not as anger but as a cry for help, distress that Anna became increasingly able to respond to. Importantly, she found the new interactions with Lilly deeply satisfying.

Therapy with Anna needed to be based on an acknowledgment of the significant attachment-related trauma that she had experienced, and the impact that this had on her personality development and adaptation. Becoming a parent offered both risk and opportunity for the development of Anna's capacity to understand her infant's needs, and to rework her own identity in the face of few positive early experiences.

Trauma-focused interventions – general principles

Intervening in the early months of an infant's life is central to preventing repetition of early trauma and relationship failure, and in promoting healthy attachment behaviour in the caregiver. The traumatised caregiver can be supported in developing a capacity to read and respond to her infant's communication, to gain a capacity to reflect on the infant's inner experience, and to gain confidence in her ability to support the infant manage strong emotions. The literature on infant–parent psychotherapy describes this as a process of supporting the parent in their thinking about the infant, which is crucial in the establishment of an organised attachment relationship and the basis of early emotional interaction (Lieberman and Van Horn, 2009). A key focus is on developing the parents' capacity to reflect on the way in which early trauma has impacted their parenting and their management of strong emotions. Parents can be supported to rework their understanding of themselves as parents and to develop positive interactions with their infant. Direct coaching of emotional interaction between parent and infant can be supported by video feedback.

Slade describes a clinical approach where infants and parents are worked with together, where the therapist has a role in modelling reflectiveness, giving voice to infant experience, and supporting the parent in the development of a reflective stance, hypothesising, and wondering about the inner world of the infant (Slade, 2006). The interactions observed in the session between infant and parent are used as a primary source to encourage this process of mentalisation and improving the understanding of the infant's affective experience. The therapist then has a central role in holding the parent in mind – in other words, providing a container for the parent's anxiety – and providing them with an understanding of the links between the caregiver's past and those feelings currently experienced in their relationship with the infant. These approaches can also be described as attachment-based interventions, and a focus on relationships can begin with intervention during pregnancy, the crucial period of transition to parenting, as well as with infants and in early childhood.

It should be noted that these types of approaches do vary somewhat from the cognitive-behavioural and psychoeducational models and that particularly for high-risk parents, these types of approaches without a focus on emotional attunement, though they might improve infant management, may not lead to improvements in the emotional aspects of the parent–child relationship. This is particularly important when considering early intervention for parents with significant trauma such as mothers with BPD where it is simultaneously important to support better organisation of the attachment relationship as well as working on empathic functioning and responsiveness to the infant. It can be argued that it is always important to involve an infant directly as a participant in therapy given that a primary focus of intervention needs to be on infant–parent interaction and giving the infant opportunities for better self-organisation through an improved relationship with the caregiver.

Parenting with Feeling

"Parenting with Feeling" (PWF) is a reflective attachment-based parent–infant therapeutic approach developed in Australia, specifically designed for use with parents who have experienced early trauma (Newman et al., 2015). The program offers group sessions for up to eight mother–infant dyads over a 10-week period. The program is designed to both facilitate the development of parental reflective functioning and the parent's role as an attachment figure, and to improve the sensitivity and emotional availability of the parent for the infant.

Parents' own early histories of abuse and attachment-related trauma are addressed each session in a series of exercises designed to support reflection on the role of a parent and the challenges to this where early care has been deficient. Mothers are guided to focus on the way in which they wish to rework or change their models of self as an attachment figure and the experiences of being parented that they wish their child to experience and remember. This aims to support the development of a parental self-representation that can move beyond the repetition of dysfunctional patterns. Parents are also guided in improving the capacity to self-regulate and to understand the powerful "triggering" role of the infant, reminding the parent of their own childhood, and particularly how to tolerate negative affect. The program uses infant–parent interaction in a direct way and encourages parental observational skills of the infant and reflection of the inner wold of the infants. Video feedback can be utilised as part of this psychoeducational process for the parents. It is also important as a trauma-focused intervention to address unresolved traumatic issues in the history of the parent and relate these to current relationship difficulties with the infant.

The PWF program uses:

1 Reflective parenting exercises, facilitating the development of the self as an attachment figure.
2 Observation, exercises, and support for infant–parent interaction. These involve direct coaching of interactions, support in reading and responding

to infant communications and gestures, and also building a psychological model of the infant as a communicating subject.

3 Trauma-focused therapeutic interventions focused on improving understanding of parenting in the face of adversity.

This program is currently being evaluated in a longitudinal study incorporating measurement of infant attachment outcome, parent–infant interactional quality, and parental representation of self as a parent. Evaluation of the PWF program includes measurement of parenting stress and rating of the quality of observed emotional interaction and regulation in each dyad. Parents' reflective capacity can be rated on the Parent Development Interview (Slade, 2005) which explores the parents' feelings and ideas about the infant, and capacity to reflect on the inner world of the infant and infant's mental states. Preliminary results in high-risk dyads support the utility of this approach in improving the quality of interaction and in improving parents' understanding of the impact of their own trauma on their parenting and the relationship with their infant. Parents report improvement in their understanding of infant communications and in their own sense of competence as a parent.

Conclusion

Current understanding of the significance of infancy allows for increasingly complex models of developmental psychopathology and the recognition of risk factors related to the development of later mental disorder. Despite considerable variation in developmental outcomes, it is important to consider infancy, particularly the experience of trauma during infancy, as a time of heightened neuro-vulnerability, when the serious effects of intergenerational trauma require focused and targeted early intervention. Traumatised parents frequently experience difficulties in thinking about themselves as an attachment figure, understanding about infant needs and emotional communication, but in extricating themselves from their own traumatic experiences of being cared for are frequently able to develop a healthier parental self-representation, which in turn significantly enhances parent–infant interaction and outcomes for the children involved.

References

Australian Institute of Health and Welfare (2017) *Child Protection Australia 2015–16. Child Welfare Series No 66*. Cat No CWS 60. Canberra, Australia: Australian Institute of Health and Welfare.

Bowlby J (1969) *Attachment and Loss, Volume 1: Attachment*. London, UK: Pimlico.

Cattane N, Ross R, Lanfredi M, et al. (2017) Borderline Personality Disorder and childhood trauma: Explaining the affected biological systems and mechanisms. *BMC Psychiatry* 17: 221. doi:10.1186/s12888–12017–1383–1382.

Cozolino L (2002) *The Neuroscience of Psychotherapy: Building and Rebuilding the Human Brain*. New York, NY: Norton.

Danese A and Lewis S (2017) Psychoneuroimmunology of early life stress: The hidden wounds of childhood trauma. *Neuropsychopharmacology* 42: 99–114.

De Bellis M (2001) Developmental traumatology: The psychobiological development of maltreated children. *Development and Psychopathology* 13: 539–564.

Fonagy P, Target M, Gergeley G, et al. (2013) The developmental roots of borderline personality disorder in early attachment relationships: A theory and some evidence. *Psychoanalytic Inquiry* 23(3): 412–459.

Fraiberg S, Adelson E and Shapiro V (1975) Ghosts in the nursery: A psychoanalytic approach to the problem of impaired mother-infant relationships. *Journal of the American Academy of Child Psychiatry* 14: 87–422.

Gunnar M and Quevedo K (2007) The neurobiology of stress and development. *Annual Review of Psychology* 58: 245–273.

Hart S (2008) *Brain, Attachment, Personality: An Introduction to Neuroaffective Development*. London, UK: Karnac.

Lieberman AF and Van Horn P (2009) Child–parent psychotherapy: A developmental approach to mental health treatment in infancy and early childhood. In: Zeanah CH (ed) *Handbook of Infant Mental Health*. New York, NY: Guilford, pp.439–449.

Lyons-Ruth K and Jacobvitz D (2016) Attachment disorganisation from infancy to adulthood: Neurobiological correlates, parenting contexts, and pathways to disorder. In: Cassiday J and Shaver PR (eds) *Handbook of Attachment: Theory, Research and Clinical Applications, Third Edition*. New York, NY: Guilford, pp.667–695.

Newman LK, Judd F, Olsson C, et al. (2016) Early origins of mental disorder – risk factors in the perinatal and infant period. *BMC Psychiatry* 16: 270. doi:10.1186/s12888-12016-0982-0987.

Newman LK, Sivaratnam C and Komiti A (2015) Attachment and early brain development – neuroprotective interventions in infant–caregiver psychotherapy. *Translational Developmental Psychiatry* 3: 28647.

Newman LK and Stevenson C (2005) Parenting and borderline personality disorder: Ghosts in the nursery. *Clinical Child Psychology and Psychiatry* 6: 385–394.

Perry BD, Pollard RA, Blakely TL, et al. (1995) Childhood trauma, the neurobiology of adaptation, and 'use-dependent' development of the brain. How 'states' become 'traits'. *Infant Mental Health Journal* 16(4): 271–291.

Schore AN (2000) Attachment and the regulation of the right brain. *Attachment and Human Development* 2: 23–47.

Schore AN (2009) Relational trauma and the developing right brain: An interface of psychoanalytic self-psychology and neuroscience. *Annals of the New York Academy of Sciences* 1159: 189–203.

Schore AN (2010) Relational trauma and the developing right brain: The neurobiology of broken attachment bonds. In: Baradon T (ed) *Relational Trauma in Infancy: Psychoanalytic, Attachment and Neuropsychological Contributions to Parent–Infant Psychotherapy*. New York, NY: Routledge, pp.419–448.

Slade A (2005) Parental reflective functioning: An introduction. *Attachment and Human Development* 7: 269–281.

Slade A (2006) Minding the baby: A mentalization based parenting program. In: Allen JG and Fonagy P (eds) *Handbook of Mentalization Based Treatment*. London, UK: John Wiley.

Stern DN (1985) *The Interpersonal World of the Infant: A View from Psychoanalysis and Developmental Psychology*. New York, NY: Basic Books.

Strathearn L (2007) Exploring the neurobiology of attachment. In: Mayes L, Fonagy P and Target M (eds) *Developmental Science and Psychoanalysis: Integration and Innovation*. London, UK: Karnac, pp.117–140.

Teicher M (2003) The neurobiological consequences of early stress and childhood maltreatment. *Neuroscience and Bio-behavioural Reviews* 27: 33–44.

Zeanah CH, Egger HL, Smyke AT, et al. (2009) Institutional rearing and psychiatric disorders in Romanian preschool children. *American Journal of Psychiatry* 166(7): 777–785.

Zeanah CH, Chesher T, Boris NW, et al. (2016) Practice parameters for the assessment and treatment of children and adolescents with Reactive Attachment Disorder and Disinhibited Social Engagement Disorder. *Journal of the American Academy Child and Adolescent Psychiatry* 55: 990–1003.

8 Institutional abuse of children – an Australian perspective

Carolyn Quadrio

Introduction

On 12 November 2012, the then Australian Prime Minister, Julia Gillard, announced a Royal Commission into Institutional Responses to Child Sexual Abuse. It was approved by the then Governor-General, Dame Quentin Bryce, on 11 January 2013. The background to this pivotal decision was widespread community and governmental concern following several highly publicised cases of institutional abuse of children, and the allegations of a senior police officer, Inspector Peter Fox, of a cover up by Catholic Church clergy in the Hunter Valley region of NSW. There were already two state inquiries underway in Australia at the time, and there had been other inquiries over the previous years; some had called for a Royal Commission of this kind, including the Senate's "Forgotten Australians" reports on children in institutional and out-of-home care (Australian Senate, 2004, 2009).

The terms of reference for the Commission were wide-ranging, but amongst other things it was to be informed by an understanding of individual cases, to focus on systemic issues, and to make findings and recommendations to better protect children against sexual abuse and to alleviate the impact on children when it occurs. It would do this by conducting private sessions and public hearings, and by undertaking a policy and research program (Budiselik et al., 2014). Institutions would include religious organisations, state care providers, not-for-profit bodies, and child service agencies.

Over the course of the Commission, it fielded more than 42,000 telephone calls; held more than 8,000 private sessions with individuals, mainly survivors; held 57 public hearings; heard submissions from relevant organisations and various churches, advocacy and survivor groups, charity and youth organisations, and numerous government agencies; published 59 research reports; and made more than 2,500 referrals to authorities. The findings of the Commission throughout its course have already had a significant impact in Australia and elsewhere (Doyle, 2017). The final report was presented to the current Governor-General, Sir Peter Cosgrove, on 15 December 2017. There has been a change in awareness and attitudes, both in the general community and within the various professional bodies and agencies that deal with these issues, more especially, religious organisations and churches, and within psychiatry and mental health more broadly.

This chapter is written from the vantage point of Australian psychiatry: it will provide an overview of those changes in awareness and attitudes as they have evolved over the past half century. It is based on the experiences of the author in working with several hundred survivors of childhood sexual abuse in institutional settings.

Prevalence

There are no firm figures for the prevalence of institutional child sexual abuse (CSA) in Australia, and the Commission has not identified a precise prevalence figure. Because child abuse and neglect are the major reasons for children being placed into institutional care, this is already a population for whom the rates of abuse will be well above those of the general community. In Australia, community rates of abuse are already high, with 34 per cent of women and 16 per cent of men reporting non-penetrative CSA, and 12 per cent and 4 per cent, respectively, reporting penetrative CSA (Dunne et al., 2003). Another Australian study found similar rates, with more than one-third of women and one-sixth of men reporting CSA (Najman et al., 2005). In another survey, 36 per cent of women reported CSA that had involved contact (Mazza et al., 2001). Studies of children entering care do indeed suggest higher rates than for the community, but mostly the figures refer to combined physical and sexual abuse. An American study reported that half the children entering out-of-home care had been abused or neglected (Nunno and Rindfleisch, 1991), and a British study reported that 80 per cent had been abused prior to entry into care (Hobbs et al., 1999).

What has been well established in prior investigations is that this very vulnerable population is then subjected to further abuse when they are placed in care. In Australia, "The Forgotten Australians Inquiry" reported that 21 per cent of children had suffered sexual abuse after they entered institutional care (Australian Senate, 2004). A landmark inquiry into the forced removal of Indigenous children had also covered this issue and found an overall rate of 17 per cent (Human Rights and Equal Opportunity Commission, 1997). In Ireland, a Commission of Inquiry found that more than half the children placed in care were subjected to sexual abuse (Ryan, 2009), while in a German study of more than a thousand leavers from both secular and religious institutions, 25 per cent reported sexual abuse during their stay, and more than a third of those were abused by multiple offenders; no difference was found between secular and religious institutions, and no religion was over-represented (Spröber et al., 2014). That finding of multiple offenders is relevant as, compared with other extrafamilial CSA, it is said to be one of the characteristics of institutional sexual abuse, as are longer duration and more severe abuse (Blakemore et al., 2017). To place this in context, however, most CSA does not occur in institutional settings: the Australian Personal Safety Survey reported that 11 per cent of CSA involved a stranger, 44 per cent a family member, 32 per cent a family friend, acquaintance, or neighbour, and "another known person" made up 15 per cent (Australian Bureau of Statistics, 2006). Although it is not specified, presumably cases of institutional abuse would be included in that last figure.

Institutional and spiritual trauma

Even outside the family, most sexual abuse of children is perpetrated by people they trust, by respected authority figures such as teachers, coaches, mentors, and clergy. A sense of betrayal is therefore inevitable in most instance of abuse. Betrayal is traumatic in itself; it is one of the fundamental aspects of the experience of sexual abuse, and one of the prime mediators of its long-term effects (Finkelhor and Browne, 1985). Betrayal involves a loss of trust and it shatters basic assumptions: the world is no longer benevolent or meaningful, or the self worthy (Janoff-Bulman, 2010). When the perpetrator is a trusted figure within the family or the community, or when institutions fail to act against sexual abuse, then the trauma of betrayal may extend well beyond the individual child. In the case of "institutional trauma" there is usually a culture of coercion and control and cover up and, in religious organisations, spiritual manipulation, all of which contribute to the traumatic impact on survivors and the community (Smith and Freyd, 2014).

In the case of abuse by a religious figure, the association with God makes the element of betrayal particularly acute and intensifies the victim's sense of powerlessness and confusion. Together with loss of faith and trust, this constitutes "spiritual trauma", which can be felt just as intensely within the family and the community or congregation (Smith, 2004). Perhaps in Australia this can be seen even at a national level, with a decline of belief in religion that may reflect the impact on the community of the increasing recognition of abuse of children in religious contexts.

Key issues

Though all children are vulnerable because of their immaturity and dependence on caretakers, those in institutional care are particularly vulnerable because of separation from family. Family dysfunction itself is a major vulnerability factor: this includes parental violence, substance abuse, imprisonment, unemployment, or mental illness. There are also individual vulnerability factors: alienation or social isolation, such as from bullying, premorbid psychological issues, and prior abuse or maltreatment (Finkelhor, 1993).

Childhood abuse causes damage across multiple domains of function so can lead to a range of psychosocial disturbances and significantly disrupt a child's developmental trajectory. These disturbances may be enduring and manifest in adult life in a range of psychiatric conditions, most often as a variant of Complex Post-Traumatic Stress Disorder, a condition which can encompass difficulties with mood and memory, deliberate self-harm and suicidality, flashbacks and nightmares, shame, guilt, and self-esteem, and relationship and sexual difficulties (Herman, 1992). Additionally, the risk of revictimisation is high in survivors: further abuse and interpersonal violence in adolescence and adult life is common, so that often there are continuing and cumulative traumas (Finkelhor, 1990).

Most children, however, do not report abuse because of shame, fear, or guilt. In institutional settings they feel particularly powerless, especially when it is evident that the abuse is systemic and when abuse involves religious figures or organisations. Disclosure is often met with negative reactions, which compound the trauma. Even in adulthood, many survivors remain reluctant to disclose abuse, most particularly men. Often disclosure is only prompted by media attention or some major triggering event (Pipe et al., 2007). In Australia, the Commission has been such an event and has prompted thousands of disclosures.

The terms "paedophile" and "child molester" are generally used interchangeably but strictly speaking are different. Paedophiles, by definition, feel personal distress about their interest and have not necessarily acted on their urges; child molesters have acted, and many are not distressed by their urges or activities. There is no generalisable psychiatric profile of a sex offender, and treatment or rehabilitation is difficult (Smallbone and Wortley, 2001). Child molesters often seek work in settings, including religious settings, where they have access to children, and where they establish themselves as worthy of a position of trust. They are often adept at identifying, targeting, and grooming vulnerable children, and they also groom families and communities. Grooming means gaining the child's compliance: it includes giving gifts and special attention, forming emotional bonds, and introducing alcohol, cigarettes, and/or drugs. Sexual talk and pornography are also used to desensitise the child. Less often compliance is gained by threats or coercion. There is usually a slow progression from non-sexual to sexual contact, so the child may have only a gradual awareness of what is happening and may later feel a sense of guilt and complicity, which can continue through adult life, especially if there is sexual arousal (Lanning, 2002).

The Christian Brothers case

In the early 1990s, the case against the Christian Brothers in Western Australia, the first of its kind in Australia, was a watershed moment in national awareness. The plaintiffs were more than 200 men, and the author was involved in assessing 31 of them. The case ran for three years, and, through their legal representatives, the church fought back vigorously. Finally, there was a settlement of around $AUD3.5 million, with some survivors receiving as little as $AUD2,000.

Aged in their 50s and 60s at the time of that action, the men had been "child migrants", chiefly from the UK, brought to Australia and placed in various residential facilities. This included one at Bindoon, in Western Australia, run by the Christian Brothers (the Christian Brothers are a worldwide religious community that is part of the Catholic Church). Bindoon was not far from Perth, but it was a very small town and rather isolated, which facilitated the development of a systemic culture of abuse. In the "care" of the Brothers, the migrant boys suffered years of neglect and severe abuse that was verbal, emotional, and physical, and sexual abuse that was often brutal.

Their adult lives were marked by high rates of alcoholism and unemployment, and difficulties with relationships that ranged from never having established any meaningful relationships to multiple relationship breakdowns. Many were living on the margins of society. It was particularly confronting to learn that some had made disclosures or complaints both during their time at Bindoon and after they left. They had reported to police, to child welfare, and to church authorities. No one wanted to know or to believe. One man recalled being told, "You ungrateful Pommy bastards; the good men of the church took you in and looked after you, and this is how you repay them!".

Women survivors

There were no girls placed at Bindoon, but there were many girls amongst the child migrants; they were placed in different institutions, such as Parramatta Girls Training School and the Fairbridge Farm Schools. There were also many girls who were not migrants but had been placed in care as "uncontrollable" children. Institutional placement of children was common up to the 1970s, and this included orphaned, abandoned, or neglected children, and those displaying disruptive or aggressive behaviour. The sexual mores of the day meant that girls who became pregnant or were otherwise known to be sexually active were prime targets for institutionalisation. There was limited awareness of CSA in services dealing with these situations, including psychiatry, and a girl's sexualised behaviour was less likely to be understood as a possible signal of abuse but rather as a behavioural problem. It could lead to her being brought before a children's court, deemed "uncontrollable", and placed in institutional care. As had occurred with the boys at Bindoon, these girls experienced a range of abuses, psychological, physical, and sexual. Their outcomes were similar: life-long problems with depression, substance abuse, and broken relationships, including, most especially for female survivors, multiple experiences of revictimisation.

The continuing violence in the lives of these women was particularly remarkable, as was the repetition of history with many instances of their children being removed. Domestic violence services in Australia were still in the early stages of development in the 1980s, and within psychiatry there was little recognition of the problem. There were many ways in which mental health services perpetuated abuse, but most particularly by pathologising the sequelae of child and partner abuse. Without a theory of trauma these sequelae, mostly depression, substance abuse, and personality disturbances, were understood as mental illness or disorder. Women survivors were usually assessed and treated within that paradigm, often with only the barest acknowledgement of their trauma history.

The best of schools

By the 1990s, there was better awareness of the reality of child abuse and its serious developmental consequences, both within the Australian community and within psychiatry. As the silence around child abuse was being broken, other institutions were exposed, including several prestigious private schools. Again, the author had the opportunity to assess a series of affected children. They were very different from the Bindoon survivors: their families were mostly intact, middle class, and well educated and, for most, the sexual abuse that had occurred at their schools was the only significant trauma they had experienced in life. Just as Scutt's seminal work showed that domestic violence in Australia was not confined to disadvantaged households (Scutt, 1983), these private school cases show that institutional child abuse respects no class differences. These assessments also provided an opportunity to understand the impact of sexual abuse specifically; that had not been possible with the Bindoon survivors who had suffered so much abuse, neglect, and deprivation that it was impossible to relate their difficulties to any single trauma or trauma type. It came as a surprise then to discover that what seemed like lesser degrees of trauma did not necessarily translate into less damage. For many of the private school cases, their lives had been shattered by an experience of sexual abuse that was time-limited and singular in terms of trauma experiences but was enduring in terms of the traumatic impact of shame and betrayal.

Usually these children had not suffered violent penetrative assaults, as had occurred at Bindoon. More often there was expert grooming that had established a close and affectionate bond with a perpetrator who, far from being feared, was usually popular and even much-loved in the school. Sometimes this perpetrator was a respected mentor or coach, sometimes he was more like the leader of a "Boys Own Adventure", organising outings, camps, and fishing trips, which he eventually laced with the thrill of alcohol, tobacco, cannabis, and/or pornography. Those illicit elements helped the perpetrator to bind the boys in secrecy and eased the transition to sexual contact, but it left them with a sense of shame and guilt over their participation in the abuse. They felt that others had been complicit too: that school staff had turned a blind eye, that parents had been blinded by their faith in the church. They came to feel betrayed by a man they had once admired; as one survivor said, "He was God on earth for us". They felt betrayed too by the school and the church and the families they had once trusted.

Shame and identity

Feelings of guilt and shame are a common response to sexual abuse, particularly in men. These feeling were prominent with the private school survivors; they seemed resistant to logic and were persistent, sometimes life-long. Shame limited their relationships, socially, and with intimate partners and with children;

many were fearful of closeness with their children. Frequently career progression too was limited by shame; one man said, "I have to keep my head down; I can't be in the spotlight because people will see who I am". Others were so wary of authority figures that they could not sustain regular employment: "I can't have a man stand over me".

Another prominent shame issue for all the male survivors was related to sexual identity. Almost universally, boys abused by men question their sexuality. They wonder why they were targeted; did the perpetrator identify them as gay, does that mean they are gay? Although social mores have changed greatly between the two generations of survivors described here, many of the younger men expressed the same fears as the older men had. One said, "It is still the worst thing that can be said about a man". These fears and doubts led to difficulties in relating to men and homophobic attitudes that limited peer and work relationships, and to extremes of either hypersexuality or sexual inhibition that were damaging to intimate relationships.

As with so many male survivors, most of those who had been abused in private schools were avoidant in their adjustment. Rarely did they seek treatment or counselling, rather they used alcohol and/or drugs to avoid or suppress thoughts, memories, and feelings, which in turn led to problems with employment and/or with the law. Others had developed a sense of anger and injustice that was expressed as irritability or aggression. Whether inhibited or angry, however, the outcome for the private school survivors was a dramatic derailing of developmental trajectory, with early drop-out from school and a pattern of underachievement that eclipsed earlier promise and led to a vicious cycle of feeling worthless and depressed, resulting in substance abuse, and so on.

Findings of the Royal Commission into Institutional Responses to Child Sexual Abuse

The Royal Commission ran for five years. At the conclusion of the Commission, a report was prepared. It consisted of a preface and executive summary, and 17 separate volumes (Royal Commission into Institutional Responses to Child Sexual Abuse, Final Report, 2017). The report chronicled the work of the Commission, their findings, and recommendations. The latter particularly focused on the need for a national investment in child safety, the need to make institutions safer, the need to advocate and to provide support and treatment services for survivors, and the need for redress and compensation. The final sections of this chapter address a number of these matters.

Prevention

The ubiquity of the problem of institutional sexual abuse of children has become evident and strong preventative measures are required. The Commission has identified the important areas where policy and practice need to develop, beginning with a "whole of community" approach to prevention which aims to change the social conditions that enable abuse to occur. This requires better services and better education of professionals working in the field, not only for survivors, but also for adults and young people who may have already offended or may be at risk of offending, defined by the Commission as those with problematic sexual thoughts and behaviours. Perhaps the most fundamental measure that can be taken is to eliminate or at least to minimise the necessity for institutional care. Indeed, some experts have suggested that out-of-home care brings little or no benefit to children compared with intervention in the home (Maclean et al., 2016). That step would mean providing better resources to assist families in distress and addressing the much broader issues of poverty, unemployment, and substance abuse (Bethea, 1999; World Health Organization, 2014).

Services and redress

The Commission has recommended measures that governments can take to redress or alleviate the impact of child sexual abuse in institutional contexts, including ensuring justice for victims through referrals for investigation and prosecution. Appropriate redress might also include a direct personal response by the institution, possibly an apology, and an assurance as to the steps the institution will take to protect against further abuse. Access to expert counselling should be available throughout a survivor's life, with redress and monetary payments to supplement existing services; a national redress scheme outlining these requirements has been recommended, and governments at both state and federal levels have agreed to participate. Improved services and more trauma-informed approaches would recognise that trauma is a powerful aetiological factor in many mental health problems, and there is a need for a more trauma-informed approach to assessment and treatment and, most critically, to prevention (Royal Commission into Institutional Responses to Child Sexual Abuse, Redress and Civil Litigation Report, 2015).

Conclusion

This chapter has traced the radical change in awareness and attitudes that has occurred over the past half century within the general community and various professional bodies and agencies that deal with these issues, most especially religious organisations and churches, and within psychiatry. Community attitudes have changed significantly over this time and there is now more acceptance and understanding, as well as moves to provide redress for victims. A quantum leap forward in this process has come about because of the Commission. It remains now for religious and secular organisations involved in the care of children, and for psychiatry and related clinical disciplines, to educate themselves and to change their culture, to become meaningfully trauma-informed about the effects of institutional child sex abuse, and to embody the principles and the work of the Commission.

References

Australian Bureau of Statistics (2006) *Personal Safety Survey, Australia 2005*. Canberra, Australia: Australian Bureau of Statistics.

Australian Senate (2004) *Forgotten Australians: A Report on Australians Who Experienced Institutional or Out-of-home Care as Children*. Canberra, Australia: Commonwealth of Australia.

Australian Senate (2009) *Lost Innocents and Forgotten Australians Revisited. Report on the Progress of the Lost Innocents and Forgotten Australians Reports*. Canberra, Australia: Commonwealth of Australia.

Bethea L (1999) Primary prevention of child abuse. *American Family Physician* 59(6): 1577–1585.

Blakemore T, Herbert JL, Arney F, et al. (2017) The impacts of institutional child sexual abuse: A rapid review of the evidence. *Child Abuse and Neglect* 74: 35–48.

Budiselik W, Crawford F and Chung D (2014) The Australian Royal Commission into institutional responses to child sexual abuse: Dreaming of child safe organisations? *Social Sciences* 3(3): 565–583.

Doyle TP (2017) The Australian Royal Commission into Institutional Responses to Child Sexual Abuse and the Roman Catholic Church. *Child Abuse and Neglect* 74: 103–106.

Dunne MP, Purdie DM, Cook MD, et al. (2003) Is child sexual abuse declining? Evidence from a population-based survey of men and women in Australia. *Child Abuse and Neglect* 27(2): 141–152.

Finkelhor D (1990) Early and long-term effects of child sexual abuse: An update. *Professional Psychology: Research and Practice* 21(5): 325–330.

Finkelhor D (1993) Epidemiological factors in the clinical identification of child sexual abuse. *Child Abuse and Neglect* 17(1): 67–70.

Finkelhor D and Browne A (1985). The traumatic impact of child sexual abuse: A conceptualization. *American Journal of Orthopsychiatry* 55: 530–541.

Herman JL (1992) *Trauma and Recovery*. New York, NY: Basic Books.

Hobbs GF, Hobbs CJ and Wynne JM (1999) Abuse of children in foster and residential care. *Child Abuse and Neglect* 23(12): 1239–1252.

Human Rights and Equal Opportunity Commission (1997) *Bringing Them Home: Report of the National Inquiry into the Separation of Aboriginal and Torres Strait Islander Children From Their Families*. Sydney, Australia: Human Rights and Equal Opportunity Commission.

Janoff-Bulman R (2010) *Shattered Assumptions*. New York, NY: Simon and Schuster.

Lanning K (2002) Criminal investigation of sexual victimization of children. In: Myers JEB, Berliner L, Briere J, et al. (eds) *The APSAC Handbook on Child Maltreatment, Second Edition*. Thousand Oaks, CA: Sage Publications.

Maclean MJ, Sims S, O'Donnell M, et al. (2016) Out-of-home care versus in-home care for children who have been maltreated: A systematic review of health and wellbeing outcomes. *Child Abuse Review* 25(4): 251–272.

Mazza D, Dennerstein L, Garamszegi CV, et al. (2001) The physical, sexual and emotional violence history of middle-aged women: A community-based prevalence study. *Medical Journal of Australia* 175: 199–201.

Najman JM, Dunne MP, Purdie DM, et al. (2005) Sexual abuse in childhood and sexual dysfunction in adulthood: An Australian population-based study. *Archives of Sexual Behavior* 34(5): 517–526.

Nunno M and Rindfleisch N (1991) The abuse of children in out of home care. *Children and Society* 5(4): 295–305.

Pipe ME, Lamb ME, Orbach Y, et al. (eds) (2007) *Child Sexual Abuse: Disclosure, Delay and Denial.* New York, NY: Routledge.

Royal Commission into Institutional Responses to Child Sex Abuse (2015) *Royal Commission into Institutional Responses to Child Sexual Abuse, Redress and Civil Litigation Report.* Sydney, Australia: Commonwealth of Australia.

Royal Commission into Institutional Responses to Child Sexual Abuse (2017) *Royal Commission into Institutional Responses to Child Sexual Abuse, Final Report.* Sydney, Australia: Commonwealth of Australia.

Ryan S (2009) *Commission to Inquire into Child Abuse.* Dublin, Ireland: The Commission to Inquire into Child Abuse.

Scutt JA (1983) *Even in the Best of Homes: Violence in the Family.* Ringwood, Victoria, Australia: Penguin.

Smallbone SW and Wortley RK (2001) *Child Sexual Abuse: Offender Characteristics and Modus Operandi. Australian Institute of Criminology, Trends and Issues in Crime and Criminal Justice.* Paper No.193. Canberra, Australia: Australian Institute of Criminology.

Smith S (2004) Exploring the interaction of trauma and spirituality. *Traumatology* 10(4): 231–243.

Smith CP and Freyd JJ (2014) Institutional betrayal. *American Psychologist* 69(6): 575–587.

Spröber N, Schneider T, Rassenhofer M, et al. (2014) Child sexual abuse in religiously affiliated and secular institutions: A retrospective descriptive analysis of data provided by victims in a government-sponsored reappraisal program in Germany. *BMC Public Health* 14(1): 282.

World Health Organization (2014) *Social Determinants of Mental Health.* Geneva, Switzerland: World Health Organization.

9 Incest that continues into adult life

Warwick Middleton

> Whether both parents are psychotic or only one of them is immaterial, for if one is, the other is living with him or her in a folie à deux.
>
> Robert Fliess, 1973, pp.227–228

Introduction

It is very likely that Robert Fliess was sexually abused by his father Wilhelm. Wilhelm was Sigmund Freud's closest male confidant, during a 13-year period from 1887 until 1900, when the relationship disintegrated in acrimony (Roazen, 1975; Middleton, 2016). Robert in time became a psychoanalyst, met with Freud to discuss his father, and subsequently moved to the USA in 1936, where he followed a path not unlike that taken by Sándor Ferenczi before him, moving to oppose the repudiation that Freud had made of his own "seduction theory". Robert Fliess characterised his father as suffering from an "ambulatory psychosis". This concept, introduced by Fliess, described a person who appeared normal in public, yet who in private was anything but, being highly sexualised, violent, and sadistic. Fliess wrote,

> When one is able to diagnose it, one sees relatively few families of one's patients that are entirely free of it … . The child of such a parent becomes the object of substantially defused aggression (maltreated and beaten almost to within an inch of his life), and of a perverse sexuality that hardly knows an incest barrier (is seduced in the most bizarre ways by the parent and, at his instigation, by others) … .
>
> (1956: p.xvii)

There has however been a long-standing reflex denial of incest, and, until the 1970s, society largely ignored the evidence, even when published (Masson, 2017). A critical mass of feminist writers and researchers, the emergence of the Dissociative Disorders field, and the psychological plight of Vietnam veterans, brought into stark focus by an unpopular war, occasioned a new and precarious focus on shamed and traumatised individuals.

Yet even as society began to establish a foothold in recognising those who had been grievously emotionally hurt by others, a backlash was already forming. The earlier any trauma starts and the longer it persists, the more traumatised an individual will be, and the more dissociated. Higher levels of dissociation render individuals more liable to incorporating elements into their account that are not historically accurate. Often lacking a functional family network, with limited financial resources, struggling with drugs and alcohol used to self-medicate, with a history of self-harming and suicide attempts, and psychiatric hospital admissions, those struggling in the wake of abuse do not find themselves in a sound position from which they can challenge their familial and/or institutional abusers, who have a vested interest in using any inconsistencies in their accounts to further discredit them.

The modern Dissociative Disorders field, along with the broader psychological trauma field, had a head-on encounter with the gathering backlash. It started with controversies over alleged "Satanic Ritual Abuse" (SRA) and evolved into a bitter debate about the authenticity of "recovered" memories of past trauma, as well as the validity of Dissociative Identity Disorder (DID). There was the formation of the "False Memory Syndrome Foundation" in the USA in 1992, and the "Australian False Memory Society" in 1993 – organisations set up to advocate on behalf of individuals who claim that they had been falsely accused of child sex abuse. In the USA, therapist's offices and trauma conferences were picketed, and multiple professional complaints and law-suits were directed at therapists. Only a small number had adverse findings made against them, but many more left the Dissociative Disorders and Complex Trauma field in the late 1990s, reasoning that the area was too high a risk to be practising in.

A number of experts have attempted to address these complexities. As long ago as 1984, Kluft perceptively wrote,

> In a given patient [with Multiple Personality Disorder, or MPD], one may find episodes of photographic recall, confabulation, screen phenomena, confusion between dreams or fantasies and reality, irregular recollection, and willful misrepresentation. One awaits a goodness of fit among several forms of data, and often must be satisfied to remain uncertain.
>
> (p.14)

In his 1989 text, Putnam made no specific mention of "Satanic" or "ritual" abuse. He did clearly state though,

> I am struck by the quality of extreme sadism that is frequently reported by most [MPD] victims. Bondage situations; the insertion of a variety of instruments into the vagina, mouth, and anus; and various forms of physical and sexual torture are common reports. Many multiples have told me of being sexually abused by groups of people, of being forced into prostitution by family members, or of being offered as a sexual enticement to their mother's boyfriends. After one has worked with several MPD

> patients, it becomes obvious that severe, sustained, and repetitive child sexual abuse is a major element in the creation of MPD.
>
> (p.49)

In 1997, Putnam also wrote,

> From my perspective, the best example of the creation of clinically and legally significant pseudo-memories involves allegations of SRA. Such allegations are defined here as claims that a vast, international, multi-generational conspiracy is practicing religious worship of Satan or the devil through rituals involving sex, death, torture, incest, human sacrifice, cannibalism, and necrophilia. With the exception of a few isolated 'copycat' incidents, there is no credible evidence that actual SRA is occurring or ever has occurred.
>
> (p.124)

Ross, looking back in 2008, reflected,

> Many, many therapists went completely off the deep end on SRA. Not a few. Lots. I met therapists who had post-traumatic stress disorder from listening to their clients' SRA stories. They believed absolutely that their clients had been the Brides of Satan in Satanic ceremonies and had eaten babies. Estimates of the number of babies sacrificed by Satanists in North America per year ran as high as 50,000. There was no evidence of course.
>
> (p.182)

Yet despite the backlash, the modern trauma field has steered a course where there is an enhanced general awareness about the necessity of not making public pronouncements about aspects of reported trauma that go beyond the authenticated data, of maintaining a respectful stance in responding to published critiques, of being very careful in respect to all aspects of maintaining appropriate boundaries, of publishing internationally authored papers in mainstream mental health journals, in conducting the necessary research in order to respond authoritatively to the propagation of myths about Complex Trauma that have little factual basis (Brand et al., 2016), and in supporting society as it finally begins to examine itself.

Ongoing incestuous abuse during adulthood

There have been regular press reports of ongoing incestuous abuse during adulthood for the last century and a half, and there have been books in the lay literature written by, or about, such victims, but aside from single case reports and incidental/anecdotal references to this spectrum of abuse, there had been, until 2013, no published systematic research about this significant spectrum of abuse. Putnam made a brief reference to the fact that, "actual abuse of adult MPD patients by family members does occur and can touch off devastating crises" (Putnam, 1989: p.296). Such matters have been rarely discussed in the great majority of subsequent texts on either dissociation or incest, though case examples have periodically appeared (Kluft, 2009). Courtois however stated that she had "now worked with a number of clients whose abuse continued into their adult years and whose abusers, mostly fathers, largely considered their daughters their property to do with as they pleased" (Courtois, 2010: p.32). She said that the prevalence of such cases is unknown. Clearly such victims had high suicidality as inferred by reference to this sort of abuse in highly suicidal DID patients (Kinsler, 1995; Kluft, 1995).

In researching this area, it is relevant to be mindful of what had happened previously when writers and clinicians had proclaimed there was a previously unresearched spectrum of abuse occurring widely in society as a result of SRA. It had been apparent, however, from early on that a significant proportion of patients with DID continued to experience sexual and other abuse beyond their 18th birthday. In a study of 62 individuals with DID, at least 13 per cent were in this category (Middleton and Butler, 1998). Contemporary studies also indicate that at least 1 per cent of the general population meet diagnostic criteria for DID (Brand et al., 2016). If, as the 1998 study suggested, approximately one in eight individuals with DID was subjected to ongoing incestuous abuse after their 18th birthday, this would equate to one in 800 in the general population having experienced this form of ongoing abuse.

The Austrian case of Josef Fritzl provided an opportunity to put systematic research in this area on a more solid footing. The case of Fritzl, who had imprisoned his daughter Elisabeth in an underground dungeon for 24 years as a sexual slave, during which time she gave birth to seven children, captured global attention, and for a time there was an increased frequency of stories of a generally similar nature appearing about such abusers in other countries. These press accounts, based on police statements and proven court findings, have been closely analysed (Middleton, 2009, 2011, 2013a, 2013c, 2013d, 2014a, 2014b, 2015a, 2015b, 2017). One such analysis of press accounts of 51 cases reported during the years 2007–2012 revealed that all but six cases demonstrated dynamics that were similar to the Fritzl case (Middleton, 2014a). By way of examples: the Sheffield "Gaffer" abused his two daughters for 30 years, making one or other of them pregnant 19 times, and producing nine children; the man from Moe, Victoria, abused his daughter for 30 years, producing four children (Smethurst, 2013); Armando Gomez from Argentina abused his daughter for 30 years, producing 10 children; Austrian Gottfried Wagner, arrested at the age of 80, had sexually abused his daughters for more than 41 years, and, Bronislaw K from Poland abused his daughter for more than 30 years, producing one daughter. He had also regularly sexually assaulted a granddaughter.

In a minority of the international cases, organised abuse was prominently reported, for example with Detlef Spies regularly prostituting his daughter and stepdaughter, and in respect to the multigenerational aspects of reported abuse in the Mohler and Mongelli families. However, the trend in the 51 cases described above suggested that the wider abuse networks associated with the father tended to go unreported in short press reports (Middleton, 2014a). Though a minority of these fathers went through the motions of concealing the ongoing incest from their wives, the longevity of the abuse made journalists disbelieving of wives who claimed not to know about such extensive events occurring in the family home, particularly where there were multiple offspring. In some cases, the wife was also a victim of extreme domestic violence, but other wives were clearly active co-abusers. Sometimes the local community clearly knew about the abuse but chose not to intervene, for example, in respect to Charles Shamblin Jr, who abused his daughter from age seven until she was 20, fathering three children in the process; Shamblin's daughter-in-law commented that the community knew what was going on, but looked the other way (Middleton, 2014a).

In a substantial number of cases the abusers however succeeded in projecting an image of domestic normality to the outside world, congruent with Robert Fliess' construct of an ambulatory psychosis. For example, John McMillan's daughter, Anne Marie Wilson, sexually abused by her father for 16 years and made pregnant six times, experienced constant death threats, as did her mother. She experienced her father as a "control freak" who never let her out of his sight, but she observed that outwardly, "We were a normal family, and my father had many friends and a good social life. No one suspected anything" (Middleton, 2014a).

A recurrent theme in a minority of cases is for the mother to escape the family home and leave behind the daughter with whom the father is particularly fixated. One such example involved Argentinian, Domingo Bullicio, who was arrested in January 2016 after allegedly raping his daughter for 22 years and fathering eight children with her. Bullicio was accused of turning his daughter Antonia into a sex slave after his wife departed with their three other children. "From the moment my mum left home I became my father's wife", she recalled. As with most such victims, she experienced her father as violent, and prone to make death threats, "He told me he would kill me if I said anything". She described also being sexually abused by an uncle. She also said that she was threatened by her father's siblings to withdraw her complaint (Couzens, 2016).

Bullicio is a typical example of the international group of incestuous abusers first described in a publication in 2013 (Middleton, 2013a). Almost without exception they were violent, used weapons to hurt or threaten their victims, and were extremely controlling, for example, warning off any potential boyfriends. When Alba Nidia Álvarez, daughter of Columbian Arcedio Álvarez, as a teenager developed a romantic attachment to a 17-year-old neighbourhood boy, her father turned up at the boyfriend's house with a gun in his hand, forcing an end to the relationship (Semana, 2009). Many fathers actually wanted their victims to bear children, with the offspring in turn being subjected to the same sort of control, and with some becoming in time sexually abused as well. Others physically attacked their pregnant victim, forcing them to miscarry. The average duration of the sexual abuse, before authorities brought an end to it, was nearly 20 years, and in the majority of cases there were incestuously fathered children, not infrequently in large numbers. Arcebio Álvarez fathered 11 such childen, Armando Gomez fathered 10 (one of whom suicided), Detlef Spies and Jose Agostina Pereira each fathered eight such childen, Armando Lucero and Josef Fritzl each fathered seven, while Raymond Gouardo fathered six.

Fritzl, despite at his trial changing his plea to "guilty", from gaol tried to pressure his daughter to send him money, "to study to be a lawyer so I can defend myself". Fritzl's sister-in-law Christine revealed that in his letters to Elisabeth, "There is never a word of regret or an apology from him" (Hall, 2010). A number, including Fritzl, and Jorge Iniestra Salas, were also charged with the murder of one or more victims. Dr Adelheid Kastner, who prepared a 130-page court evaluation of Fritzl, said he suffered serious personality problems, but was responsible for his actions; "He is aware – he says so himself – that he has an evil side. He is aware that he was born to rape. He has that partly under control. But as soon as he loosens his grip, everything erupts out" (Australian Broadcasting Corporation, 2009).

An analysis of ten Australian women who had been in treatment with the author of this chapter confirmed many of the above findings (Middleton, 2013b). The average total number of reported separate episodes of sexual abuse was 3,320, while the mean duration of abuse was in the order of 31 years, figures very similar to those reported in respect to Elisabeth Fritzl. The average estimated age at which the sexual abuse began was 2.7 years, progressing to sexual intercourse at an average age of 3.8 years. 90 per cent additionally reported severe physical abuse, with 70 per cent reporting injuries that were so severe that surgery was required. 80 per cent said that guns were used in the abuse. These incest victims also became orgasmic at a young age, typically around five or six, and the manipulation of orgasm became central to the ongoing sexual abuse, congruent with a conditioning process described by Yates (1982).

The abusive fathers of the women appeared to be little different in terms of their attitudes, propensity to violence, the chronicity of abuse, and use of extreme control, from those fathers described in the international press accounts. All the fathers were experienced as extremely controlling, 90 per cent of the women had received death threats, and 30 per cent had experienced more active attempts by their father to kill them. 70 per cent had also experienced their father encouraging them to suicide. Most of the fathers were also experienced as actively wanting their daughters to become pregnant by them. Characteristically, the father would in time want their victim to take part in sexual activities directed against the incestuously fathered offspring, further adding to shame and guilt, and allied with threats of death, hell, and so on, ensuring silence on the part of the women. The majority were aware that their father had been incestuously abused himself, and nearly all knew that their father had experienced an extremely dysfunctional upbringing; 40 per cent thought their father had DID himself. The majority also knew or suspected that their mother had also been sexually abused as a child.

The effect of chronic abuse and domination by the father on the development of selfhood was extreme: all ten women experienced the presence of their father as a separate personality within them, nine felt that their body did not belong to them, and eight felt "fused" with their father. Eight women experienced their father as taking an active role in the creation of dissociative identity states within them, and most were aware of their father actively inducing dissociative switching between these identity states named by them. As with the international group of fathers, all ten women experienced their father and/or other abusive family members as obsessed with pornography. All were subjected to being made the subject of pornographic pictures, and all were sexually abused within a network that their father was a member of. Such networks included child prostitution, groups of the father's friends, church associated groups, or multigenerational assortments of family members. All reported that their mother directly observed the sexual abuse, while for 70 per cent she was an active participant in the sexual abuse. Illustrative of the multi-generational dimension of this abuse, 70 per cent reported being sexually abused by a grandparent, with one being abused by both grandparents. Outwardly, nearly all fathers maintained gainful employment and stable marriages, and 60 per cent of them were closely associated with a church.

Trauma-informed approaches

By far the majority, if not all, individuals whose incestuous abuse extended from childhood into adulthood meet the diagnostic criteria for DID. Although treatment is informed by the International Society for the Study of Trauma and Dissociation Guidelines for DID (2011), there is much that is encountered with this group on which these guidelines are silent (Kluft, 2017; Middleton, 2017).

First, and most critically, therapists and other health professionals need to have an awareness of this type of abuse, as the history is generally not likely to be volunteered. Therapists need to be mindful of the need to establish the reasons for chronic extreme fear, serious suicidality, and an extreme propensity for shame, as well as reasoning that those individuals with complex or very fragmented forms of DID usually have identifiable traumas that have invoked such extreme versions of dissociation.

It is also important to note that the women have intense and ambivalent attachments to the perpetrator, a connection that continues even after death. This knowledge needs to be considered when a therapist learns that a patient is still being abused, such that early attempts to simply insist that the abuse must stop for therapy to continue may be unhelpful and will usually prematurely terminate the treatment.

Patients who have undergone such repeated abuses from an early age are not experienced in developing their own boundaries with others either. The issue of boundaries in therapy is therefore crucial and must be addressed at the beginning of treatment and throughout. These issues need to be sensitively approached, and the maintenance of sexual and other boundaries should be clearly modelled by therapists. Unfortunately, this does not always occur, and patients with this level of difficulty are often vulnerable to being abused by therapists.

It is also important to note that while feeling bad and shameful, these patients have had little if any love or support in their lifetimes, and they have a high need for acceptance and empathic connection. Therapists must repeatedly attempt to demonstrate that they understand what has happened to them, and how devastating the abuse was, and to bear witness to and not turn away from the events; the therapist must be able to demonstrate that they are able to empathically deal with the perverse and sadistic experiences that their patient has endured.

This type of patient has also been conditioned not to trust others, and to subdue emotional responses on the one hand, whilst on the other they are acutely aware of all of their therapist's facial expressions. Therapists in turn must be acutely aware of the relevance of these moment-to-moment emotional interchanges between themselves and the patient. They must also be comfortable enough to discuss material that the patient has never before discussed in detail with any other. This often involves the way that sexuality was conditioned from an early age, while their abuser shamed them for the very responses that they had themselves orchestrated. Generally speaking, these abuse victims respond positively to precise information that demonstrates that their responses, which they believed were immensely shameful, are in fact identical to the responses of others brought up in similarly abusive environments.

These patients also invariably have one or more dissociative identity states or internal "alters" that are based around aspects of the abusive father. They represent the compartmentalisation of the various utterances and behaviours that characterised the father, and they incorporate various memories of trauma involving the father. Despite superficial resemblances, they are not the father; in fact, they are psychological parts of the patient that carry particularly difficult loads and need to be afforded the respect that comes with fully appreciating their burdens. All alters have been created around the compartmentalisation of memories, affects, and functions, and they need to be treated with equal respect. All alters have important roles and the meaning of their functioning may involve paradoxes, for example, an alter associated with self-harm may represent a dynamic where self-harm and the associated release of tension is seen as preferable to the unchecked building of suicidal ideation; individuals within this spectrum of abuse are understandably particularly prone to self-harm and suicide.

Treatment invariably also means attempting a reshaping of the life landscape, effecting separation from the father and other abusers, as well as dealing with the multiple issues that such abuse has caused to marital and other relationships, and those issues that are likely in time to be investigated by police. It is a poignant point of emerging trust, but also of extreme vulnerability on the part of the patient, when a therapist sits with a patient and her husband and reveals to him for the first time that sexual abuse by her father continued throughout their marriage until the time of his death, or a therapist sits with a patient and her adult daughter and reveals to the daughter that she was fathered by her grandfather.

Conclusion

As a therapist and researcher, the author of this chapter has seen many victims in this spectrum and has also had contact with a number of their abusive parents. It is apparent from this experience that the Fliess description of "ambulatory psychosis" fits well the profile of the abusive father, and that, despite its hidden nature, this form of extreme ongoing incestuous abuse occurs relatively frequently, and repeatedly overlaps with one or more forms of organised abuse.

With respect to treatment, there can logically be no short-term resolution of the effects of severe abuse that has frequently spanned much, if not all, of a lifetime, and filled an individual's formative years. There is substantial variability in whether patients in this group can reach "escape velocity", and progressively build sufficient selfhood for a safe alternative life, away from their abusers, or whether they will remain at long-term risk of re-abuse, and the self-harm and suicidality that accompanies this. Despite decades spent in a hellish existence, some can and do build sufficient boundaries, find occupational and relationship success, and, with therapy, deal with their shame and fear to the extent that they find a growing capacity to have trusted partners and friends, and to risk sharing their vulnerability.

References

Australian Broadcasting Corporation (2009) Fritzl 'born to rape', psychiatrist tells court. Available at: tinyurl.com/y9m7at99.

Brand BL, Sar V, Stavropoulos P, et al. (2016) Separating fact from fiction: An empirical examination of common myths about dissociative identity disorder. *Harvard Review of Psychiatry* 24(4): 257–270.

Courtois CA (2010) *Healing the Incest Wound, Second Edition*. New York, NY: Norton.

Couzens G (2016) Dad 'fathered eight children with his daughter' during 22-year reign of terror. *Mirror*. Available at: tinyurl.com/y95wt23f.

Fliess R (1956) *Erogeneity and Libido: Addenda to the Theory of the Psychosexual Development of the Human. Psychoanalytic Series: Volume One*. New York, NY: International Universities Press.

Fliess R (1973) *Symbol, Dream, and Psychosis, with Notes on Technique. Psychoanalytic Series: Volume Three*. New York, NY: International Universities Press.

Hall A (2010) Cellar monster Josef Fritzl begs his rape victim daughter for cash … to fund his legal training. *Daily Mail*. Available at: tinyurl.com/ybff6lrw.

ISSTD (2011) Guidelines for treating dissociative identity disorder in adults, Third Revision. *Journal of Trauma and Dissociation* 12(2): 115–187.

Kinsler PJ (1995) A story for Marcie. *Dissociation* 8(2): 100–103.

Kluft RP (1984) Treatment of multiple personality disorder. *Psychiatric Clinics of North America* 7: 9–29.

Kluft RP (1995) Six completed suicides in dissociative identity disorder patients: Clinical observations. *Dissociation* 8(2): 104–111.

Kluft RP (2009) A clinician's understanding of dissociation: Fragments of an acquaintance. In: Dell PF and O'Neill JA (eds) *Dissociation and the Dissociative Disorders: DSM-V and Beyond*. New York, NY: Routledge, pp.599–624.

Kluft RP (2017) Weaponized sex: Defensive pseudo-erotic aggression in the service of safety. Special (double) Issue. *Journal of Trauma and Dissociation* 18(3): 249–283.

Masson J (2017) End note. A personal perspective: The response to child abuse then and now. Special (double) Issue. *Journal of Trauma and Dissociation* 18(3): 476–482.

Middleton W (2009) *Oedipus, adulthood and attachment to abusing fathers.* Plenary paper for conference, "Trauma, Mentalisation and Dissociative Processes: Translating Theory into Practice", The Royal Australian and New Zealand College of Psychiatrists Section of Psychotherapy Conference. Crowne Plaza Hotel, Surfers Paradise, Australia.

Middleton W (2011) *'Always daddy's little girl': Incestuous abuse during adulthood.* Invited plenary paper, World Congress for Psychotherapy, "World Dreaming", Sydney Convention and Exhibition Centre, Darling Harbour, Sydney, Australia.

Middleton W (2013a) Parent–child incest that extends into adulthood: A survey of international press reports 2007–2011. *Journal of Trauma and Dissociation* 14(2): 184–197.

Middleton W (2013b) Ongoing incestuous abuse during adulthood. *Journal of Trauma and Dissociation* 14(3): 251–272.

Middleton W (2013c) Ongoing incestuous abuse during adulthood. *European Society for Trauma and Dissociation Newsletter* 3(3): 9–12.

Middleton W (2013d) Response to Commentary by Adah Sachs on, "Parent–child incest that extends into adulthood: A survey of international press reports", and, "Ongoing incestuous abuse during adulthood". *Journal of Trauma and Dissociation* 14 (5): 580–583.

Middleton W (2014a) Parent–child incest that extends into adulthood: A survey of international press reports, 2007–2012. In: Sar V, Middleton W and Dorahy M (eds) *Global Perspectives on Dissociative Disorders: Individual and Societal Oppression.* London, UK: Routledge, pp.45–64.

Middleton W (2014b) Nicht endender Inzest: die Fritzl-Analogie. *Zeitschrift für Psychotraumatologie und ihre Anwendungen* 12(4): 34–42. (Unending incest: The Fritzl analogue. Invited paper for journal special issue ZPA).

Middleton W (2015a) Tipping points and the accommodation of the abuser: The case of ongoing incestuous abuse during adulthood. *International Journal for Crime, Justice and Social Democracy* 4(2): 4–17.

Middleton W (2015b) *Child sexual abuse: Organised and unending.* Plenary paper, presented at ISSTD Bi-National Regional conference, "Broken Structures, Broken Selves: Complex Trauma in the 21st Century". Westin Hotel, Sydney, Australia.

Middleton W (2016) Wilhelm Fliess, Robert Fliess, Ernest Jones, Sandor Ferenczi and Sigmund Freud – ISSTD President's editorial. *Journal of Trauma and Dissociation* 17(1): 1–12.

Middleton W (2017) Extreme adaptations in extreme and chronic circumstances: The application of 'weaponized sex' to those exposed to ongoing incestuous abuse. Special (double) Issue. *Journal of Trauma and Dissociation* 18(3): 284–303.

Middleton W and Butler J (1998) Dissociative identity disorder: An Australian series. *Australian and New Zealand Journal of Psychiatry* 32: 794–804.

Putnam FW (1989) *Diagnosis and Treatment of Multiple Personality Disorder.* New York, NY: Guilford.

Putnam FW (1997) *Dissociation in Children and Adolescents: A Developmental Perspective.* New York, NY: Guilford.

Roazen P (1975) *Freud and His Followers.* New York, NY: Knopf.

Ross CA (2008) *The Great Psychiatry Scam: One Shrink's Personal Journey.* Richardson, TX: Manitou.

Semana (2009) The daughter of the Colombian monster. *Semana*. Available at: tinyurl.com/lk7ofzn.

Smethurst S (2013) The worst case of child abuse Australia has ever seen: A father raped his daughter for 30 years and fathered four children. *Australian Women's Weekly* October edition, pp.132–133.

Yates A (1982) Children eroticized by incest. *American Journal of Psychiatry* 139: 482–485.

10 Aboriginal Australia – trauma stories can become healing stories if we work with therapeutic intent

Judy Atkinson

> We are the product of our childhoods. The health and creativity of a community is renewed each generation through its children.
>
> Bruce Perry, 2004, p.3

Introduction

Trauma may be experienced and carried, like a virus, across multiple generations. This is no more evident than in the work done with Aboriginal women incarcerated for violence in the Alice Springs Prison, in remote Central Australia, as they make their "loss history" maps and give context to the trauma passed down across generations. For some, naming their own family and community connections to the Coniston Massacre of 1928, the last sanctioned massacre of Aboriginal peoples (Elder, 2003), is of particular relevance to this process.

This chapter will initially focus on the work done in the Alice Springs Prison, how listening to and learning from the challenges of the women imprisoned there has helped delineate the pathways necessary to move forward, to heal the layered generational trauma of their fractured lives. Although Aboriginal people comprise only 2 per cent of the Australian adult population aged 18 and over, Aboriginal women make up 34 per cent of the national female prison population (Australian Bureau of Statistics, 2016), and, in Alice Springs, 89 per cent of the female prison population (Northern Territory of Australia, Department of Attorney-General and Justice, 2017). All of these women have histories of being violated in various ways before their behaviour in response to trauma brought them to prison. They inherit the aggression and hostility of a colonial past, massacres, starvation, subjugation, and the systemic racism, oppression, and poverty embedded in their present lives. Aboriginal women in Central Australia are at extreme risk of death or injury due to male violence, "identified as among the most victimised by intimate partner violence in the world" (Kerr, 2016: p.3).

Consideration will then be given to "symptom as history" to help contextualise Aboriginal experiences that continue to occur as a consequence of colonialisation, and contribute to mental and emotional distress, physical ill-health, spiritual and cultural disharmony, substance misuse, and escalating incarceration and suicide rates (Dudgeon et al., 2014; Zubrick et al., 2014).

It is then explained that "behaviour is language" when looking at the lives of two Aboriginal children and their families, demonstrating the responsibility to listen to and reflect upon what may be communicated through behaviour. The stories the children tell through their "behaviour" helps deepen the understanding of how two people living in the same situation, having similar experiences, can exhibit two very different reactions to the same trauma. In such circumstances, workers with trauma-specific skills are required, capable of responding to symptoms which are perplexing and distressing unless contextualised within the greater generational trauma story. This also means having an understanding of the concepts of developmental and Complex Trauma.

A trauma-integrated service response to the needs of these children and their families, so essential for healing, is finally described.

Stories from a prison

The Kunga Stopping Violence Program in the Alice Springs Prison supports Aboriginal women who are generally incarcerated for violent behaviour. In mid-2015, the program coordinator requested the development of an educational pre-release package, which would run for four weeks, from 9am to 3pm, five days a week, twice yearly, to help the women examine their offending behaviours. The first program was designed as an, "Anger–Violence–Boundaries–Safety Package" (AVBS), which concluded with an exploration of issues related to grief and loss.

By 2017, it became clear that the violence perpetrated by the women was almost always in response to the trauma that they had seen and suffered as children and were subsequently experiencing in adult life. It was decided that some major changes needed to be made to the course, and to the approach taken by staff: there would be no more direct instruction, no "PowerPoint" presentations, and no "teaching" the women how they could change their behaviour. Rather, emphasis was to be placed on the development of conversations, the program starting with grief, loss and trauma, and then finishing with the AVBS modules.

Importantly, the women were told that they would be supported to construct their "loss history maps". This meant sitting with each woman, outside a small classroom to ensure privacy, to help them map their stories from birth to the present, and it meant sitting beside each of the women when they painted, or did their story books, engaging in conversations that took them deeper and deeper into those stories. Though the women generally have English as a third or fourth language, painting, it was clear, was both a language in and of itself, and a deep meditative or mindfulness practice, a safe way to reflect on their lives and circumstances, and to choose what they felt ready to disclose. The process was graded and gentle, and it provided a therapeutic space within which the women could feel more and more comfortable.

The work was, however, often very painful as it became clear that multiple layers of trauma were part of a "lived experience" which led to the situations which took them to prison. The complexity of the trauma stories cannot be adequately captured in words. Trauma, though, started early in their lives, for some, even before birth, as a result of traumatised parents living in distressing social circumstances. Alcohol was often a major factor in their early childhood, with care-givers who drank, and in their experiences of intimate partner violence (Kerr, 2016). In the situation of domestic violence, as women fought back, their risk of serious injury or death increased, as did the risk of injury to their assailant. Kerr points out that women were identified as the aggressor in physical violence in 47 per cent of the fights identified (Kerr, 2016), generally after years of violent assaults, unresolved within the policing system. In one case, carefully reviewing many years of police records, a woman suffered 13 years of violence at the hands of her male partner, with him repeatedly accusing her of infidelity, while he was the guilty party. After forcing her to drink with him on multiple occasions she eventually picked up a weapon and attacked him. She had endured undiagnosed Complex Trauma (Kerr, 2016).

The work has taken the women more profoundly into an understanding of themselves and how they came to be adults. Their depth of honesty, even in their shame and grief, was humbling. As they gained insight, they began to look at new ways to help themselves escape the trauma spiral.

But prisons are not the safest or the most suitable places for such change to happen, and no matter what their intentions, when they leave prison these women may re-experience considerable difficulty, being drawn back into the distressed behaviour of family members, where all have been failed by local services (Atkinson, 2015–2018).

"Symptom as history" – being trauma-informed

It is only in recent years that the impacts of trauma on, and within, Aboriginal populations, from earliest colonial times to the present, have begun to be accepted and understood (Dudgeon et al., 2014). The findings of the landmark Adverse Childhood Experiences (ACE) study in the USA are also relevant to Aboriginal Australians (Felitti et al., 1998). Expanding upon this work, Van der Kolk wrote about the effects on children, that adverse experiences lead to them feeling unsafe, to struggle with grief, shame, and self-destructive behaviours, to have difficulties at school, and in youth to show early substance abuse, aggression, and suicidal ideation (Van der Kolk, 2007). In Australia, Aboriginal youth suicides are twice the national rate (Australian Bureau of Statistics, 2010). In adults, the long-term sequelae of adverse childhood experiences include higher rates of heart, liver, and lung disease, diabetes, and cancer (Felitti et al., 1998). Adverse childhood experiences also lead to higher rates of both juvenile detention and adult incarceration (Van der Kolk, 2007). For many Aboriginal people, the pathway to incarceration begins in early childhood within the complex generational trauma and the distressed behaviour of Aboriginal family and community lives. For Aboriginal Australians, the ACE study directly questions the previous policies of all Australian states, of the forced removal of Aboriginal children, investigated under the "Bringing them Home Report" (Human Rights and Equal Opportunity Commission, 1997).

Mapping such impacts provides clear evidence of "symptom as history". Working to understand symptoms as cause and effect opens an uncomfortable and often highly resistant space for much of white Australia, and an unsafe, painful, and sometimes shameful place for many Aboriginal people.

The British prison hulks sailed into Sydney Cove in 1788, and the worlds of the peoples on the lands now called Australia were overturned. The diseases incubated in the slums of England were introduced to the local Gadigal people and spread quickly through coastal communities. The Gadigal were previously healthy, with more than enough to eat, but, as they were forced off their land, starvation also resulted. The University of Newcastle is presently mapping massacre sites, with the first recorded killings on 1 September 1794 at Sydney Cove, and the last, the Coniston Massacre on Warlpiri lands and peoples, from August to October 1928 (University of Newcastle, 2017). Deaths through epidemics, starvation, and massacres have long-lasting impacts, including the passing down of traumatic memories, both consciously and unconsciously, the stories told to and held deeply within many generations (Atkinson, 2002). As colonial law was implemented, a pyramid of structural power controls also resulted in loss of sovereignty and territory, cultural genocide, and enforced assimilation through extensive policies of forced child removals (Human Rights and Equal Opportunity Commission, 1997).

It is additionally important to link the colonisation of Australia with other colonisations internationally, for example, on the North and South American continents, Hawaii, Africa, and in New Zealand, providing evidence that this is not just an Australian story, and that symptoms are history across the world. Salzman and Halloran describe the destruction of cultural worldviews which sustained Indigenous peoples for millennia, a collective experience across diverse cultures and peoples: the Yup'ik of Alaska, the Navajos and Athabaskan Indians of North America, Hawaiian Natives, Maori in New Zealand, and Aboriginal Australians, all having experienced similar physical, social, behavioural, and psychological symptoms, including high rates of suicide, alcoholism, accidental and intentional deaths, and layers of grief, loss and trauma (Salzman and Halloran, 2004).

Harold Napoleon wrote "Yuuyarag – the Way of the Human Being" at a time when he was in Fairbanks prison. He writes of the time before westerners arrived, when "The Yup'ik people were alone in their riverine and the Bering Sea homeland, they and the spirit beings that made things the way they were … they were free and secure" (Napoleon, 1991: p.4). They were ruled by the customs, traditions, and spiritual beliefs that provided meaning to their lives and were shaped by these and the environment in which they lived. They knew this world as a spirit entity, complete and old. Napoleon believes that the all-encompassing experiences of the "Great Death in Alaska" on those who survived, as whole communities died through influenza introduced by missionaries, explains in large part the persona of the children, grandchildren, and great-grandchildren who were alive when he wrote his paper. He says for the 13 years he worked at his job as Executive Director of the Association of Village Council Presidents, struggling to provide services and programs to his people, "Something in my soul, in my background, in my family's and village's history, had preconditioned me to internalise and personalise every perceived defeat" (Napoleon, 1991: p.2). He began to drink as he went to meetings in Anchorage, Juneau, and Washington. Here, he says, everybody drank, and he soon became alcoholic. He says his world ended in June 1984 with the death of his son, due directly to his alcoholism. His years in gaol have been spent grieving, not only for his son, "But for all the others who have died in this long night of our alcohol-induced suffering. I have also spent that time looking into my own soul and the souls of my fellow Native people" (Napoleon, 1991: p.3).

He believes his people, in trying to suppress, deny, or ignore the unbearable trauma, acted it out on those around them. The symptoms of this deeply buried historic trauma manifest when under the influence of alcohol or drugs. The pent-up anger, guilt, sorrow, frustration, and hopelessness explodes into violence on self and others. The sufferers and their families are then driven deeper into the cycle of guilt and blame, and further traumatic distress (Napoleon, 1991). He could have been writing about Australia.

Muid has called this historic trauma, "The collective emotional and psychological injury, in the life of an individual or of a community, both over the life span and across generations" (Muid, 2006: p.36). As a result, it needs to be understood that, for Aboriginal peoples, trauma is both individual and collective wounding at multiple levels. This collective trauma, this "soul wounding" (Duran et al., 1998), covers a range of symptoms: losing relationships to land and kin, substance misuse, violence, incarceration, suicide, physical illness, and premature death. In Alice Springs Prison, three generations of women, a grandmother, a mother, and a granddaughter were all serving sentences at the same time. Another on remand was the third generation to be removed as a child and placed into state care. Her mother on release from state care at 16 soon fell pregnant and gave birth to the young woman. She was then raised by her grandmother, who died when she was 13. This triggered the need to find her mother, but during that search she re-experienced domestic violence at the hands of inappropriate partners; she was placed on remand for refusing to give evidence against her assailant.

Documentation of the Coniston Massacre in Australia shows how experiences of trauma across colonial history are layered and can be mapped in the history of a country. Levine writes of this through the work of the cultural anthropologist, Merida Blanco, who studied the effects of colonial domination in South America (Levine, 2007). Blanco believed that damage occurred over five generations. In the first generation, the men are killed, imprisoned, or enslaved; in the second, many of the men turn to alcohol and drugs as their cultural identity is damaged, and their self-worth eroded; in the third, social trauma and lost connection to earlier generations results in increasing spousal assault and other forms of domestic violence; in the fourth, abuse moves from spousal assault to child abuse; and finally, in the fifth generation, the cycle repeats itself, as trauma begets violence begets trauma. Prisons and the increasing incarceration rates are evidence of symptom as history, of the colonial construct which continues in the countries, on the lands and in the minds and the hearts of peoples who were colonised. Until work can be done to reverse these many injustices, embedded trauma will not be healed.

Kreig (2009) outlines the signs and symptoms of trauma in Aboriginal Australian populations that must be considered in any health, education, and legal responses to recovery: a deep mistrust of self and others, even within the family; self-directed violence, including suicide and risk-taking behaviour; substance misuse; unremitting grief, shame, and humiliation; intergenerational conflict; violence against women; role diffusion, including sexual abuse and boundary violations; cultural genocide; and loss of traditional values. Such symptoms can only be understood within the context of Aboriginal experiences of colonial history.

These are the psychological consequences of a generation now trapped in a choice between different forms of failure. The reality is clear from the statistics. Incarceration rates are not just a sign of the oppressor, but a breakdown in the social structures of the oppressed. The extraordinary rates of Aboriginal child removals are not just the toxicity of national child removal policies, but also reflect a breakdown in family systems, reinforced by the institutions and policies of the state. A fundamental problem is that the complexity and depth of the collective trauma has been profoundly underestimated. Escalating child removals, suicides, and imprisonment indicate the wounding of whole social groups, subject to overt and covert physical, structural, and psychosocial abuse and violence, over long periods, the wounding being multi-layered, complex, and comprehensive.

A vignette – "Billy" and "Betty" – behaviour is language

The behaviours of Aboriginal children Billy, seven, and Betty, eight, are reflective of children with transgenerational and developmental trauma, where symptom is history, and behaviour needs to be viewed as a type of communicative language. Billy and Betty demonstrate how children process differently the violence they witness and experience on a regular basis.

Billy and Betty live in a situation where their father, who has an acquired brain injury from a prison fight, regularly attacks their mother with a knife. She has been stabbed numerous times, the police have been called, and the mother has been taken to hospital in ambulances repeatedly; police and ambulance sirens trigger reactive behaviour in both children. They express their traumatic distress in difference ways, however; Billy is seen as deserving of punishment, a "flogging" at home or an expulsion from school, while Betty's behaviour is seen as not only acceptable but, in fact, praiseworthy.

Billy has a fixation on knives and he is always scheming to get his hand on a knife, with which he will try to attack others. During these episodes, his eyes will roll back for a second, and then, with an intense glazed look on his face, he will aggressively attack, with no memory of what he has done afterwards; he dissociates. Billy re-creates the behaviour of his father, who has held the family captive with knife attacks on Billy's mother, each time with respite only when he returns to prison. While his father is away, Billy is safer with his fixation on knives, and he involves himself in repetitive traumatic "play" or traumatic "acting out". These difficulties will remain unresolved until he receives therapeutic help, to resolve the drive to repeat the traumatic imprints of his father's behaviour on his mother. Behaviour is language, as he tells us that his world is very unsafe.

His sister has a different language in trying to make sense of the world in which she lives. She is obsessed with funerals and her play is about funerals. She knows the words of all the hymns sung at funerals. She will hitchhike to any funeral she hears about, sometimes 100 kilometres away from where she lives, without the knowledge of her mother or the school. She participates respectfully in all the funeral protocols. In free play, she will have as many of the other children as she can "play funerals", including making coffins and running a full funeral ceremony, which she will conduct. Betty also visits cemeteries where she washes the plastic flowers and cleans up around the graves. Aboriginal Elders and non-Aboriginal people speak about her as a respectful, good child. She is however also involved in repetitive play, trying to make sense of death and dying, as she sees her mother "dying" when the ambulance comes, yet again.

There is within both their stories intense fear and anxiety, expressed in different ways. When there is trauma in a child's life, the survival part of the brain is activated. This part of the brain is driven by fear, and it overrides the learning brain, interfering with usual development. As a result, the child focusses on danger and survival, rather than on trust and learning. Billy creates danger that he can control by repetitive play. Betty seeks resolution of what for her is inevitable, death and funerals.

Complex or developmental trauma results in fractured attachments in which the world feels unsafe, unreliable, and unpredictable. Physical and psychological development is arrested. Emotional regulation becomes unbalanced, here with Billy's aggression and Betty's focus on death and dying. Both children have difficulties in understanding what happens to them, and how it has come about; they lack a continuous and predictable sense of self, both also feeling shame and guilt, while also trying to make sense of the world in which they live. While they are Aboriginal children with a traumatic memory that is embedded in their country, they are responding as human beings to trauma that is generational and ongoing.

Trauma-integrated service systems

In response to the specific needs of Billy, Betty, and their mother, a trauma-integrated services approach was instigated. While the police, ambulance, and hospital provided immediate emergency responses to the injuries of the mother, this family needed other integrated services.

Attempts were made to keep both children at school, in non-judgmental care, while trying to understand how what was happening in the home was intruding into the school environment. Billy's behaviour was seen to be much more problematic, however teachers also held concern for Betty's increasing absences. The mother began to regularly visit the school. During those visits, when she acknowledged that she was indeed "flogging" Billy for his bad behaviour, the principal took the opportunity to explain why flogging would not help, because Billy had no memory of his behaviour.

The school also worked to get a doctor to visit in order to assess the health needs of the children, and both parents were invited to be part of these assessments. The father did not attend. The doctor, an Aboriginal woman who had been alerted to the situation, asked the mother an important question, "Do you think he [the husband] deserves you?". The response being, "No, but I feel sorry for him". The doctor also asked, "Do you think your children are harmed by seeing you stabbed?". These two questions, and the discussion that followed, resulted in the mother overriding her previously held loyalty to her husband so that she could start to put the needs of her children first.

Child Protection had received numerous mandatory reports about the children, and finally they were asked to act. The child protection worker invited the mother to work with her to find a place where she and her children would be safe. This meant looking for supported accommodation in another location and a house became available that was close to a school, shops, and public transport. The worker then helped to get the family settled into the new location and the previous school worked with the new school to enable a safe transfer of the children. Counselling services were also put into place, and the mother was provided support from her local Aboriginal community service.

Conclusion

The family presented in this vignette eventually did well. Most families do not. Trauma-informed care and practice depends on an integration of service systems, so that children, families, and social groups receive the trauma-specific services that they need.

The first thing that is required is a nuanced understanding of both developmental and transgenerational trauma in Aboriginal populations. "Symptom as history" requires acknowledging and understanding the generational impacts of trauma across history: epidemics, starvations, massacres, which came with the prison hulks; enforced institutional discrimination and racism; government policies and practices of economic disadvantage and social exclusion; and the extensive historical and continuing child removals. The symptoms are clear with multiple life stressors resulting in significant physical health issues, mental and emotional health issues, substance misuse, and family breakdown with violence and abuse on partners and children. Multiple layers of grief, loss and trauma seep through the souls and cultures of people so affected.

It is also vitally important to recognise that behaviour is a language; it speaks louder than words. Children with grief, loss and unresolved trauma act out their pain in and out of schools as they try to make sense of the worlds in which they live. They may be suspended or expelled from school. These are the first steps toward detention or prison. Yet solutions are clear: when the women in prison constructed their "loss history" maps it allowed them an important life review, and an understanding of cause and effect influencing the actions that took them to prison. Choices were made to move away from relationships which triggered their "offending" behaviour. In the situation of Billy and Betty, the mother made choices to relocate, moving beyond the violence affecting her and her children. Organisational support for her moved beyond a trauma-informed approach into a trauma-integrated service systems response.

What is required is culturally competent workers, building relationships of care and support, enhancing self-sufficiency and self-governance, helping heal family and community relationships (Atkinson, 2013). The work undertaken with the women of the Alice Springs Prison is a powerful example of what can be done. The response to the needs of the mother of Billy and Betty demonstrates clear positive outcomes, for the woman, in support of her needs to be free from violence and her choice to protect her children from further traumatic injury.

References

Atkinson J (2002) *Trauma Trails: Recreating Song lines. The Transgenerational Effects of Trauma in Aboriginal Australia.* Melbourne, Australia: Spinifex Press.

Atkinson J (2013) *Trauma-informed services and trauma-specific care for Indigenous Australian children. Resource sheet no. 21.* Produced for the Closing the Gap Clearinghouse. Canberra, Australia: Australian Institute of Health and Welfare, and Melbourne, Australia: Australian Institute of Family Studies.

Atkinson J (2015–2018) *Kunga Stopping Violence Reports – Multiple.* Alice Springs, Australia: Central Australian Aboriginal Legal Aid Service (unpublished).

Australian Bureau of Statistics (2010) *Suicide in Australia.* Canberra, Australia: Commonwealth of Australia.

Australian Bureau of Statistics (2016) *Prisoners in Australia.* Canberra, Australia: Commonwealth of Australia.

Dudgeon P, Milroy H and Walker R (2014) *Working Together: Aboriginal and Torres Strait Islander Mental Health and Wellbeing Principles and Practices, Second Edition.* Canberra, Australia: Commonwealth of Australia.

Duran E, Duran B, Brave Heart MYB, et al. (1998) Healing the American Indian soul wound. In: Danieli Y (ed) *International Handbook of Multigenerational Legacies of Trauma.* New York, NY: Plenum Press, pp.341–354.

Elder B (2003) *Blood on the Wattle.* Sydney, Australia: New Holland Publishers.

Felitti VJ, Anda RF, Nordenberg D, et al. (1998) Relationship of childhood abuse and household dysfunction to many of the leading causes of death in adults. *American Journal of Preventive Medicine* 14(4): 245–258.

Human Rights and Equal Opportunity Commission (1997) *Report of the National Inquiry into the Separation of Aboriginal and Torres Strait Islander Children from their Families.* Canberra, Australia: Commonwealth of Australia.

Kerr J (2016) *A Descriptive Analysis of the Characteristics, Seriousness and Frequency of Aboriginal Intimate Partner Violence in the Northern Territory, Australia: A Strategy for Targeting High Harm Cases*. Unpublished Masters' Thesis. Oxford, UK: Oxford University.

Kreig A (2009) The experience of collective trauma in Australian Indigenous communities. *Australasian Psychiatry* 17 Suppl 1: S28–S32.

Levine P (2007) *Trauma Through a Child's Eyes*. Berkeley, CA: North Atlantic Books.

Muid O (2006) *Then I Lost my Spirit: Analytical Essay on Transgenerational Theory and its Application to Oppressed People of Colour Nations*. Ann Arbor, MI: UMI dissertation Service ProQuest.

Napoleon H (1991) *Yuuyaraq: The Way of the Human Being*. Fairbanks, AK: Center for Cross-Cultural Studies.

Northern Territory of Australia, Department of the Attorney General and Justice (2017) *Northern Territory Correctional Services and Youth Justice Annual Statistics 2015–2016*. Darwin, Australia: Criminal Justice Research and Statistics Unit.

Perry B (2004) *Maltreatment and the Developing Child: How Early Childhood Experience Shapes Child and Culture*. Margaret McCain Lecture Series, Inaugural Lecture, London Convention Centre. London, UK.

Salzman M and Halloran MJ (2004) Culture, meaning, self-esteem and the re-construction of the cultural worldview. In: Greenberg J, Koole SL and Pyszczynski T (eds) *Handbook of Experimental Existential Psychology, First Edition*. New York, NY: Guilford Press, pp.231–246.

University of Newcastle (2017) *Colonial Frontier Massacres 1788–1872*. Available at: c21ch.newcastle.edu.au/colonialmassacres/contact.php.

Van de Kolk BA (2007) The developmental impact of childhood trauma. In: Kirmayer LJ, Lemelson R and Barad M (eds) *Understanding Trauma: Integrating Biological, Clinical and Cultural Perspectives*. New York, NY: Cambridge University Press, pp.224–241.

Zubrick SR, Shepherd CCJ, Dudgeon P, et al. (2014) Social determinants of social and emotional wellbeing. In: Dudgeon P, Milroy H and Walker R (eds) *Working Together: Aboriginal and Torres Strait Islander Mental Health and Wellbeing Principles and Practice, Second Edition*. Canberra, Australia: Commonwealth of Australia, pp.93–112.

11 The mental health of refugees and people who seek asylum

Derrick Silove and Sarah Mares

Introduction

The 1951 United Nations Convention relating to the Status of Refugees defined a refugee as a person holding a well-founded fear of persecution based on race, religion, nationality, membership of a social group or adherence to a political opinion (United Nations High Commissioner for Refugees, 2010). The 145 signatory countries to the Convention and the later Protocol in 1967 committed themselves to provide refugees with physical and legal protection, a path to citizenship, and access to the same civil, political, economic, social, and cultural rights enjoyed by native nationals. Important additional protections highlighted in the Convention are the right to cross national borders to seek refuge, an act that should be regarded as a right and not a crime, and freedom from forced repatriation to places of danger, the non-refoulement provision. Although Australia has not adopted a bill of rights, the nation is signatory to a number of international instruments that are directly relevant to the treatment of persons displaced by persecution, including the United Nations Declaration of Human Rights, the International Covenant on Civil and Political Rights, the Convention against Torture and Other Cruel, Inhuman and Degrading Treatment or Punishment, and the Convention on the Rights of the Child.

The modern term, asylum seeker, refers to those persons seeking protection from persecution who arrive in the host country without a refugee visa. For the past 30 years, Australia has implemented a two-tier policy that distinguishes between refugees and asylum seekers. Refugees screened and accepted overseas are admitted under the off-shore program according to annual quotas. These people receive a progressive program of resettlement support including access to a well-developed network of torture and trauma rehabilitation services and are entitled to future citizenship. In contrast, asylum seekers, including adults and children arriving by boat or air without formal refugee status, are subjected to a range of restrictions, including indefinite detention.

Australian psychiatrists and psychologists have taken a lead role in assisting both refugees and asylum seekers. They have helped develop a network of torture and trauma services around the country, providing psychotherapy and rehabilitation to refugee survivors of abuse and trauma. In relation to asylum seekers, they have taken an active role in clinical services, research, awareness raising, and the provision of expert reports.

Asylum seekers and refugees respond primarily to "push factors", fleeing conditions of persecution, victimisation, and political violence, in contrast to regular migrants who are attracted to the new country by "pull" factors such as employment opportunities or family reunion. Many displaced persons have taken courageous stands against oppression in their homelands, bringing with them values of humanism and social commitment that enrich the fabric of Australian society. In addition, asylum seekers and refugees come from a wide range of backgrounds and traditions, their presence contributing to the diversity of Australia's multicultural society. Some have however experienced extensive traumas and losses that have lasting psychological impacts and require access to specialist trauma-informed mental health services.

Historical perspective

Prior to the 1951 Refugee Convention, the distinction between migrants and refugees was less clear-cut, both in Australia and internationally. As a consequence, many people arriving in Australia as migrants in the past would today be regarded as refugees or asylum seekers. The first European settlement in Australia involved the forced removal from their homeland of people often convicted of minor transgressions. After enduring dangerous sea journeys to a remote and unknown land, they were held in conditions of confinement and deprivation, denied basic human rights, and often subjected to harsh punishment.

The European invasion also had profound impacts on Aboriginal communities, resulting in conflict, mass loss of life, and forced displacement of Indigenous people from their traditional lands and country, the source of their identity, and ancient culture. Lack of resolution of the collective trauma of Australia's Indigenous people continues to leave its mark on society today (Dudgeon et al., 2010). However, the lessons that should have been learned from exclusionary policies imposed on Indigenous people have not been translated into those applied to modern day asylum seekers.

Over the course of European settlement, push factors have played an important role in several waves of migration to Australia. A combination of religious restrictions as well as political and economic pressures led German Lutherans to migrate to South Australia in the 1830s. Less than two decades later, the potato famine in Ireland led to the mass forced displacement of 30,000 people to Australia. During the same era, 50,000 West Pacific Islanders (Kanakas) were coerced by "blackbird" traders to settle in Northern Queensland where they worked under harsh conditions as indentured labourers. Later, large numbers of that community were forced to return to their islands, rupturing established families and ties in Australia.

During the mid-century gold rush, Chinese immigrants were subjected to racist-inspired riots, resulting in expulsions, injuries, and deaths. The underlying culture of xenophobia continued through to Federation in 1901, with one of the first acts of the new national parliament being the adoption of the Immigration Restriction Act that prohibited the movement of so-called non-whites into Australia. This culture of ethnocentrism set the stage for what became known as the White Australia Policy which restricted settlement to European migrants until the 1970s.

In the aftermath of World War II, Australia contributed to the International Displaced Persons Scheme by resettling more than 170,000 Europeans, including 17,000 Jewish survivors of the Nazi Holocaust. From the late 1940s onwards, the slogan "populate or perish" gained wide acceptance, opening the doors to large numbers of migrants from the UK, Ireland, and Europe, including people who would today be regarded as refugees. In the 1970s, the Whitlam Labour government finally abandoned the White Australia Policy, paving the way for the acceptance of more than 200,000 Southeast Asian people displaced by the Indochinese wars, the largest Australian intake of a refugee population from a non-European region of the world. The term "boat people" first entered the national lexicon during this time (Phillips and Spinks, 2013). The Asian refugees were afforded a model resettlement program including access to language classes, income and work support, education, health, and housing. A population study, 20 years after the first settlers arrived, indicated that the majority of Vietnamese had recovered from the traumatic stress reactions they had experienced prior to and soon after migration (Steel et al., 2002).

Displaced people – Australia's response in the context of a global crisis

To locate Australia's refugee and asylum seeker policy within a wider perspective, it is important to examine trends in the flow of displaced persons at a global level. In 1992, when Australia first implemented a policy of mandatory detention of boat people, 23 million people were listed as being "of concern", that is, probable refugees, by the United Nations (United Nations High Commissioner for Refugees, 1993). This number has steadily escalated, with steep increases occurring around the turn of the century and again in 2012. The global refugee population now stands at a record 65.6 million people (United Nations High Commissioner for Refugees, 2017), the increase being an outcome of protracted conflicts in the Middle East, the Greater Horn of Africa, and regions of Asia. The most recent upheaval has involved a million Rohingya fleeing ethnic cleansing in Burma.

The geographical distribution of refugees is important in judging the contribution made by Australia to addressing this global crisis. More than four-fifths of refugees are either internally displaced within their own countries or have crossed borders to neighbouring countries. Almost all of the major host nations are low or middle-income countries in the developing world. Of the top ten recipient countries, together hosting 60 per cent of recently displaced populations, only one, Germany, is an economically developed nation.

Australia's off-shore or annual quota program admits between 12,000 and 20,000 refugees who have had permanent visas granted overseas, representing far less than 1 per cent of the total world refugee population (Phillips and Spinks, 2013). Periodically, the number is increased by special programs, for example, supporting family reunion, women at risk, and, more recently, Syrian refugees. As previously indicated, permanently resettled refugees receive a range of resettlement and social services as well as eligibility for full Australian citizenship after a period of residency.

In the late 1980s, the Australian Government introduced a major shift in refugee policy. From then onwards, asylum seekers arriving without established refugee visas were subject to stringent policies of deterrence and restriction. People arriving by air have generally been granted temporary visas to reside in the community, although with restrictions in access to income support, education, and health services. Since 1992, however, all people arriving by boat have been subject to mandatory, indefinite detention. Asylum seekers can now be detained until the government makes a final determination to either grant refugee status and release them into the community, or to force repatriation or deportation elsewhere, a process that may take many years. The onus is placed on the individual to prove refugee status, which is often difficult without corroborating evidence. Asylum seekers and those found to be refugees may also be held indefinitely if they are deemed a risk to the community. Prior to 1992, detention centres only held people who had overstayed their visas, foreign nationals who had committed crimes, and others who were deemed not to qualify to remain in Australia.

The new policy of deterrence applied to asylum seekers required a substantial and costly expansion of the network of detention centres which were extended to off-shore facilities, for example, Christmas Island, an Australian territory situated close to Indonesia. A turning point came in late 2001 when a Norwegian ship, the MV Tampa, was refused entry to Australian waters after rescuing more than 400 mainly Afghan asylum seekers from a sinking boat off Christmas Island. The so-called "Pacific Solution" was then introduced, and after a brief repeal of the provision in 2008, was re-introduced and made more stringent in 2013. Current provisions mandate that all boat people are transported to detention centres located in neighbouring island countries of Nauru and Papua New Guinea (Manus Island). These persons are prohibited from ever resettling in Australia. Yet, the number of boat people who have arrived in Australia is modest, approximately 70,000 since 1976, when judged in the context of the world refugee population. It is clear, therefore, that at a global level, low-income countries with the least resources and capacity to do so carry by far the major responsibility for caring for refugees and asylum seekers. At the same time, countries with high levels of resources, such as Australia, have imposed increasingly harsh restrictions on the relatively small number of asylum seekers reaching their borders, and in the process are expending a large quantum of funds that could be used to support the major recipient countries or to offer increased resettlement and support services to existing displaced populations within Australia.

The global mental health challenge

Over the past 30 years, a growing body of epidemiological studies has documented the mental health status of refugees from diverse cultural backgrounds (Porter and Haslam, 2005; Steel et al., 2009). Rates of mental disorder vary across studies, but most estimates of the prevalence of Posttraumatic Stress Disorder (PTSD) and Depression range from 15 to 30 per cent (Steel et al., 2009). A conservative figure of 15 per cent for PTSD translates into a population of approximately 10 million refugees and asylum seekers worldwide with this diagnosis. Refugees often experience mental health problems other than PTSD and Depression, including complicated grief, anxiety, somatic symptoms, and anger (Silove and Bryant, 2006). Moreover, campaigns of terror, which many refugees have experienced, use torture, rape, and abduction of children to intimidate and subjugate the entire population and undermine political opposition at a society-wide level. As a result, the traumas of persecution and mass violence tend to have a multiplier effect, extending beyond the individual survivor to the family and the wider community.

High rates of distress have also been identified amongst refugee children who make up more than 50 per cent of displaced populations, and these problems are particularly marked in those seeking asylum (Fazel and Stein, 2002; Weine et al., 2004; Fazel et al., 2012; Bryant et al., 2018). In assessing children's mental health, attention needs to be given to age and developmental stage, coping ability, access to an effective caregiver, usually the parent, and the availability of wider family and social supports (Lustig et al., 2004; Lau et al., 2018). Unaccompanied minors are particularly vulnerable although some show remarkable resilience and resourcefulness (Hodes et al., 2008; Bronstein et al., 2013; Jakobsen, 2018; Norredam et al., 2018).

Conceptual issues

Several conceptual models have been proposed to encompass the complex psychosocial responses of refugees exposed to a sequence of disruptions, traumas, and stressors through the course of their displacement experiences. Although concepts of trauma and PTSD are of central interest, some critics have cautioned against the imposition of these western concepts onto culturally distinct communities that hold their own views of suffering and healing (Summersfield, 1999). The challenge is to achieve a balance between focusing on trauma-related mental disorder in the individual and promoting community resilience at a wider level (Betancourt, 2011).

The "Adaptation and Development After Persecution" (ADAPT) model attempts to reconcile the psychosocial and clinical perspectives by focusing on the support systems that are eroded during the sequential phases of forced displacement, which includes exposure to conflict and trauma, uprooting, flight, temporary refuge in deprived situations (refugee camps, detention centres), and, for some, final resettlement (Silove, 2013). The five key psychosocial systems that are disrupted include those that support security and safety; interpersonal bonds and networks; justice; roles and identities; and the capacity to pursue activities that confer existential meaning, including in the domains of culture, religion, spirituality, ideology, and political and social beliefs and values. From a systems perspective, a cascade of influences impact on these psychosocial pillars and hence on the capacity for refugees to adapt. At the most general level, geopolitical factors such as international refugee policy, the role of the United Nations, and contemporary national politics interact to exert a major influence on the conditions that impact on refugee mental health and well-being. At the local level, important influences include levels of xenophobia in the community, internecine conflict within refugee populations, the level of family and kinship support, and the availability of helping agencies and services. A key principle promoted by the ADAPT model is that the effective repair of the five core psychosocial pillars is essential to enable refugees to overcome trauma-related mental distress; the more successful the recovery program, the less the need for individual interventions such as psychotherapy. Nevertheless, there will always be a minority of people whose traumatic stress reactions are so severe and disabling that they are not able to take advantage of social opportunities for self-directed recovery without individual interventions. In general, however, repair of the social environment is the best remedy for most refugees and clinical services for traumatic stress should focus on the minority with the greatest needs (Silove, 2005; Kronick, 2018).

Adaptation and Development After Persecution (ADAPT) framework

Psychosocial systems undermined in the process of seeking asylum include:

- those that support safety and security,
- interpersonal bonds and networks,
- justice,
- roles and identities,
- existential meaning, including the right to pursue cultural, religious, spiritual, ideological, political, and social beliefs and values.

Australia's approach to trauma-affected refugees

Australian psychiatrists and psychologists have long worked with survivors of persecution, including Holocaust survivors, dissidents escaping Eastern Bloc countries during the cold war, and refugees exposed to torture. In the 1980s, a seminal report commissioned by the NSW state government identified widespread unmet mental health needs amongst refugees from a range of ethnic backgrounds (Reid and Strong, 1987). The impetus created led to the establishment of the state-wide refugee trauma and torture service, the NSW Service for the Treatment and Rehabilitation of Torture and Trauma Survivors (STARTTS), now one of the largest and most comprehensive agencies of its kind in the world. A network of similar services soon became established across Australia and New Zealand.

From the outset, services were grounded in a humanistic philosophy, adopting a comprehensive approach to care which paid attention to issues of culture, human rights, trauma and ongoing postmigration stresses, including acculturation and resettlement needs. Cultural issues extend beyond language to the modification of concepts such as trauma and PTSD to ensure they make sense within each relevant group. In most services, bicultural counsellors are employed who play an integral role in all aspects of the agency.

Clinical experience indicates that many trauma and torture survivors find it difficult to recount their trauma stories at the outset of therapy, requiring time to build trust in the therapist. The interaction itself is key to the healing process, the therapist spending time creating a relationship with the patient that reverses the abuse of power, erosion of dignity, and dehumanisation that are core to the torture experience. Individual psychotherapy and the judicious use of medications are implemented within a broader program of rehabilitation which may include referral for physical health issues, occupational therapy, social work, and intervention with families. In this way, a trauma-informed care model is embedded within a multidisciplinary and multimodal approach to interventions.

Services also play a major role at the community level, in advocacy, awareness raising, education, support for other agencies (schools, the police, ethnic community organisations), and advising on policy formulation. To ensure successful acculturation and resettlement, torture and trauma services liaise with a range of relevant agencies including migrant support services, English-language training, work preparedness, social services, education, medical and mental health services, as well as housing and legal assistance.

Research into the impact of Australia's asylum policy

Service providers encounter specific challenges in providing care for asylum seekers subject to restrictive policies in the community and particularly for those in detention. Early in the implementation of the policy of deterrence it became apparent to mental health professionals that many of the restrictions imposed on asylum seekers worsened their symptoms of PTSD, Depression, and other forms of mental distress, undermining any therapeutic efforts to assist this population.

Apart from restrictions on accessing services and material support, asylum seekers living in the community are denied direct contact with families overseas and are prohibited from ever achieving family reunion in Australia. Legal proceedings to test their refugee claims are often protracted, complicated, and difficult to understand, particularly for people whose memories are affected by severe traumatic stress reactions. During the process of pursuing refugee claims, asylum seekers are marginalised in the community and live in constant fear of forced repatriation. Some of the first studies focusing specifically on asylum seekers were conducted in Australia. These investigations confirmed that conditions of insecure residency and restrictions in access to services added to the effects of past trauma in generating severe and persisting symptoms of PTSD and Depression (Silove et al., 1997, 1998).

Asylum seekers held in detention are subject to prison-like conditions with limited access to the outside world, including to personal and legal supports. For some, conditions in detention trigger memories of trauma and torture in political prisons and other situations of previous confinement, thereby intensifying their posttraumatic stress reactions. Many inmates do not speak English, compounding their sense of isolation and disorientation.

Over the 30 years of implementation of the detention policy, there have been widely publicised episodes within immigration centres of violence, including riots, burning of facilities, conflict with guards, accounts of abuse and harsh treatment, and repeated acts of suicide, self-injurious behaviours, and hunger strikes (Silove et al., 2000). In the off-shore detention centres on Manus Island and Nauru, tensions with members of the Indigenous population have also been a source of inter-communal violence, rioting, injuries, and deaths. Detained children are routinely called by number, not by name, and many have witnessed protests, violence, and public acts of self-harm. Most detention facilities and not equipped to provide adequate facilities for schooling, play, or recreation (Mares, 2016a).

In spite of logistic and administrative obstacles, Australian psychiatrists and psychologists have taken a lead in documenting the impact of detention on asylum seekers (Silove et al., 1997; Steel et al., 2006). Without exception, available data indicate that adult and child detainees manifest high rates of mental disorder (Mares, 2016b). In general, the longer the period of detention, the greater the deterioration in mental health of both adult asylum seekers (Steel and Silove, 2001; Steel et al., 2006) and their children (Mares and Jureidini, 2004; Steel et al., 2004; Mares, 2016a). Within families, the extreme alienation, insecurity, and mental distress experienced by adults impacts on their capacity to provide adequate care and protection to their children (Mares et al., 2002; Mares and Zwi, 2015; Mares, 2016b). Recent analyses of data collected under the auspices of the Australian Government have confirmed these adverse social and mental health effects of detention (Young and Gordon, 2016).

Even years after release, asylum seekers continue to experience posttraumatic stress symptoms directly related to the detention experience (Steel et al., 2006). These people often report that traumatic memories of the detention experience such as witnessing public suicidal acts, exposure to riots, and other forms of violence are as distressing as pre-migration traumas related to war and persecution. The cost of the disability caused by detention extends to Australian society as a whole, given that by far the majority of asylum seekers held in immigration facilities are ultimately granted resettlement visas.

These research findings have been timely in providing crucial evidence for use by successive national commissions of inquiry into detention undertaken by the Australian Human Rights Commission (Human Rights and Equal Opportunity Commission, 2004; Australian Human Rights Commission, 2014). Both

Australian and international agencies such as the United Nations High Commissioner for Refugees have been highly critical of the policy, pointing out that conditions in detention violate a range of fundamental rights, including to dignity, privacy, freedom of association and movement, and access to adequate services (Human Rights and Equal Opportunity Commission, 2004; Australian Human Rights Commission, 2014; Gottesman, 2016; Mares, 2016b).

Recent events

A recent judicial ruling in Papua New Guinea found that the Manus Island detention centre was illegal, a turning point that led to the subsequent closure of the facility. This development provoked a humanitarian crisis in late 2017 when 600 asylum seekers refused to leave the centre, preferring to live without water, food, and services than to be resettled within the island community, a protest motivated by fear of further conflict with the Indigenous population. However, the closure has generated some impetus to arrange resettlement of detainees from Nauru in other countries. A small number have been resettled in the USA, but Australia has refused offers from New Zealand to accept others from this group. Legal action throughout 2018 triggered by a severe deterioration in the health of many children and adults on Nauru, and statements by leading medical bodies, resulted in most children and families being moved temporarily from Nauru to Australia. There remains no permanent settlement solution for most single men or children and families despite the majority being found to be refugees.

Professional concerns

Some practitioners, including psychiatrists, have resigned from their positions in detention health facilities, making public their strong concerns about the traumatic effects of prolonged detention, the safety and well-being of asylum seekers, including children, and the compromised health care standards within detention centres (Essex, 2016; Sanggaran et al., 2016). Recognising the challenges and ethical risks involved for professionals, the local professional body representing psychiatrists in Australia and New Zealand has developed guidelines for those working in detention (Royal Australian and New Zealand College of Psychiatrists, 2016, 2017). The guidelines make numerous recommendations including that asylum seekers should be granted conditional community release wherever possible, that detention should be only a measure of last resort and for the shortest period possible, and that certain groups, particularly children, pregnant women, and those with mental illness, should never be detained.

In 2015, the Australian Government introduced the Border Force Act which made it a criminal offence for health and other workers employed in detention centres to make public statements concerning their observations of conditions in these facilities (Dudley, 2016). This provision was only repealed after a High Court challenge led by medical professionals. Mounting evidence regarding the negative impact of detention on mental health appears to have influenced the public statements made by policy-makers. No more do they deny that detention is injurious to mental health, instead defending the policy as necessary to protect borders, curtail people smugglers, and prevent deaths at sea (Mares, 2016a).

A vignette – "OM"

A 28-year-old single man, "OM", fled a Middle Eastern country with his mother and female cousin after being subjected to repeated harassment, discrimination, and vilification because of his family's religious beliefs. OM had been targeted by vigilante groups who repeatedly apprehended him, humiliated him, and, on one occasion, subjected him to torture in a warehouse, the abuse only ending when he promised to give up his religion.

With minimal resources, the family passed through various countries, being repeatedly harassed by immigration officials and exploited by people smugglers. Eventually, they arrived by boat in Australia in the hope of joining the small group of resettled compatriots who shared their religious faith. The family group was held in several detention centres, including at an off-shore facility. In a riot at that centre, OM's cousin was raped repeatedly and sustained severe injuries. Ultimately, after extensive advocacy, she was transferred for medical care to mainland Australia, accompanied by OM and his mother, who were both still held in detention. Later, the mother and cousin were released into community detention because of the latter's deteriorating mental health, leaving OM on his own in the detention centre.

After six years in detention, OM embarked on several hunger strikes, nearly dying on the last occasion. When he was interviewed by a psychiatrist, he was found to show symptoms of severe PTSD, experiencing intrusive memories of past trauma in his homeland, and in detention, high levels of arousal, sleeplessness, poor concentration, and avoidance and withdrawal. He indicated that he had lost all faith in the authorities and, although he wished to live, would rather die than remain in detention. He expressed anger and disbelief that a civilised country such as Australia could treat him and his family in this way.

Conclusions

Australia exemplifies some of the best and the worst models of reception and care for people displaced by mass violence and persecution. The off-shore program provides comprehensive support for refugees selected for permanent residency prior to arrival, and research has indicated the success of this approach. Services for torture and trauma survivors established throughout Australia have led the world in providing comprehensive programs of care including psychotherapy, pharmacotherapy, and a range of rehabilitation and community-focused programs.

In contrast, the steadfast and harsh policy of deterrence applied to asylum seekers has impacted adversely on the mental health of persons fleeing persecution, damaging Australia's reputation as a humanistic society that welcomes refugees within its midst. The policy is at odds with a trauma-informed model of care that has been adopted throughout Australia in dealing with people exposed to violence. Instead, extensive funds have been expended on border security arrangements and on building and managing large detention centres in Australia and in the region, the sole purpose being to deter a relatively small number of vulnerable people from seeking protection. These resources could be better used to assist in peace-building programs aimed at preventing large flows of refugees, supporting developing nations who take the greatest responsibility for hosting refugees, or creating supportive arrangements to accept more asylum seekers and refugees within Australia.

In the past 30 years, mental health workers and their professional organisations have played major roles in awareness raising, advocacy, research, service provision, development, and training aimed at mitigating the adverse mental health effects of the ongoing asylum policy. In so doing, professionals have confronted difficult ethical dilemmas, for example, in deciding whether or not to work in detention centres given the risk of inadvertent collusion with a system that has been shown to cause mental distress amongst inmates.

Ultimately, however, the responsibility for providing humane care for displaced people reaching our shores rests with the Australian society as a whole. Our society does not appear to have learned from the lessons of the past, particularly in relation to the devastating effects of policies of exclusion, displacement, and dispossession applied to our own Indigenous population. Confronting that history may act as a restraint on mainstream Australian society from condoning the use of harsh methods to deter asylum seekers in the misguided belief that such measures are necessary to safeguard the sovereignty of our nation.

References

Australian Human Rights Commission (2014) *The Forgotten Children: National Inquiry into Children in Immigration Detention*. Sydney, Australia: Australian Human Rights Commission.

Betancourt TS (2011) Attending to the mental health of war-affected children: The need for longitudinal and developmental research perspectives. *Journal of the American Academy of Child and Adolescent Psychiatry* 50: 323–325.

Bronstein I, Montgomery P and Ott E (2013) Emotional and behavioural problems amongst Afghan unaccompanied asylum-seeking children: Results from a large-scale cross-sectional study. *European Child and Adolescent Psychiatry* 22: 285–294.

Bryant RA, Edwards B, Creamer M, et al. (2018) The effect of post-traumatic stress disorder on refugees' parenting and their children's mental health: a cohort study. *The Lancet Public Health* 3: e249–e258.

Dudgeon P, Wright M, Paradies Y, et al. (2010) The social, cultural and historical contexts of Aboriginal and Torres Strait Islander Australians. In: Purdie N, Dudgeon P and Walker R (eds) *Working Together: Aboriginal and Torres Strait Islander Mental Health and Wellbeing Principles and Practice, First Edition*. Canberra, Australia: Australian Government Department of Health and Ageing, pp.25–42.

Dudley M (2016) Helping professionals and Border Force secrecy: Effective asylum-seeker healthcare requires independence from callous policies. *Australasian Psychiatry* 24: 15–18.

Essex R (2016) Healthcare and clinical ethics in Australian offshore immigration detention. *The International Journal of Human Rights* 20: 1039–1053.

Fazel M and Stein A (2002) The mental health of refugee children. *Archives of Disease in Childhood* 87: 366–370.

Fazel M, Reed RV, Panter-Brick C, et al. (2012) Mental health of displaced and refugee children resettled in high-income countries: Risk and protective factors. *The Lancet* 379: 266–282.

Gottesman I (2016) Refugee and migrant crisis: The deficient global response. *The Lancet* 388: 633–730.

Hodes M, Jagdev D, Chandra N, et al. (2008) Risk and resilience for psychological distress amongst unaccompanied asylum seeking adolescents. *Journal of Child Psychology and Psychiatry* 49: 723–732.

Human Rights and Equal Opportunity Commission (2004) *A Last Resort: National Enquiry into Children in Immigration Detention*. Sydney, Australia: Human Rights and Equal Opportunity Commission.

Jakobsen M (2018) *Mental health of unaccompanied refugee minors: A longitudinal study from arrival in Norway to outcome of the asylum procedure*. Dissertation presented to the Faculty of Medicine, University of Oslo. Oslo, Norway: University of Oslo.

Kronick R (2018) Mental health of refugees and asylum seekers: assessment and intervention. *The Canadian Journal of Psychiatry* 63(5): 290–296.

Lau W, Silove D, Edwards B, et al. (2018) Adjustment of refugee children and adolescents in Australia: outcomes from wave three of the Building a New Life in Australia study. *BMC Med* 16(1): 157. doi:10.1186/s12916-018-1124-5

Lustig SL, Kia-Keating M, Knight WG, et al. (2004) Review of child and adolescent refugee mental health. *Journal of the American Academy of Child and Adolescent Psychiatry* 43: 24–36.

Mares S (2016a) Fifteen years of detaining children who seek asylum in Australia – evidence and consequences. *Australasian Psychiatry* 24: 11–14.

Mares S (2016b) The mental health of children and parents detained on Christmas Island: Secondary analysis of an Australian Human Rights Commission data set. *Health and Human Rights Journal* 18(2): 219–232.

Mares S and Jureidini J (2004) Psychiatric assessment of children and families in immigration detention: Clinical, administrative and ethical issues. *Australian and New Zealand Journal of Public Health* 28: 520–526.

Mares S, Newman L, Dudley M, et al. (2002) Seeking refuge, losing hope: Parents and children in immigration detention. *Australasian Psychiatry* 10: 91–96.

Mares S and Zwi K (2015) Sadness and fear: The experiences of children and families in remote Australian immigration detention. *Journal of Paediatrics and Child Health* 51: 663–669.

Norredam M, Nellums L, Nielsen RS, et al. (2018) Incidence of psychiatric disorders among accompanied and unaccompanied asylum-seeking children in Denmark: a nation-wide register-based cohort study. *European Child and Adolescent Psychiatry* 27(4): 439–446.

Phillips J and Spinks H (2013) *Boat arrivals in Australia since 1976*. Canberra, Australia: Parliament of Australia. Available at: aph.gov.au/About_Parliament/Parliamentary_Departments/Parliamentary_Library/pubs/BN/2012–2013/BoatArrivals.

Porter M and Haslam N (2005) Pre-displacement and post-displacement factors associated with mental health of refugees and internally displaced persons: A meta-analysis. *Journal of the American Medical Association* 294: 602–612.

RANZCP (2016) *Guidance for Psychiatrists Working in Australian Immigration*. Available at: ranzcp.org/Files/Resources/College_Statements/Practice_Guidelines/PPG-12-Guidance-for-psychiatrists-working-in-Austr.aspx.

RANZCP (2017) *The Provision of Mental Health Services for Asylum Seekers*. Available at: ranzcp.org/Files/Resources/College_Statements/Position_Statements/ps46-pdf.aspx.

Reid J and Strong T (1987) *Torture and Trauma: The Health Care Needs of Refugee Victims in NSW. A Report to the Western Metropolitan Health Region of the NSW Department of Health*. Sydney, Australia: Cumberland College of Health Sciences.

Sanggaran J-P, Haire B and Zion D (2016) The health care consequences of Australian immigration policies. *PLoS Medicine* 13: e1001960.

Silove D (2005) The best immediate therapy for acute stress is social. *Bulletin of the World Health Organization* 83(1): 75–76.

Silove D (2013) The ADAPT model: A conceptual framework for mental health and psychosocial programming in post-conflict settings. *Intervention: International Journal of Mental Health, Psychosocial Work and Counselling in Areas of Armed Conflict* 11(3): 237–248.

Silove D, Sinnerbrink I, Field A, et al. (1997) Anxiety, depression and PTSD in asylum-seekers: Associations with pre-migration trauma and post-migration stressors. *The British Journal of Psychiatry* 170(4): 351–357.

Silove D, Steel Z, McGorry P, et al. (1998) Trauma exposure, postmigration stressors, and symptoms of anxiety, depression and post-traumatic stress in Tamil asylum-seekers: Comparison with refugees and immigrants. *Acta Psychiatrica Scandinavica* 97(3): 175–181.

Silove D, Steel Z and Watters C (2000) Policies of deterrence and the mental health of asylum seekers. *Journal of the American Medical Association* 284: 604–611.

Silove D and Bryant R (2006) Rapid assessments of mental health needs after disasters. *Journal of the American Medical Association* 296: 576–578.

Steel Z and Silove DM (2001) The mental health implications of detaining asylum seekers. *The Medical Journal of Australia* 175: 596–599.

Steel Z, Silove D, Phan T, et al. (2002) Long-term effect of psychological trauma on the mental health of Vietnamese refugees resettled in Australia: A population-based study. *The Lancet* 360: 1056–1062.

Steel Z, Momartin S, Bateman C, et al. (2004) Psychiatric status of asylum seeker families held for a protracted period in a remote detention centre in Australia. *Australian and New Zealand Journal of Public Health* 28: 527–536.

Steel Z, Silove D, Brooks R, et al. (2006) Impact of immigration detention and temporary protection on the mental health of refugees. *The British Journal of Psychiatry* 188: 58–64.

Steel Z, Chey T, Silove D, et al. (2009) Association of torture and other potentially traumatic events with mental health outcomes among populations exposed to mass conflict and displacement: A systematic review and meta-analysis. *Journal of the American Medical Association* 302(5): 537–549.

Summerfield D (1999) A critique of seven assumptions behind psychological trauma programs in war-affected areas. *Social Science and Medicine* 48(10): 1449–1462.

United Nations High Commissioner for Refugees (1993) *Populations of Concern 1992*. Available at: popstats.unhcr.org/en/overview.

United Nations High Commissioner for Refugees (2010) *Convention and Protocol Relating to the Status of Refugees*. Geneva, Switzerland: UNHCR.

United Nations High Commissioner for Refugees (2017) *Global Trends: Forced Displacement in 2016*. Available at: unhcr.org/globaltrends2016.

Weine S, Muzurovic N, Kulauzovic Y, et al. (2004) Family consequences of refugee trauma. *Family Process* 43: 147–160.

Young P and Gordon MS (2016) Mental Health screening in immigration detention: A fresh look at Australian Government data. *Australasian Psychiatry* 24: 19–22.

12 Humanising responses to people who have experienced sexual violence

Jackie Burke

Introduction

Humanising the responses provided by the helping professions to people who have experienced mental health difficulties can optimise recovery from a wide range of disorders. This chapter will focus on people who have experienced sexual violence and will articulate the importance of providing humanised responses to assist the recovery of those affected.

The term sexual violence can be understood to encompass all forms of non-consensual sexual activity including unwanted sexual touching, acts of indecency, indecent assault, childhood sexual assault or abuse, sexual assault, and rape. In the discussion of data, the terminology used by the original authors will be retained. Otherwise, the terms childhood sexual assault or sexual violence will be applied.

Sexual violence – history

In 1896, Sigmund Freud proposed that sexual violence was much more prevalent than generally accepted. Many of his female patients had told him of the incest that they had suffered, most frequently at the hands of their fathers, and Freud suggested that repressed memories of sexual assault in childhood were a necessary precondition for "Hysteria", the predominant female neurosis of the time (Masson, 1998). What has since become known as the "Seduction Theory" may well have been the Western world's first realisation that sexual assaults against children occurred not only frequently, but that they were damaging. Freud recanted his theory within a year, instead publishing work hypothesising that children sexually idealise their opposite sex parent and manufacture false memories of sexual encounters with parents during childhood (Masson, 1998). There has been significant debate on the topic ever since, both regarding whether Freud believed his revised theory involving the "Oedipus complex", or whether he remained convinced about the prevalence of childhood sexual assault. There has also been debate about the reasons for his recanting, but it seems likely that the bourgeois social climate of Vienna at the time contributed significantly.

The impact of Freud's recanting was significant and enduring (Herman, 1992). Dominant social notions that sexual violence was a rare and relatively harmless phenomenon remained for many decades. Henry Wigmore, for example, argued in 1934 that women and children were essentially predisposed to bring allegations of sexual abuse against good men (cited in Eastwood et al., 2006), and it was not until the 1970s that ideas about sexual violence began to change. When feminist scholars deconstructed men's violence against women, they, like Freud, noted the often severe psychological and social impacts of sexual violence (Burgess and Holmstrom, 1974; Brownmiller, 1975). Such scholarly investigations of sexual violence, occurring at a time of rising feminist thinking, challenged the dominant beliefs about sexual violence. The prevalence and impact of sexual violence became visible, and it became possible to conceptualise recovery from such events. At around the same time, increasing recognition of the severe ill effects of war in returned Vietnam veterans led to a growing understanding of the mental health impacts of trauma, and resulted in the inclusion of the diagnosis of Posttraumatic Stress Disorder (PTSD) in the Diagnostic and Statistical Manual of Mental Disorders, the DSM (American Psychiatric Association, 1980). Today it is understood that sexual violence is one of the events most likely to result in PTSD (Kessler et al., 1995).

Prevalence of sexual violence

Measuring the prevalence of childhood sexual assault is challenging. Australia currently has no systematised national approach to the measurement of either the prevalence or the incidence of this crime. Given knowledge about under-reporting (Roesler and McKenzie, 1994; O'Leary and Barber, 2008), differing definitions of what constitutes abuse, and the practical and ethical challenges of measuring this phenomenon, existing prevalence estimates are imprecise. The Australian Institute of Family Studies recently reviewed data on the prevalence of childhood sexual abuse and concluded that boys experience penetrative sexual assault at rates of 1.4 to 7.5 per cent, and non-penetrative sexual assault at rates of 5.2 to 12 per cent, whereas girls experience penetrative sexual assault at rates of 4 to 12 per cent, and non-penetrative assaults at 14 to 26.8 per cent (Australian Institute of Family Studies, 2017).

Australia's largest national survey of personal safety is administered every four years, producing the nation's most reliable estimates of the prevalence of sexual assault experienced by adults. Analysis of the data from the most recent administration of this survey revealed that, since the age of 15 years, 1.5 million women in Australia have experienced sexual assault, and a total of 87,800 women reported experiencing a sexual assault in the year prior to the survey (Cox, 2016). Additionally, 15 per cent of all Australian women reported having been sexually assaulted by someone they knew, three-quarters of these women reported that the most recent assault occurred in a private residence, and one in six women had not told anyone about the sexual assault they experienced (Cox, 2016).

Adult men experience sexual violence much less frequently than women, with one in 22 men reporting experiences of sexual assault since the age of 15 years (Cox, 2016). Despite the clear gender disparity in relation to sexual violence, men who experience these crimes are impacted no less severely than women and deserve to receive the same humanised responses when they seek support.

Impact of sexual violence

Knowledge about the psychological ramifications of sexual violence has improved markedly since the inclusion of PTSD within the DSM. According to the DSM-5, symptoms of PTSD include traumatic intrusions, avoidance, nervous system dysregulation, and alterations to cognition and mood (American Psychiatric Association, 2013).

Traumatic intrusions are involuntary recollections of traumatic events, presenting as emotional, sensory, or narrative memories, either singly or in combination. The experience of intrusions is often frightening, due to their unpredictability, almost like a repetition of the traumatic event, rather than a recollection. People often feel as if they are "right back" where the trauma happened, and many are fearful of going insane. Intrusions are a common feature of trauma and arise in response to internal or external stimuli. They occur in consciousness, when they are referred to as flashbacks, and occur during sleep as distressing dreams and nightmares.

External cues including people, places, activities, topics of conversation, objects, or situations, and internal cues such as thoughts, emotions, and body sensations that in some way resemble or remind people about traumatic events, become feared stimuli and are avoided. Through the process of generalisation, people who have experienced sexual violence perpetrated by a man may, for example, seek to avoid contact with all men, because the resemblance between any man and the specific man who perpetrated the sexual violence is sufficient to produce a reaction. In this way, trauma arising from sexual violence can reduce tolerance for the experiences of everyday life. Social disengagement, including withdrawal from employment or study, and isolation both from and within relationships, are common results of this avoidance, which is ultimately very limiting.

Research suggests that when a person is unable to effect resolution of a traumatic event utilising the natural activation of their nervous system, a pattern of dysregulated arousal results (Van der Kolk, 2015). For many people who have experienced sexual violence, dysregulated arousal in the sympathetic nervous system will produce symptoms such as irritability, heightened anger or anxiety, hypervigilance, exaggerated startle response, problems with sleep, concentration, and/or reckless behaviour (American Psychiatric Association, 2013). Sometimes trauma results in a pattern of dysregulated parasympathetic nervous system response instead (Ogden et al., 2006). The DSM-5 articulates clearly the challenges of acute or chronic sympathetic nervous system arousal, but the shame, disengagement, and chronic inability to motivate the self that is associated with dysregulation of the parasympathetic nervous system is less well articulated.

Negative alterations to cognitions and mood occurring since the traumatic event include negative beliefs about the self, others, or the world in general, distorted cognitions about the causes or consequences of the traumatic exposure, feelings of isolation from others, diminished interest in activities that were previously pleasurable, a diminished ability to experience positive emotions, and/or a persistent negative emotional state. Though practitioners have noted for many years the prevalence of negative cognitions relating to self in people who have experienced sexual violence, a recent study found that the degree of negative cognitions about self in the initial aftermath of sexual violence predicts overall severity of PTSD some months later (Carper et al., 2015).

Service responses to people who have experienced sexual violence

Many criticisms have been made about the utility of PTSD in describing the impact of a broad range of traumatic experiences. In 1992, Judith Herman proposed that the criteria were inadequate to describe the more complex psychological sequelae that follow prolonged or repeated traumatic events such as ongoing childhood sexual assault, domestic violence, and lengthy combat deployment (Herman, 1992). Herman and others have also noted that when experiences of interpersonal trauma are complex, that is when they occur during childhood, are repeated, remain unresolved for many years, and especially when they are perpetrated by a trusted other, presenting symptoms may include: significant problems with affect or mood regulation; chronic and maladaptive distress tolerance attempts, including deliberate self-harm; serious disruptions in the sense of self, including self-loathing and extreme forms of dissociation; suicidal ideation; and relational difficulties (Herman, 1992; Courtois, 2014; Van der Kolk, 2015). Herman coined the term "Complex Post-Traumatic Stress Disorder" (C-PTSD), to refer to this complex symptom constellation (Herman, 1992). If helping professionals understand this presentation, they are more likely to recognise that those presenting with a wide array of difficulties may have been traumatised. This is particularly important if abuse was perpetrated early in life, when memories of such abuse may be pre-verbal, and beyond recall. Without this knowledge, the modern DSM classification system encourages a patient with this presentation to be diagnosed with many "comorbid diagnoses", potentially obscuring the major aetiological factors.

Failure to recognise a history of sexual violence, or to comprehend the traumatic nature of sexual violence, can lead to inadvertent transgressions against people who have experienced sexual violence. Such transgressions not only include inaccurate diagnoses, but also punitive responses, such as the requirement to stop behaviours that are in fact coping strategies intended to deal with or to communicate severe distress. Application of such inappropriate and ineffective treatment or service provision protocols also have the effect of re-traumatising the person and replicating the dynamics of abuse. Inefficient collaboration between services and fragmented responses to the diverse needs of people who have experienced sexual violence are also common. The effects of Complex Trauma can often lead to behaviours that may be seen as "manipulative", and interpersonal difficulties often present significant challenges in relating with helping professionals, requiring sustained and repetitive work. Meeting these complex needs is inherently challenging, but possible, when they are understood as the impacts of severe trauma.

The revised diagnostic criteria of PTSD in the latest edition of the DSM, along with the inclusion of a Dissociative Subtype of PTSD, and separate criteria for PTSD in children under seven years of age, is a partial response to the call of traumatologists for better articulation of the differences in PTSD according to the type and timing of traumatic events (American Psychiatric Association, 2013). There is, however, still a great deal of work to be done to ensure that this highly influential system of categorising mental health disorders adequately conveys the severity and diversity of impacts that can result from experiences of sexual violence, to help foster a humanised response to people who have experienced sexual violence.

Social responses to sexual violence

In addition to punitive responses from the helping professions, there is a culture in Australia that is dominated by views that blame people who have experienced sexual violence for their own victimisation, while simultaneously excusing the violence of perpetrators. Social norms that reward hyper-masculine behaviour, including the disrespectful treatment of people with less social power, are major drivers of sexual violence against women and children (Our Watch et al., 2015). The same dynamic also explains the higher prevalence of sexual violence against people who face greater social disadvantage, including people with disability (Australian Institute of Family Studies, 2008).

One of the manifestations of this inequitable gender dynamic is social subscription to a diverse range of myths relating to the causes and consequences of sexual violence. Notions that women "ask" for sexual violence by the way they dress, the amount of alcohol they drink, or behaviours such as walking alone at night, as well as false claims of experiences of sexual violence, are some of the myths that dominate contemporary Australian society. The social impacts of these myths contribute to poor public comprehension of what constitutes sexual assault (Cox, 2016), and low reporting and conviction rates for sexual assault in every Australian jurisdiction (Lievore, 2004).

Justice responses to sexual violence

Australians view establishing justice as integral to their ability to heal from sexual violence (Clark, 2010). Only a small proportion of sexual violence cases, are, however, subjected to scrutiny by Australian criminal justice systems

(Criminal Justice Sexual Offences Taskforce, 2005), and those that do enter the criminal justice system are subject to high attrition rates. Lievore's analysis suggests that most cases of sexual violence cease to progress whilst being investigated by police; that prosecutors also frequently make decisions that cases should not progress to court; that the proportion of defendants who plead guilty is low in comparison with other crimes; that sexual offences result in a higher number of acquittals than other crimes; and that despite rising numbers of sexual offence charges in recent years, conviction rates have remained steadily low (Lievore, 2004). Taken together, these data suggest that Australian criminal justice systems struggle to hold perpetrators of sexual violence accountable or to offer redress to those who have been subjected to sexual violence.

Trials relating to sexual offences in almost all cases require endurance from the violated person. Numerous reports over recent years have drawn attention to the need for reform in terms of evidentiary processes, questioning of the complainant, duration of court processes, and access to information about the complainant (Victorian Law Reform Commission, 2004; Criminal Justice Sexual Offences Taskforce, 2005). Enduring such a trial is likely to result in exacerbation of traumatic impacts, making recovery more difficult.

Recovery and justice for those who have experienced sexual violence is challenged by the actions of social disbelief and blame, a lack of trauma orientation in the helping professions, and inadequate responses from the justice system. People who have experienced sexual violence, especially those with a complex and cumulative experience, receive inadequate help, which often compounds their fear, self-blame, and shame. The need for a more humanised response is clear. Two models that offer promise in such responses are the Recovery Model, and trauma-informed approaches.

A humanised response to people who have experienced sexual violence

The Recovery Model

The Recovery Model (RM) is a philosophy underpinning treatment for mental illness, rather than a treatment itself. Originating in the USA in the 1970s (Mental Health Coordinating Council, 2009), the model focusses on the person and their potential to recover functioning and satisfaction in life, rather than seeking to directly treat a disorder. Representing a significant departure from the paternalism of psychiatry, the RM views the potential for recovery as innate, rather than a product of treatment. It preferences the term consumer, attempting to move away from more biomedical constructs, giving power to the person in need to choose what outcomes might signal success and which interventions might help. The model further privileges the views of the consumer and their social networks in the design and delivery of services.

The RM focusses on changing dysfunction, disability, impairment, and disadvantage. Working in this way with people who have experienced sexual violence could mean that the effects of social attitudes and stigma, negative impacts of the ramifications of avoidance including unemployment, and the consequences of being subjected to violence may be targeted. Recovery approaches take the focus away from the problem, and instead foster actions that will help the person feel more in control. This focus on empowering the help-seeker, and keeping them in control, are both effective frames for working with people who have experienced sexual violence, because they oppose the dynamics of experiences in which autonomy and control are taken away.

The language of the RM is being increasingly used within policy and programs delivered to people with serious mental health issues (Jacob, 2015), and many of the central tenets of the RM have been shown to be effective in helping people recover from mental illness (Warner, 2010).

An important aspect of the RM is that a full recovery is not expected. This principle however does not fit well when working with people who have experienced sexual violence. The DSM-5 states that complete recovery from PTSD is expected for approximately half the individuals who receive the diagnosis (American Psychiatric Association, 2013). Though the trajectory may be longer, recovery from prolonged, repeated, or otherwise complex sexual violence, including childhood sexual assault, is also common, and the possibility of a full recovery should not be underestimated when working with such people.

Trauma-informed approaches

Trauma-informed approaches are systemic in nature, providing guidance not only for direct work with traumatised people, but also for the structure and functions of the organisation delivering services. Trauma-informed approaches emerged in the late 1990s and early 2000s, when it was discovered that mental health and drug and alcohol service providers had little awareness of the traumatic histories of their clients (Harris and Fallot, 2001). These professionals were among the first to call for a redesign of human services to better meet the needs of severely traumatised people.

Trauma-informed approaches highlight the importance of understanding the role that violence and victimisation play in the lives of service users, and the need to deliver services in a more appropriate, effective, and acceptable way. Though there are several different conceptualisations of trauma-informed care (Quadara and Hunter, 2016), there is a shared focus on the following important components: awareness of the prevalence of trauma histories and their impacts, prioritising safety for service users, a commitment to work in ways that empower service users, interagency collaboration, and acknowledgement of diverse socially and culturally-based needs. These strategies together seek to promote recovery and to minimise the potential for re-traumatisation.

Trauma-informed approaches have gained momentum in the UK, Canada, New Zealand, Australia, and the USA (Quadara and Hunter, 2016), and evidence of the effectiveness of these approaches in decreasing symptoms, substance abuse, mental health difficulties, impulsive behaviours, and incarceration are emerging (Moses et al., 2003; Morrisey et al., 2005). A growing number of guidelines for implementing trauma-informed approaches in different settings are also available (Jennings, 2004; Whittemore and Knafl, 2005; Hopper et al., 2007; Covington, 2008; McLindon and Harms, 2011; Kezelman and Stavropoulos, 2012; Mental Health Coordinating Council, 2013).

It is important to differentiate trauma-informed approaches, which seek to understand and appreciate the relevance of trauma and enable adjunct services to be provided effectively to people who have experienced trauma, from the delivery of services that seek to resolve the trauma specifically. The latter services are usually termed trauma-specific, and this signifies that the therapeutic approaches used are known to be effective in responding to the needs of people suffering effects of trauma. Trauma-specific models include Sensorimotor Psychotherapy (Ogden and Fisher, 2015); Trauma-focused Cognitive Behaviour Therapy (Australian Centre for Posttraumatic Mental Health, 2007); Exposure Therapy (Foa et al., 2000); the Conversational Model (Meares, 2004); Eye Movement Desensitisation and Reprocessing (Shapiro and Forrest, 2016), Dialectical Behaviour Therapy (Linehan, 1993); and therapies stemming from Narrative approaches (Bird, 2004).

Whilst the RM and trauma-informed approaches offer much useful guidance to professionals assisting those who have experienced sexual violence, four additional principles are recommended.

Principles of a humanised response to recovery from sexual violence

1. Recognition that Complex Trauma is inadequately described in the authoritative literature

Until a formal categorisation of disorder that articulates the impacts of complex experiences of sexual violence is available, people who experience prolonged, repeated sexual violence, especially during childhood, will continue to be misdiagnosed and accorded comorbidity. As Van der Kolk has noted, the prevalence of multiple diagnoses in people with PTSD is not true comorbidity, but distinct aspects of the primary problem (trauma) which is not adequately described within the DSM classification system (Van der Kolk, 2005). Understanding that prolonged, or repeated trauma, especially during childhood, gives rise to a complex version of PTSD, or Complex PTSD (Herman, 1992), allows helping professionals to respond to these impacts in a way that situates the problem within the traumatic events and the person/s who perpetrated them, rather than blame the person who experienced sexual violence for their own suffering, and subject them to inappropriate diagnoses and treatments.

2. *Use of appropriate language*

The language used in assisting people who have experienced sexual violence is important. Using terms like "victim" or "survivor" to denote people who have experienced sexual violence conveys that a person is defined by the detrimental impacts of the traumatic event or events that they have experienced. The term victim is no longer commonly used in research and therapeutic lexicons, although the term survivor is still very commonly used. Although "survivor" attempts to highlight the positive aspects of having survived a traumatic event or events, it nevertheless defines a person by that experience. An alternative that prioritises personhood is desirable. Experiences of sexual violence can have lasting and devastating impacts upon people's lives, but the personhood of those who experience sexual violence is never absent from the event, the impacts of the event, their recovery, or the life they lived before, during, or after sexual violence. For this reason, two preferred terms are offered: person who has experienced sexual violence or person who has been subjected to sexual violence.

3. *Recognise the importance of the personhood of the helping professional*

When victimisation occurs within an interpersonal context, healing is facilitated most effectively within an interpersonal relationship. The potential power of a positive relationship with a helping professional in this context is profound. An aware, astute, and humanised response can offset the impacts of social stigma and assist in the establishment of both safety and recovery. In contrast, an ill-informed, authoritative approach compounds the damage. The personhood of the helping professional is therefore of critical importance. Recent discoveries about the functioning of mirror neurons (Corballis, 2015), and Polyvagal Theory (Porges, 2011), illustrate how important the helping professional's self is to the ability of their client to regulate their emotions and nervous system. The self of the helping professional is then as important as the tools and strategies they use to assist recovery.

People who have experienced repeated sexual violence have out of necessity developed finely tuned abilities to discern the mood of a perpetrator to predict with some accuracy the likely timing of offending and to take whatever actions are possible to evade or minimise harm from such perpetration. The helping professional's own mood, stress level, and emotional experience may be discerned with great accuracy by such people. The helping professional's ability to regulate their own emotions is fundamental to being attuned and emotionally available to assist such a person. Helping professionals must be predictable, and compassionate, not just with words and body language, but also with a nervous system that is well regulated despite the pressures of life. Such predictable self-regulation assists the person who has experienced sexual violence to regulate their own emotions, and to recover.

4. Have the courage to innovate

The provision of human responses to people who have experienced sexual violence requires that courage is embodied, and that innovation is embraced. Though many therapeutic models offer an evidence base for the treatment of PTSD, there is much less of an evidence base for the skills and techniques required to treat those who have been subjected to significant and/or repeated sexual violence and who suffer with C-PTSD. Many clinicians are primarily trained in the structured treatments, like Cognitive Behaviour Therapy, and will naturally want to apply this form of treatment to those who present to them, even if they have experienced sexual violence. This therapy and many other traditional talking therapies require the person who has experienced sexual violence to bring a fully functioning cortex to the therapeutic endeavour. Severe trauma interrupts the availability of cortical functioning and therefore such therapies require traumatised people to do what cannot be done. Using more human, somatically or relationally-focused therapies that do not require a fully functioning cortex, and therefore do not place people who have experienced sexual violence in this double bind, requires that a best practice approach should be used rather than an evidence-based approach.

Conclusion

People who have experienced sexual violence often face health, social, and justice responses that deter their recovery. A more appropriate, humanised response which facilitates healing is necessary, and for which there is a significant body of research. Attending to the principles offered by the RM is helpful: the person is the expert in their recovery, the healing potential is innate, the helping professional is an aid to that healing potential, work is done to empower the person, and the focus is on offsetting the negative impacts of sexual violence. Trauma-informed and trauma-specific approaches focus on understanding the impact of trauma, prioritising safety, fostering collaboration, and responding to the diverse social and cultural contexts of people who have experienced sexual violence. In addition, providing a humanised response entails listening to people who have experienced sexual violence in a way that prioritises their experiences over the authoritative literature, and seeking to resolve suffering in the most efficient and the most ethical manner possible. The helping professional's attention to language and self-regulation, and the courage to innovate, are important ingredients to assist recovery from experiences of sexual violence, including those that occurred during childhood.

References

American Psychiatric Association (1980) *Diagnostic and Statistical Manual of Mental Disorders, Third Edition*. Washington, DC: American Psychiatric Publishing.

American Psychiatric Association (2013) *Diagnostic and Statistical Manual of Mental Disorders, Fifth Edition*. Arlington, VA: American Psychiatric Publishing.

Australian Centre for Posttraumatic Mental Health (2007) *Australian Guidelines for the Treatment of Adults with Acute Stress Disorder and Posttraumatic Stress Disorder*. Melbourne, Australia: Australian Centre for Posttraumatic Mental Health.

Australian Institute of Family Studies (2008) *Sexual assault and adults with a disability. ACSSA Issues* 9. Available at: aifs.gov.au/publications/sexual-assault-and-adults-disability/prevalence-sexual-assault-adults-disabilities.

Australian Institute of Family Studies (2017) *The prevalence of child abuse and neglect. CFCA Resource Sheet*. Available at: aifs.gov.au/cfca/publications/prevalence-child-abuse-and-neglect.

Bird J (2004) *Talk That Sings: Therapy in a New Linguistic Key*. Auckland, New Zealand: Edge Press.

Brownmiller S (1975) *Against Our Wills: Men, Women and Rape*. New York, NY: Simon and Shuster.

Burgess AW and Holmstrom LL (1974) Rape Trauma Syndrome. *American Journal of Psychiatry* 131(9): 981–986.

Carper TL, Mills MA, Steenkamp MM, et al. (2015) Early PTSD symptom sub-clusters predicting chronic posttraumatic stress following sexual assault. *Psychological Trauma: Theory, Research, Practice, and Policy* 7(5): 442–447.

Clark H (2010) 'What is the justice system willing to offer?' Understanding sexual assault victim/survivors' criminal justice needs. *Family Matters* 85: 28–37.

Corballis MC (2015) Theory of mirror neurons. In: Wright J (ed) *International Encyclopedia of the Social and Behavioural Sciences, Second Edition*. London, UK: Elsevier Health Sciences, pp.582–588.

Courtois C (2014) *It's Not You, It's What Happened to You: Complex Trauma and Treatment*. Dublin, Ohio: Telemachus Press.

Covington S (2008) Women and addiction: A trauma-informed approach. *Journal of Psychoactive Drugs, SARC Supplement* 5: 377–385.

Cox P (2016) Violence against women in Australia: Additional analysis of the Australian Bureau of Statistics' Personal Safety Survey 2012. *ANROWS Horizons, Revised Edition*. Available at: anrows.org.au/publications/horizons-0/PSS.

Criminal Justice Sexual Offences Taskforce (2005) *Responding to Sexual Assault: The Way Forward*. Available at: justice.nsw.gov.au/justicepolicy/Documents/cjsot_report.pdf.

Eastwood C, Kift S and Grace R (2006) Attrition in child sexual assault cases: Why Lord Chief Justice Hale got it wrong. *Journal of Judicial Administration* 16(2): 81–91.

Foa EB, Keane TM, and Friedman MJ (2000) Guidelines for the treatment of PTSD. *Journal of Traumatic Stress* 13: 539–588.

Harris M and Fallot RD (2001) *Using Trauma Theory to Design Service Systems*. San Francisco, CA: Jossey Bass.

Herman J (1992) *Trauma and Recovery*. New York, NY: Basic Books.

Hopper E, Bassuk E and Olivet J (2007) *Shelter from the Storm: Creating Trauma-informed Homeless Services*. Washington, DC: US Department of Health and Human Services.

Jacob KS (2015) Recovery model of mental illness: A complementary approach to psychiatric care. *Indian Journal of Psychological Medicine* 37(2): 117–119.

Jennings A (2004) *Models for Developing Trauma-informed Behavioral Health Systems and Trauma-specific Services*. Alexandria, VA: National Association of State Mental Health Program Directors, National Technical Assistance Center for State Mental Health Planning.

Kessler RC, Sonnega A, Bromet E, et al. (1995) Posttraumatic Stress Disorder in the National Comorbidity Survey. *Archives of General Psychiatry* 52: 1048–1060.

Kezelman C and Stavropoulos P (2012) *The Last frontier: Practice Guidelines for Treatment of Complex Trauma and Trauma-informed Care and Service Delivery*. Sydney, Australia: Adults Surviving Child Abuse.

Lievore D (2004) *Prosecutorial Decisions in Adult Sexual Assault Cases: An Australian Study*. Available at: aic.gov.au/publications/tandi/tandi291.

Linehan M (1993) *Cognitive-Behavioral Treatment of Borderline Personality Disorder*. New York, NY: The Guilford Press.

McLindon E and Harms L (2011) Listening to mental health workers' experiences: Factors influencing their work with women who disclose sexual assault. *International Journal of Mental Health Nursing* 20(1): 2–11.

Masson JM (1998) *The Assault on Truth: Freud's Suppression of the Seduction Theory*. New York, NY: Pocket Books.

Meares R (2004) The Conversational Model: An outline. *American Journal of Psychotherapy* 58(1): 51–66.

Mental Health Coordinating Council, Being Mental Health and Wellbeing Consumer Advocacy Group (2009) *Recovery Oriented Service Self-Assessment Toolkit (ROSSAT)*. Sydney, Australia: Mental Health Coordinating Council.

Mental Health Coordinating Council (2013) *Trauma-informed Care and Practice: Towards a Cultural Shift in Policy Reform Across Mental Health and Human Services in Australia – A National Strategic Direction. Position paper and recommendations of the National Trauma-Informed Care and Practice Advisory Working Group*. Sydney, Australia: Mental Health Coordinating Council.

Morrisey JP, Ellis AR, Gatz M, et al. (2005) Outcomes for women with co-occurring disorders and trauma: Program and person level effects. *Journal of Substance Abuse Treatment* 28(2): 121–133.

Moses DJ, Glover Reed B, Mazeli R, et al. (2003) *Creating trauma services for women with co-occurring disorders: Experiences from the SAMHSA Women with Alcohol, Drug Abuse and Mental Health Disorders who have Histories of Violence Study*. Available at: researchgate.net/publication/252171592_Creating_Trauma_Services_for_Women_with_Co-Occurring_Disorders.

Ogden P and Fisher J (2015) *Sensorimotor Psychotherapy: Interventions for Trauma and Attachment*. New York, NY: WW Norton and Company.

Ogden P, Minton K and Pain C (2006) *Trauma and the Body*. New York, NY: WW Norton and Company.

O'Leary PJ and Barber J (2008) Gender differences in silencing after childhood sexual abuse. *Journal of Childhood Sexual Abuse* 172(2): 133–143.

Our Watch, ANROWS and VicHealth (2015) *Change the Story: A Shared Framework for the Primary Prevention of Violence Against Women and their Children in Australia*. Available at: ourwatch.org.au/getmedia/0aa0109b-6b03-43f2-85fe-a9f5ec92ae4e/Change-the-story-framework-prevent-violence-women-children-AA-new.pdf.aspx.

Porges SW (2011) *The Polyvagal Theory: Neurophysiological Foundations of Emotions, Attachment, Communication and Self-regulation*. New York, NY: Norton.

Quadara A and Hunter C (2016) *Principles of Trauma-informed Approaches to Child Sexual Abuse: A Discussion Paper.* Sydney, Australia: Royal Commission into Institutional Responses to Child Sexual Abuse.

Roesler TA and McKenzie N (1994) Effects of childhood trauma on psychological functioning in adults sexually abused as children. *Journal of Nervous and Mental Disease* 182(3): 145–150.

Shapiro F and Forrest M (2016) *EMDR: The Breakthrough Treatment for Overcoming Anxiety, Stress and Trauma, Second Edition.* New York, NY: Basic Books.

Victorian Law Reform Commission (2004) *Sexual Offences Final Report.* Available at: lawreform.vic.gov.au/sites/default/files/VLRC_Sexual_Offences_Final_Report.pdf.

Van der Kolk B (2005) Developmental trauma disorder: Toward a rational diagnosis for children with Complex Trauma histories. *Psychiatric Annals* 35(5): 401–408.

Van der Kolk B (2015) *The Body Keeps the Score.* New York, NY: Penguin Books.

Warner R (2010) *Does the scientific evidence support the recovery model?* Available at: pb.rcpsych.org/content/34/1/3 DOI 10.1192/pb.bp.109.025643.

Whittemore R and Knafl K (2005) The integrative review: Updated methodology. *Journal of Advanced Nursing* 2(5): 546–553.

13 Recognising and understanding the experience of trauma in the context of domestic violence

Agi O'Hara

Introduction

Considering the frequency with which reference is made in the media to domestic violence, and the statistic that on average one woman dies every week in Australia as a result of such violence (Bryant and Cussen, 2015), it seems reasonable to believe that the phenomenon is a modern-day epidemic. In fact, the media focus represents the public recognition of the previously hidden but long-standing reality of domestic violence. It is now well accepted that, "Domestic and family violence is a crime. It includes any behaviour, in an intimate or family relationship, which is violent, threatening, coercive or controlling, causing a person to live in fear" (NSW Ministry of Health, 2016: p.2). Domestic violence is intimidating and abusive, and can include physical, sexual and psychological violence, verbal and emotional abuse, social or spiritual isolation, and financial deprivation.

It is also widely acknowledged that women are statistically more likely to be victims of domestic violence and this is overwhelmingly at the hands of their male partners. "In 2012, an estimated 17% of all women aged 18 years and over (1,479,900 women) and 5.3% of all men aged 18 years and over (448,000 men) had experienced violence by a partner since the age of 15" (Australian Bureau of Statistics, 2013). The statistics relating to males highlights the fact that domestic violence occurs across all demographics, "regardless of age, gender, race, sexuality, wealth and geography" (Hester et al., 2012: p.3). Despite incomplete statistics, it is also apparent that the rates of domestic violence in Indigenous people are much higher than in non-Indigenous people. Reports comparing domestic violence statistics for urban versus rural contexts in NSW reveal that, "19 out of the top 20 NSW Local Government Areas for domestic violence are in rural or regional NSW" (Grech and Burgess, 2011: p.5), the majority of which also have high Indigenous populations. Furthermore, Australia's National Research Organisation for Women's Safety reports, "that Indigenous women … are five times more likely to be homicide victims than non-Indigenous people, and … 35 times more likely to be hospitalised than non-Indigenous people" (Phillips and Vandenbroek, 2014: p.10). It can be assumed that many of the homicides are a result of domestic violence as international studies reveal that "40-70% of female murder victims were killed by their husbands or boyfriends" (We Will Speak Out, 2009: p.2).

In this chapter, the focus will be on domestic violence within adult relationships. Domestic violence that is intergenerational or involves other pairings of relatives is also a significant issue but is beyond the scope of this chapter. It is also beyond the scope of this chapter to detail the experiences of domestic violence in other contexts, for example, violence in gay and lesbian relationships. The trauma associated with violence and the subsequent impact on psychological and physical health detailed in this chapter will however still be relevant, irrespective of the variations in relationship contexts.

The pronouns "he" and "she" will be used to refer to the perpetrator and victim, respectively, for ease of reading, but does not imply that victims are always female but perpetrators always male. It should also be noted that the term victim has been used as it is common parlance in the field, but those who have suffered at the hands of others should not be so simplistically labelled, much as a sufferer of Schizophrenia should not be labelled "schizophrenic".

Background

The current prominence of domestic violence in the media is the culmination of many decades of community and political advocacy. Flood and Pease cite Bush in emphasising that the, "public recognition of men's violence against women as a 'social problem' has been a major achievement of the women's movement" (Flood and Pease, 2009: p.136). It is also important to recognise that it was the specifically targeted domestic violence protest movement of the 1970s that located, "violence against women and children as occurring within a society where male dominance is normalised and men feel entitled to use violence to maintain their privileged position ... [and] systems and institutions, such as the 'family' and 'marriage', have served to maintain this dominance" (Women's House Shelta collective, 2009: p.7).

What has changed historically is not the incidence of domestic violence, but the attitude to it, such that violence in the home is no longer minimised and considered "just a domestic", a private matter that people do not want to talk about or interfere in, let alone report. Instead, domestic violence is recognised as a significant public health issue. As a result, there are now state and national campaigns, domestic violence policies, and funding initiatives, with many millions of dollars spent to raise awareness, provide support, and reduce the incidence of domestic violence in Australia.

The death of Luke Batty in suburban Melbourne in 2014, at the hands of his father, who had for years physically violated his mother Rosie Batty, captured the attention of the public. The community's emotional connection with Rosie's trauma galvanised the grass roots advocacy that she started. Through her Luke Batty Foundation, the "Never Alone" campaign played a significant role in raising awareness of the impact of domestic violence on children. The political impact of her work resulted in Rosie becoming Australian of the Year in 2015 and brought about significant government policy changes. In 2016, Rosie also helped launch "Justice for Kids", a five-step plan involving early intervention, enhanced support, and legal and financial initiatives. Her request to the, "Never Alone supporters to sign the 'Justice for Kids' petition and demand the government to put safety first in family law" (Never Alone Luke Batty Foundation website, 2017) resulted in 11,000 signatures in just seven days and, "A year after the launch of the plan, the Federal Government announced a comprehensive review of the family law system, including some key measures to address safety issues" (Never Alone Never Luke Batty Foundation website, 2017).

It is also important to note that the domestic violence protest movement has brought about significant advancements in the mental health and legal fields. The greater awareness and understanding among health and legal professionals about the impact of domestic violence has led to the acceptance of the diagnosis of the Battered Woman Syndrome (BWS). Medically, within The Diagnostic and Statistical Manual of Mental Disorders, Fifth Edition (DSM-5) (American Psychiatric Association, 2013), it is a subcategory of Posttraumatic Stress Disorder (PTSD). In the Tenth Edition of the International Classification of Diseases (ICD-10-CM) (World Health Organization, 1992), domestic violence is identified using a series of codes that delineate specific abuses including physical, sexual, psychological, and unspecified maltreatment. Legally, BWS is seen as "a construct used to explain how repeated domestic violence affects women" (Nedim, 2015). Prior to the acceptance of the diagnosis of BWS, there had been no adequate means by which the trauma and fear resulting from living in a violent relationship could be considered mitigating circumstances for a victim assaulting or murdering her violent partner. "Recent studies [reveal that] more than a fifth of all homicides occur between intimate spouses, and that the majority of women imprisoned for murder have, at some stage, been victims of domestic violence" (Craven, 2003: p.1). Despite the potential legal benefits derived from the use of BWS, it is seen by some to pathologise the experiences of women, and to incorrectly imply that the condition is common to all women who are in physically violent relationships.

Theoretical explanations of domestic violence

Many theoretical perspectives for the aetiology of domestic violence exist, but the majority are inadequate in explaining intimate partner violence. Psychological explanations usually focus on either individual pathology or socially learned behaviour. The former sees "violence as stemming from personal weaknesses, failures, abnormality or disorders of the perpetrators" (Jansen, 2005: p.6), and that deficits are found "in the ego structure of the violent man, which cause him to lose control of anger" (Peters et al., 2002: p.256). However, such personal deficits do not lead to the expression of anger in other contexts, for example, at work or with friends, so this is not an adequate explanation for the violence in their intimate relationships. Social learning theories suggest that

> Men who beat their wives either do so because they have been targets of parental abuse as children, or that they might have experienced their fathers abuse their mothers and are therefore inclined to repeat such a violence in their own adulthood. The same perspective also suggests that female children who experience their mothers being beaten might end up in abusive relationships themselves
>
> (Jansen, 2005: p.6)

Such explanations, though apparently relevant for many, do not account for the reality that not all males who witness domestic violence as children go on to perpetrate violence as adults, and that many women whose mothers were violated by their male partners do not tolerate abusive behaviours in their adult relationships. Feminist theories focus on the domination and repression of women, and perceive domestic violence as based on "universal, structural and hierarchical inequality based on gender … [that] violence is used as a corrective measure to ensure the upholding of male authority, and is considered a functional, and not dysfunctional, affirmation of a patriarchal social order" (Green cited in Jansen, 2005: p.6). Although feminist theories offer a compelling explanation for male perpetrated violence in heterosexual relationships, they do not account for violence perpetrated by men and women in same-sex relationships, nor women's violence in heterosexual relationships. Control theory suggests that some individuals have a need for power and control and use threats of force and or violence as a means of controlling the behaviour of others (Hyde-Nolan and Juliao, 2012). Although this describes the dynamic at play, it offers no explanation as to why such a need for power and control exists in certain individuals.

Focusing on the nature of early experiences of nurture and the development of attachment to primary caregivers may offer a more generally applicable explanation of intimate partner violence. Whereas, "Men who have strong attachments to significant others and fear negative reactions from these individuals are less likely to abuse their wives" (Hyde-Nolan and Juliao, 2012: p.10), [for others] "unmet dependency needs in childhood persist into adulthood, often accompanied by a sense of rage that one's needs were not met. As a result, the search to fulfil dependency needs as an adult becomes both desperate and demanding" (Hyde-Nolan and Juliao, 2012: p.6). This, and other attachment-related theories, may help to explain the relevance of developmental and relational deficits within the perpetrator, and how these might impact on future relationships.

The dynamics of domestic violence

The build-up to physical violence may be slow and gradual over several years, but the psychological and emotional abuse often emerges early in the relationship. By the time the physical violence has begun the victim's self-esteem and ability to identify options available to her have been eroded by the criticism, belittling, and humiliation to which she has been subjugated. The forced isolation from friends and family prevents opportunities for the victim to gain support and clarity about what is happening to them. When leaving is not considered an option, the victim's focus is on trying to identify a pattern in the perpetrator's violent behaviour. Craven (2003) cites Walker in suggesting that domestic violence follows a cyclical pattern, beginning in stage one with the build-up of tension, during which there is verbal and emotional abuse, and sometimes lower levels of violence, such as slapping or pushing. Victims frequently develop a myriad of strategies to anticipate and avoid situations that might "provoke" the perpetrator, or ways to try to appease and calm him, if violence cannot be avoided. Despite the strategies, the violence recurs in the second stage, and often escalates over time. The victim feels powerless to stop the violence, and many victims experience a form of learned helplessness, as nothing they do seems to make a difference to the outcome. Craven (2003), citing Walker again, suggests that it is

> At this time that a victim's sense of fear and perceptions of danger [are] at their height as [is] the risk of death or serious injury. The discharge of tension in the second stage … would invariably lead to a third phase of "loving contrition" in which the batterer would exhibit conciliatory behaviours and may attempt to convince the victim of their intentions to change.
>
> (Craven, 2003: pp.2–3)

The manipulation in the third "honeymoon" stage is initially effective in offering hope to the victim, who may love their partner, and desperately want to believe that the violence will cease. However, the feeling of hope is short-lived, and the build-up of tension begins again, often with briefer periods between the stages over time, so there becomes very little reprieve from the violence. The victim loses confidence in her ability to make the right decision, and sometimes her decision-making is negatively influenced by the responses of others to her situation. Through ignorance and projected fears, family and friends may advise her to try harder to please him, to not break up the family, to think of the children, who according to them would be better off in an intact family, and to consider the social consequences, sometimes pleading that she not bring shame on the family.

> Abused women risk being stigmatized in the general community, paradoxically for being both home wreckers and for not leaving their abusive partners. In the first case, women are made responsible for keeping families together, regardless of the individual cost. In the second case, women who are subjected to male violence are made responsible for solving this difficult social problem by the individual act of leaving.
>
> (Enander, 2010: p.6)

Attitudes toward domestic violence

A great many myths and unhelpful generalisations still prevail, despite the media focus on domestic violence. Each offers the opportunity to deny the reality of domestic violence in all social contexts, particularly one's own. If the myth that domestic violence only occurs in particular cultural or ethnic groups or only among lower socio-economic groups is accepted, then abusive behaviours enacted by those who do not fit the stereotype will be minimised or ignored. Many people, including women who are in abusive relationships, believe that all violent men come from violent homes, or that all violent men are psychiatrically ill. If these characteristics are not present in the abuser, then the coercive, controlling, demeaning, and invalidating behaviours are often perceived to be an excessive though "normal" expression of relationship conflict. Family and friends may ascribe blame and responsibility equally to both the victim and the perpetrator. Mention is made of her "nagging", her "inability to control the kids", and her "less than acceptable house-keeping standards" as provocations for the abusive behaviour. The behaviours are not considered to be domestic violence until there is a threat of, or actual, physical violence. Unfortunately, even when physical violence occurs, it is often blamed on excessive alcohol consumption, or excused because the violent man couldn't help it, he had just suddenly "lost control". These justifications ignore the fact that only "forty-one percent of domestic assault incidents in NSW were flagged by police as alcohol-related" (Grech and Burgess, 2011: p.4), and violent men are frequently controlled enough to take care not to hit partners where injuries show. Although there is conflict in all relationships and dysfunctional patterns of communication are common, coercive, demeaning, abusive, and violent behaviours are not acceptable methods of solving conflict. Rather they are a deliberate means of maintaining power and control.

Responsibility for entering into, or remaining in, a violent relationship is sometimes still ascribed to the victim and echoed in the sentiments that some women actually seek out abusive men, and women only get beaten up when they "ask for it". Although it is difficult to believe that any woman would consciously seek to be violated or specifically seek a violent partner, it has been suggested that not all women are equally able to recognise behaviours that might flag that a potential partner is controlling, manipulative, not respectful of boundaries, and may end up being violent. Benstead offers the metaphor of a "shark cage" to explain why this might be the case (2011). The "bars" in the shark cage represent a boundary or basic human right, and a bar is added into a protective cage each time a woman is taught through words and actions that a particular behaviour is unacceptable. Some of these include being controlled, threatened, shouted at, called names, being hit, or touched in ways that cause discomfort. When the bars have been well constructed, abusive people find it difficult to get close enough to hurt their targets. Unfortunately, some people have inadequately constructed shark cages, thereby not recognising or not being able to defend against the abusive people they encounter. This could be due to their primary caregivers sometimes modelling an acceptance of inappropriate behaviours, perhaps due to their own inadequate shark cages, or themselves behaving inappropriately.

Misunderstanding women's experience of domestic violence – the issue of leaving

Perhaps the most harmful generalisation in the context of domestic violence is the mistaken belief that if the relationship is so bad the woman should or could just leave. Embarrassment and shame often prevent disclosure of the violence. Not leaving may also appear to be the most effective safety strategy, as threats of death to herself or her children are very real. "The end of the relationship does not necessarily equate with an end to violence exposure … violence has been found to continue after separation and may actually increase in severity and lethality" (Holt et al., 2008: p.800). We Will Speak Out, citing Lees, also suggest that, "Women are at greatest risk of homicide at the point of separation or after leaving a violent partner" (2009: p.4). Many women fleeing violent relationships have no relatives or friends with whom they can stay and require housing. If fortunate they are able stay in refuges, but others end up homeless due to the inadequate number of beds available or the woman's unsuitability, for example, due to drug and alcohol problems. Cramer and Carter (2002) offer the statistic that domestic violence is the most significant contributor in 40 per cent of women becoming homeless.

Language, culture, and religious issues

The inability to consider leaving may also be exacerbated if there are language difficulties, for example, if English is not her first language, and if she is unaware of the community resources that are available for women experiencing violence. If she comes from a small, close-knit community, or one that is a marginalised social, religious or cultural group, she could be more worried about the impact on her community, than herself, if the violence was made public. She might also feel shame not only in relation to herself, but also to her community. There may also be beliefs, attitudes, and imperatives specific to her religion that are misappropriated and manipulated by the perpetrator and may intensify her reluctance to reveal her experience of violence. Fortunately, domestic violence has become a critical focus in many religious communities, and there is now a greater understanding of the pivotal role that all religious leaders can play in preventing an acceptance of domestic violence.

The trauma of domestic violence

Disempowerment and disconnection from others are part of the experience of psychological trauma (Herman, 1998). In the context of domestic violence, they are acutely felt, due to the deliberate manipulation by the perpetrator. Isolation from family and friends may initially be through subtle means, perhaps by promoting the belief that the relationship is so special and valued that limiting contact with others would enable a deepening of the relationship. In time, however, the manipulation and control become blatant and contact with family and friends may be forbidden, with threats of violence. Isolation enables the continuation of violence, and the woman is left powerless to prevent it.

Herman suggests that,

> Methods of establishing control over another person are based upon the systematic, repetitive infliction of psychological trauma … . Methods of psychological control are designed to instil terror and helplessness and to destroy the victim's sense of self in relation to others … . Fear is also increased by inconsistent and unpredictable outbursts of violence … . The ultimate effect of these techniques is to convince the victim that the perpetrator is omnipotent, that resistance is futile.
>
> (1992: p.77)

She becomes emotionally dependent on the abuser, "The more frightened she is, the more she is tempted to cling to the one relationship that is permitted: the relationship with the perpetrator" (Herman, 1992: p.81). Paradoxically, some victims return to the violent relationship, after having left it, due to empathy for the perpetrator, fear that friends and family would abandon him, and that she is the only one who can love and understand him. For others, it is the fear of the consequences that force her to return. It has been estimated that it can take between five and seven attempts at leaving a violent relationship before a woman can permanently leave.

Even if she has escaped the relationship and the violence has ended, the shame and guilt carried by victims sometimes prevents them from reconnecting with friends and family. Victims have experienced unspeakable acts and can generally never return to how it had been prior to the trauma, particularly in relation to trust. Feeling different, and assuming that nobody would understand, may lead to further disconnection from friends and family, unless a woman is able to get support from health professionals who can demonstrate their understanding of the impact of her traumatic experiences.

The impact of domestic violence is both physical and psychological. Physical effects include headaches, chest and/or back pain, heart palpitations, hyperventilation, startle-reaction to noise, light, and touch, and gastrointestinal abnormalities. The psychological consequences can include depressive and anxiety symptoms, panic attacks, drug use, dissociation, suicidal ideation, and posttraumatic stress responses. The latter may include intrusive memories of the violence, hypervigilance, avoidance of people or places associated with the violence, and feeling emotionally flat and isolated. The traumatic reactions are experienced both whilst in the relationship and, for some, after leaving the violent relationship. These responses are exacerbated if there are children involved, who can also become victim to the manipulation and intimidation of the perpetrator. The impact of domestic violence on children is dependent on many factors including their age and the severity of violence. Children are not only traumatised by seeing or hearing the violence and sensing their mother's fear, prior to her leaving the relationship, but they may sometimes be used as hostages as a means of ensuring the mother's return to the home, or they may be interrogated and involved in spying on their mother. They are told that their parents would be together, if not for the mother's behaviour, undermining her and encouraging negative opinions of her mothering ability, as a way of breaking down the mother–child bond (Tomison, 2000). The children may also experience mental health symptoms such as anxiety and depression, but a worrying possibility is that, for some young people, the experience of violence profoundly impacts their understanding of what is acceptable behaviour. This may lead to use of violence in later relationships, leading to a, "transferral of violence across generations, as children become parents themselves" (Trauma, Loss and Grief Network, 2016).

Trauma-informed responses and services

Professionals, family, and friends need to understand that despite their best intentions in trying to offer suggestions and action strategies, it is unhelpful to ask questions that try to ascertain the reasons for the violence as this may inadvertently suggest that the violence is somehow the fault of the victim. The focus needs to be on listening and support, and not criticism, if she says she still loves her partner. It is helpful to criticise the violent behaviour and let her know that no-one has the right to abuse her, but not to personally criticise her partner, as this is likely to make her want to defend him. Information about available services and resources should be provided, but it is not appropriate to advise or pressure her to leave, as this will reduce her confidence in making her own decisions.

An ideal trauma-informed domestic violence service would cater to the physical and psychological needs of the victim and her children, as well as involve the perpetrator in an intervention program. Trauma-informed treatments for victims recognise that traumatic memories initially intrude and bring with them feelings such as fear, anxiety, helplessness, shame, guilt, and anger. The victim is assisted to learn strategies to help understand, contain, and challenge these feelings and manage the memories, eventually having the ability to focus and defocus from them, at will. Rebuilding her self-esteem and her ability to reconnect with others is a primary goal, and it is important for her to construct meaning and a coherent narrative of her experiences of the trauma, ascribing responsibility for the violence with the perpetrator (Herman, 1992).

Programs for perpetrators are still controversial because of inadequate research into their long-term efficacy, however ignoring perpetrator rehabilitation inevitably results in further violence to other women, even if the original partner has managed to leave the relationship. Intervention programs for the perpetrator need to challenge his beliefs that enabled his violence and provide strategies to assist him to manage his anger, thereby minimising the likelihood of future violence. Perpetrator programs such as "Taking Responsibility" run by Relationships Australia also contact and support former or current partners and encourage them to attend courses and seminars relating to their experiences of violence. This contact, if desired by the victim, also acts as a means of monitoring the behaviour of the perpetrator if he and the woman are still in a relationship. The program "Aims to assist men who have hurt someone they love and are ready to take responsibility for their use of violent, controlling or abusive behaviours … . It also helps strengthen attitudes and skills necessary for respectful, fair and loving relationships with female partners and children" (Relationships Australia website, 2017).

A vignette – "Jane" and "Michael"

From the very beginning of their relationship, Michael was far more attentive than previous partners, wanting to know where Jane was when they weren't together. He was very charming, and, at first, she was flattered and excited by the attention he gave her. Everyone liked him initially, but they spent very little time with friends and family. When they did socialise, Michael was critical of Jane, and seemed to dominate the conversation, so that Jane seemed uncharacteristically quiet and subdued. He became angry if she spoke for too long on the phone to her friends or family. He also became moody, and frequently belittled her, and the arguments became more frequent. She tried very hard to please him, to anticipate what might annoy him, but she found herself constantly "walking on eggshells". Jane hoped that becoming pregnant might make him happy, but she was unaware that 30 per cent of domestic violence begins in pregnancy (We Will Speak Out, 2009). He was furious when she was tired and couldn't do the things he wanted, particularly if she wasn't interested in having sex. Her first physical experience of violence was when she was five months pregnant, when Michael punched her in the stomach, saying that he would not allow "the kid" to wreck his life. He apologised the next day, saying that he had had a few drinks and that he would never hurt her again. But a few months later when baby Tom had been crying for some time, he became furious, yelled at her, pushed her against the wall, and punched her in the face, threatening to kill Tom if she didn't find a way to keep him quiet. There were many such incidents over the next five years, and she was terrified for both herself and Tom. Sometimes he was in the room when Michael hit her, and Tom would cry and plead for Michael to stop hurting his mummy. She felt guilty about what Tom was witnessing, but felt paralysed by fear, that Michael would kill them both if she told anyone, or tried to leave, so nobody knew what was going on. The fear and anxiety affected her health, and she went to see her General Practitioner (GP) about her frequent headaches and weight loss. Her GP became very concerned about the drastic changes in her appearance and demeanour and asked her about her relationship. Jane burst into tears, and slowly revealed the whole story. She was provided with information about domestic violence helplines, and the GP called the local women's health centre so that Jane could see a counsellor later the same day. She was encouraged to call her sister, who collected her and Tom. The counsellor provided information about taking out an Apprehended Violence Order (AVO), creating a safety plan, and several future appointments were arranged to help Jane begin to work through the trauma she had experienced. Jane and her sister went to the police to take out the AVO, to prevent Michael having any contact with them, until long-term arrangements could be made.

Conclusion

Jane was very fortunate to have the support of her family, who provided both her and Tom a safe place to stay. Although they had many questions, they did not pressure her to speak about her experiences, focusing instead on giving her the security of a loving family, and a safe and predictable environment. Strategies to overcome the experience of violence must be individualised as some victims find it very difficult to speak about their experiences. When they do, they may choose not to use medical or mental health labels such as BWS or even PTSD to describe the long-term consequences. For these women, there is stigma attached to the labels, and a belief that they afford the perpetrator extra power and satisfaction if they were to acknowledge the extent of psychological harm (as opposed to the physical harm) that the perpetrator may have caused them (Herman, 1992).

Recovery from trauma is a slow and non-linear process. There is no ordered or predictable course that accounts for all responses. Issues of trust and safety are likely to be processed many times but remain unresolved for many women. A successful trauma recovery process would be one in which it is, "Possible to recognize a gradual shift from unpredictable danger to reliable safety, from dissociated trauma to acknowledged memory, and from stigmatized isolation to restored social connection" (Herman, 1992: p.155).

References

American Psychiatric Association (2013) *Diagnostic and Statistical Manual of Mental Disorders, Fifth Edition.* Arlington, VA: American Psychiatric Publishing.

Australian Bureau of Statistics (2013) *4906.0 – Personal Safety, Australia, 2012.* Canberra, Australia: Australian Bureau of Statistics.

Benstead U (2011) 'The Shark Cage': The use of metaphor with women who have experienced abuse. *Psychotherapy in Australia* 17(2): 70–76.

Bryant W and Cussen T (2015) *Homicide in Australia: 2010–11 to 2011–12; National Homicide Monitoring Program Report.* Canberra, Australia: Australian Institute of Criminology.

Cramer H and Carter M (2002) *Homelessness: What's Gender Got To Do With It?* London, UK: Shelter.

Craven Z (2003) *Battered Woman Syndrome. Australian Domestic and Family Violence Clearinghouse Topic Paper.* Sydney, Australia: Australian Domestic and Family Violence Clearinghouse.

Enander V (2010) "A fool to keep staying": Battered women labelling themselves stupid as an expression of gendered shame. *Violence Against Women* 16(1): 5–31.

Flood M and Pease B (2009) Factors influencing attitudes to violence against women. *Trauma, Violence, and Abuse* 10(2): 125–142.

Grech K and Burgess M (2011) *Trends and Patterns in Domestic Violence Assaults: 2001 to 2010. Crime and Justice Statistics Bureau Brief.* Sydney, Australia: NSW Bureau of Crime Statistics and Research.

Herman J (1992) *Trauma and Recovery*. New York, NY: Basic Books.

Herman J (1998) Recovery from psychological trauma. *Psychiatry and Clinical Neurosciences* 52 (Suppl) (S1): 145–150.

Hester M, Williamson E, Regan L, et al. (2012) *Exploring the Service and Support Needs of Male, Lesbian, Gay, Bi-sexual, Transgendered, Black and Other Minority Ethnic Victims of Domestic and Sexual Violence. Report prepared for Home Office SRG/06/017.* Bristol, UK: University of Bristol.

Holt S, Buckley H and Whelan S (2008) The impact of exposure to domestic violence on children and young people: A review of the literature. *Child Abuse and Neglect* 32: 797–810.

Hyde-Nolan M and Juliao T (2012) *Theoretical basis for family violence*. Available at: samples.jbpub.com/9780763780340/80340_ch02_final.pdf.

Jansen K (2005) *Abuse and suffering: A feminist perspective on domestic violence, bodies, and battered women's coping strategies in Mauritius*. Available at: bora.uib.no/bitstream/handle/1956/1877/Hovedfagsoppgaven%20final%20pdf%20test%20Karine.pdf?sequence=1.

Nedim U (2015) *Battered Woman Syndrome: A help or hindrance?* Sydney Criminal Lawyers blog. Available at: sydneycriminallawyers.com.au/blog/battered-woman-syndrome-a-help-or-hindrance/.

Never Alone Luke Batty Foundation website (2017) *Family Law Reform*. Available at: https://lukebattyfoundation.org.au/about-us/our-achievements/.

NSW Ministry of Health (2016) *NSW Domestic and Family Violence Blueprint for Reform 2016–2021: Safer Lives for Women, Men and Children*. Sydney, Australia: NSW Ministry of Health.

Peters J, Shackelford TK and Buss DM (2002) Understanding domestic violence against women: Using evolutionary psychology to extend the feminist functional analysis. *Violence and Victims* 17(2): 255–264.

Phillips J and Vandenbroek P (2014) *Domestic Violence in Australia – An Overview of the Issues*. Canberra, Australia: Parliamentary Library.

Relationships Australia website (2017) *Taking Responsibility – A Course for Men*. Available at: relationshipsnsw.org.au/support-services/.

Tomison AM (2000) *Exploring Family Violence: Links between Child Maltreatment and Domestic Violence. National Clearing House Issues Paper No. 13*. Melbourne, Australia: Australian Institute of Family Studies.

Trauma, Loss and Grief Network (2016) *Stepping up for Kids: Understanding and Supporting Children Who Have Experienced Family and Domestic Violence*. Available at: earlytraumagrief.anu.edu.au/resource-centre/abuse-neglect-violence.

We Will Speak Out (2009) *Domestic violence statistics*. Available at: wewillspeakout.org/wp-content/uploads/2013/03/domestic-violence-statistics-2009.pdf.

Women's House Shelta collective (2009) *Domestic Violence and Child Protection: Best Practice from a Feminist Perspective*. Brisbane, Australia: Women's Community Aid Association QLD LTD.

World Health Organization (1992) *The ICD-10 Classification of Mental and Behavioural Disorders: Clinical Descriptions and Diagnostic Guidelines*. Geneva, Switzerland: World Health Organization.

14 Trauma-informed care in the context of alcohol and other drug use disorders

Katherine Mills and Maree Teesson

Introduction

A history of trauma exposure is almost universal among clients of Alcohol and Other Drug (AOD) Services. Consequently, rates of Posttraumatic Stress Disorder (PTSD) and other trauma-related conditions are elevated in this population. Despite this, the possible relevance of trauma to substance use, and the potential impact of trauma upon treatment, go largely unrecognised in this sector. In this chapter, the extent of trauma exposure and PTSD among people with AOD use disorders is outlined, and the nature of the relationship between these conditions is discussed. This is followed by an examination of the issues surrounding the implementation in this area of a trauma-informed approach, and a brief overview of the research regarding trauma-focused treatment options for clients with AOD use disorders.

Prevalence of trauma exposure and PTSD among people with AOD use disorders

More than 80 per cent of clients of Australian AOD services report having experienced a traumatic event in their lifetime, most commonly having been physically or sexually assaulted, witnessed a serious injury or a death, been threatened with a weapon, or held captive (Mills et al., 2005; Dore et al., 2012; Kelly et al., 2016; Goodhew et al., 2016). Most clients have experienced multiple traumas, and more than half have experienced trauma during childhood (Mills et al., 2005; Dore et al., 2012; Kelly et al., 2016; Goodhew et al., 2016). It is therefore unsurprising that up to two-thirds have been found to suffer from PTSD (Kingston et al., 2017), which is associated with a more severe clinical profile and poorer treatment outcomes (Mills et al., 2005, 2007). Trauma exposure, comorbid PTSD, and AOD problems are also disproportionately high among Indigenous Australians (Nadew, 2012; Lee et al., 2014). In a sample of people from remote Aboriginal communities in Western Australia, 96 per cent reported a history of trauma exposure, 55 per cent met diagnostic criteria for PTSD, and, of these, 91 per cent also met diagnostic criteria for an Alcohol Use Disorder (Nadew, 2012).

The most common AOD use disorder found among individuals with PTSD is Alcohol Use Disorder, at 24 per cent; however, only 5 per cent of people with an Alcohol Use Disorder have PTSD (Mills et al., 2006). When looking specifically at people with AOD use disorders, PTSD is most commonly found among those with Opioid, Sedative, and Amphetamine Use Disorders, at 33 per cent, 29 per cent, and 24 per cent, respectively, and is most strongly associated with these disorders (Mills et al., 2006).

Regardless of whether a person goes on to develop PTSD, or any other mental health disorder, traumatic events are often life-changing, and can redefine a person's views about themselves (for example, feeling weak, bad, or worthless), the world around them (for example, the world is not safe), and how they relate to it (for example, people cannot be trusted). These beliefs may be particularly well-entrenched in those who have experienced childhood trauma.

Prolonged or repeated trauma, particularly in childhood, has been proposed to result in a complex presentation that includes not only PTSD symptoms, but also other symptoms reflecting disturbances in emotion regulation, interpersonal relations, attention and consciousness, belief systems, somatic experience, and level of organisation (Cloitre et al., 2011). Childhood trauma has also been consistently found to have strong and enduring associations with all classes of mental disorders across the lifespan (Anda et al., 2006; Kessler et al., 2010; Norman et al., 2012a; Mersky et al., 2013).

The US Adverse Childhood Experiences study has been pivotal in improving the level of understanding of the impact of child trauma on development and long-term outcomes relating to physical health, mental health, and to psychosocial function (Anda et al., 2006). Adverse childhood experiences (ACEs) were found to be associated with increased rates of alcohol abuse and illicit drug use, an earlier age of onset of illicit drug use, and overall poorer mental health (Dube et al., 2002, 2003, 2006). Indeed, ACEs were found to account for one-half to two-thirds of all serious problems with drug use (Dube et al., 2003). A dose–response relationship was also observed, whereby the risk of occurrence and severity of each of the AOD outcomes described increased with the number of adverse events experienced (Dube et al., 2002, 2003, 2006). For example, for each additional event experienced, the odds of developing an illicit drug problem increased by 30–40 per cent (Dube et al., 2003). A similar pattern emerged from more recent analysis of data from the second Australian National Survey of Mental Health and Wellbeing: one-third of adults who reported exposure to childhood trauma developed an AOD use disorder (predominantly alcohol and cannabis), a rate nearly three times that of adults who had never experienced trauma (13 per cent), and 1.3 times that of people who had only experienced trauma in adulthood (23 per cent) (Barrett et al., 2015).

The relationship between trauma, PTSD, and AOD use – theoretical perspectives

No single theory can explain the nature of the relationship between trauma, PTSD, and AOD use, but research suggests that self-medication of trauma symptoms may play a significant role in the development and maintenance of AOD use disorders (Darke, 2013). Empirical research examining the temporal sequencing of conditions has found that the onset of trauma exposure and PTSD symptoms predates the onset of AOD use disorders in at least half of cases (Chapman et al., 2012). However, AOD use also confers an increased risk of trauma exposure, re-traumatisation, and, consequently, PTSD (Mills et al., 2008). Both AOD use disorders and PTSD may also share common underlying risk factors. It is most likely, however, that there are multiple pathways leading to co-occurring AOD use disorders and PTSD, and irrespective of how they come to co-occur, once established, each serves to maintain and exacerbate the other.

Research has also documented an association between improvements in PTSD symptoms and subsequent improvements in AOD use (Hien et al., 2010). The reciprocal relationship, however, is not observed; the relevant literature generally demonstrates that there is usually little change in PTSD symptomology even following dramatic improvements in substance use. On the contrary, PTSD symptoms may worsen in the absence of substance use, making it difficult for people to sustain abstinence (Read et al., 2004). Knowledge and awareness of a client's trauma history is therefore crucial and helps inform the development of the most suitable treatment approach.

The relationship between trauma, PTSD, and AOD use – neurobiology

Research suggests that the development and maintenance of trauma-related symptoms and problems related to AOD use may be partially explained by structural and functional abnormalities in common neurobiological pathways, particularly those relating to the stress response and reward pathways. These neuroadaptations may interact with epigenetic and environmental influences, predisposing a person to psychiatric disorders, AOD use disorders, or both (Brady and Sinha, 2005; Norman et al., 2012b; Stephens and Wand, 2012). It has been suggested that exposure to trauma in critical periods of brain maturation, such as childhood or adolescence, may have particularly long-lasting impacts, or may even permanently alter stress responsivity, which may explain the association between childhood trauma and the development of AOD use and other psychiatric disorders in adulthood (De Bellis, 2002).

Both PTSD and AOD use have been associated with cortico-limbic changes, particularly hyperactivity of the amygdala, hypo-activity of the prefrontal cortex, and changes in hippocampal volume – brain structures integrally involved in the mediation of stress-induced sensitisation of the startle response, memory, and executive functioning (Brady and Sinha, 2005; Norman et al., 2012b; Stephens and Wand, 2012). Collectively, the evidence suggests that dysregulation of these cortico-limbic structures may impair a person's ability to regulate intrusive trauma-related and craving-related thoughts, and inhibit repetitive maladaptive behaviours, including habitual substance use (Goldstein and Volkow, 2011; Gilmore et al., under review).

Of relevance is that acute and chronic stress activates several neurotransmitter systems and neuroendocrine axes. Research to date has focused predominantly on the hypothalamic–pituitary–adrenal (HPA) axis, extra-hypothalamic corticotropin-releasing factor (CRF), and the noradrenergic system, all of which are involved in the pathophysiology of the stress response, PTSD, and AOD use disorders (Brady and Sinha, 2005; Norman et al., 2012b; Stephens and Wand, 2012). Stressors, including the physiologic stress invoked by AOD use and withdrawal, activate the HPA axis, resulting in the release of a succession of hormones including CRF, adrenocorticotropic hormone (ACTH), and glucocorticoids, including cortisol. Excess cortisol normally binds to glucocorticoid receptors to terminate the stress response and maintain homeostasis. Both PTSD and AOD use disorders have been associated with dysregulation of this negative-feedback loop, leading to elevated levels of CRF and cortisol, and hypersensitivity of glucocorticoid receptors (Stephens and Wand, 2012). Elevated levels of CRF have been implicated in the pathophysiology of Anxiety, Affective, and AOD use disorders. Among people with PTSD, elevated CRF, particularly in the amygdala, has been shown to potentiate fear-related behavioural responses (for example, symptoms of hyperarousal). Increased cortisol also enhances the reinforcing properties of some drugs (and worsens the severity of withdrawal symptoms) through interactions with the dopaminergic reward pathway, functioning to perpetuate behaviours that will maintain high cortisol levels in a feed-forward system (that is, repeated AOD use) (Brady and Sinha, 2005; Coffey et al., 2008). These actions may, in turn, influence vulnerability to, and maintenance of, AOD use disorders. Glucocorticoids are also implicated in the promotion of habit-based learning, through their impact on the hippocampus, amygdala, and prefrontal cortex. Alterations in the biological mechanisms described help to explain attempts to self-medicate PTSD symptoms in those with AOD use disorders, increases in vulnerability to the development of AOD use disorders, worsening of PTSD symptoms during withdrawal, and the difficulties experienced when trying to break the cycle.

Implementing trauma-informed care in AOD settings

The high rates of trauma exposure and PTSD among people with AOD use disorders, and the fundamental role that trauma symptoms may play in a person's recovery, have led experts to advocate for a "trauma-informed" approach to care provision (Elliott et al., 2005; Marsh et al., 2012). In relation to AOD services, trauma-informed care has been described as,

> a service delivery approach whereby programs, (i) recognise the high rates of exposure to trauma in the patient populations they serve; and, (ii) provide a safe environment and services that accommodate the needs of patients presenting with a history of significant trauma.
>
> (Killeen et al., 2015: p.235)

It also involves understanding the potential impact of trauma on AOD services and the need to, "create treatment environments that are more healing and less retraumatising" (Killeen et al., 2015: p.235). At a minimum, all practitioners working with AOD clients should, (i) have an awareness of the extent of trauma exposure among their clients; (ii) understand the consequences of trauma exposure and its potential to impact on recovery; (iii) be able to recognise the signs and symptoms of PTSD and other trauma-related disorders; and, (iv) integrate that knowledge into their practice (Mills, 2015).

Recognising the high rates of trauma exposure

It is recommended that practitioners and services operate on the assumption that all clients have experienced trauma, a "universal precautions" approach. However, this does not negate the need to assess clients individually, and trauma exposure should be routinely assessed by suitably trained practitioners. Incorporating some questioning into most initial assessments signals that this is a standard process important in both understanding why people present and in determining appropriate treatment pathways.

Prior to questioning in this area, practitioners should however seek the client's permission to do so. Trauma exposure and AOD use disorders are both characterised by a loss of control, and practitioners must do their best to help the client re-establish a sense of control, and to reduce the power imbalance inherent in the helper–helped relationship. Questioning also needs to be sensitive, and should not be pursued if the client does not wish to proceed (Marel et al., 2016). Practitioners should also clearly communicate the reasons for asking these questions. It may not be obvious to the client that gaining a better understanding of their history may help to contextualise their current situation, and inform their treatment planning, and they may not be aware of the potential interplay between trauma symptoms and AOD use (Elliott et al., 2005; Marsh et al., 2013).

Clients may also feel uncomfortable answering trauma-related questions due to their personal nature. Client discomfort may also be associated with distrust of others in general (and of service providers in particular), a history of having their boundaries violated, or fear that the information could be used against them (Elliott et al., 2005). Before conducting a trauma assessment, it is important to advise the client of any restrictions on confidentiality and acknowledge that talking about traumatic events can be distressing. Even clients who want to talk about their trauma history may underestimate the level of emotion involved (Najavits, 2004). However, studies have also found that although some people may become upset when talking about these events, talking about the trauma does not overwhelm or retraumatise the majority of people, and, on the contrary, most people describe the process as a positive experience (Jaffe et al., 2015).

It is also vitally important not to "dig" for information that is not forthcoming, as this may result in destabilisation (Najavits, 2004). For people who have experienced interpersonal trauma, pressure from an authority figure may imitate the interpersonal dynamics that were evident in an abusive relationship and exacerbate trauma symptoms. In some situations, it may be more beneficial to raise the issue of trauma some weeks after the initial assessment interview, once the client feels safer and a therapeutic relationship has been developed (Marsh et al., 2013).

Creating a safe environment

Creating a safe environment relates to both the physical setting and the atmosphere of a service. Physical surroundings, practitioner approaches, programs and procedures can all be modified to create a space that is safe and welcoming, and where the likelihood of re-traumatisation is minimised. A safe physical environment is one that is free from the risk of harm. It is one in which there is, (i) sufficient space for comfort and privacy; (ii) an absence of exposure to violent or sexual material (for example, magazines left in the waiting area, television programs or films viewed in common areas); and, (iii) sufficient staffing to monitor the behaviour of others that may be perceived as intrusive or harassing (Elliott et al., 2005). These needs cannot be over-emphasised for a client group with high rates of trauma exposure and related conditions, who are frequently hypervigilant, have significant issues with trust, and are prone to re-victimisation.

Practitioner approaches, programs, and procedures

Clients who have experienced trauma may be physically and mentally "on guard". Ensuring that clients have enough personal space, and the use of slow, calm movements, and a gentle tone of voice, may be useful in reducing this hypervigilance. It is also important to create an environment in which clients feel that, should they wish to, they can talk about their trauma, and their reactions to it, without judgment (Marel et al., 2016). People who have experienced trauma often feel a great deal of shame and guilt either in relation to the trauma itself or how they reacted to the trauma. Praising clients for their resilience in the face of adversity is important, even if past adaptations and ways of coping, such as AOD use, are now causing problems. Understanding AOD use as an adaptive response can help to reduce a client's guilt and shame, and provides a framework for developing new skills to better cope with symptoms (Elliott et al., 2005).

Many common procedures and practices used in AOD services may potentially retraumatise. For example, aggressive or confrontational group techniques can trigger memories of past abuse, are counterproductive, and may lead clients who have been exposed to trauma to revert to previous coping strategies, for example dissociating or shutting down, and further AOD use. This may then lead to the client being labelled as "treatment-resistant", with consequent feelings of failure and self-blame.

A structured program in which clients know what to expect can be particularly helpful for those experiencing hypervigilance (Marel et al., 2016). In addition, clients should be advised what to expect in terms of their progress through treatment. As previously noted, it is not uncommon for trauma symptoms to increase when substance use is reduced or ceased. Preparing the client for these reactions and normalising them may make them easier to manage. Psychoeducation about common reactions to trauma and symptom management has also been found to be of some benefit to AOD clients who have experienced trauma (Mills et al., 2014). Normalising symptoms may also help to alleviate some of the shame and guilt felt about not recovering from the trauma sooner.

If a client does become distressed by trauma symptoms, it is important that avoidance or suppression of thoughts or feelings is not encouraged, as avoidance symptoms, rather than re-experiencing symptoms, have been associated with the perpetuation of trauma-related symptoms (Pineles et al., 2011). Similarly, avoidance or suppression may also intensify feelings of guilt and shame. For those who have experienced abuse, it may closely re-enact the experience of being told to keep quiet about it (Elliott et al., 2005). This does not mean that clients should be pushed to revisit events or disclose information if they are not ready to do so. Rather, it means that it is understandable that the person may be upset by thoughts and feelings that may arise, and that they should be allowed to engage with them in order to help process the trauma emotionally (Marel et al., 2016). Ideally, clients will have developed good self-care skills, and will have skills to regulate their emotions, before they delve into their own traumatic experiences, or are exposed to the stories of others, however, choice and control should be left to the client (Elliott et al., 2005). Notwithstanding, even in the absence of details of a client's trauma, practitioners can assist them in the use of anxiety management techniques such as breathing retraining, progressive muscle relaxation, and grounding techniques, to help manage their symptoms (Marel et al., 2016).

Barriers to providing trauma-informed care

Despite its intuitive appeal, trauma-informed care has not been adopted in most AOD services. There are several reasons for this. First, despite the pervasiveness of trauma exposure and PTSD among AOD clients, and the potential impact on treatment, both are largely unrecognised at the service level. Very few services systematically assess for a history of trauma exposure among their clients, with most preferring to put the onus on the client to raise the issue. However, for a multitude of reasons, including shame and an inability to trust, most clients are unlikely to volunteer information about their past trauma experiences unless specifically asked (Schlenger et al., 2004).

The reluctance to assess for trauma is in large part related to concerns regarding client safety, specifically, fears regarding the ability of AOD clients to manage the emotions that may be elicited. Although well-intentioned, this practice is likely to be doing more harm than good; it is worth repeating that though some people may become upset when talking about these events, talking about the trauma does not overwhelm or retraumatise the majority of people, and most people describe the process as a positive experience, when it is conducted in an empathic manner.

Second, service providers are understandably concerned about their capacity to respond. Trauma training is not a core feature of most certification courses, and it is estimated that less than two-thirds of Australian AOD workers have undergone some form of trauma training (Ewer et al., 2015). There are also concerns regarding the potential impact of client trauma on the wellbeing of practitioners themselves. A survey of Australian AOD workers found that close to 20 per cent met criteria for secondary traumatic stress, also known as vicarious traumatisation. The symptoms of secondary traumatic stress mimic those of PTSD and relate to the emotional distress that arises from hearing firsthand about the trauma experiences of others. Importantly, the findings from this survey suggest that the likelihood of practitioners developing secondary traumatic stress can be reduced through the management of caseloads, and the provision of adequate and appropriate training and support (Ewer et al., 2015).

Finally, until recently, there was very little empirical evidence to guide treatment responses. There is, however, a growing body of evidence that supports the use of integrated trauma treatments for PTSD and AOD use disorders; that is, the treatment of both disorders at the same time by the same clinician (Killeen et al., 2015; Roberts et al., 2015).

A vignette – "Julie"

Julie, 33, presented to her local AOD service, seeking to undertake withdrawal, with a view to entering a residential rehabilitation program. She first started using cannabis at 13, before experimenting with a range of other drugs. By her early 20s, Julie was using both cannabis and heroin every day. She had completed year 12 with average grades, but, because of her drug use, had not been able to hold down a job. Although Julie had achieved brief periods of abstinence over the years, she had difficulty maintaining this over the long-term.

Following admission, Julie underwent a standard intake assessment and a routine case formulation. During the assessment, she was asked whether she had ever experienced any traumatic events in her life. Julie reported several assaults, including rape, in the context of her drug use, as well as having been a passenger in a car accident in which her boyfriend was killed. Although Julie had talked about the assaults and the accident with police, she had never sought any counselling. In fact, she said that she tried not to think or talk about these events.

Julie's case manager organised a follow-up appointment with one of the service psychologists the next day to undertake a more comprehensive assessment of Julie's mental health. The psychologist explained that she was hoping to get a better understanding of the impact of these traumatic events on her life, emphasising that Julie did not have to talk about anything that she did not want to, and could take a break at any time. Julie agreed to the assessment but didn't feel that there was much to tell; Julie initially reported experiencing only a few PTSD symptoms in relation to these events. Later in the session though, given the opportunity to talk about her childhood, Julie revealed that she had thought that many of her symptoms were a result of something else: she reported having been sexually abused by a relative over several years from the age of 12, after which she started using marijuana. This was the first time Julie had disclosed the trauma to anyone, apart from her mother, who had not believed her; Julie sobbed, and the psychologist just sat quietly with her. The psychologist thought that her mother's refusal to believe Julie might be an important source of additional trauma, and that her psychologist "bearing witness" to both the trauma and the betrayal was an important part of the treatment. Julie went on to say that the sexual abuse had a profound effect on her ability to maintain relationships.

When asked whether she noticed any change in her symptoms in relation to changes in her drug use, she stated that this was one of the most challenging aspects of staying drug-free. The psychologist normalised these reactions and encouraged her to talk with ward staff if she was having difficulty managing them. Julie also gave permission for the psychologist to let the other ward staff know that her symptoms might get worse during withdrawal because she had used drugs to help her cope with a range of traumatic experiences, and to be mindful of this. The psychologist also went through some anxiety management techniques with Julie, and organised for a follow-up appointment, to further discuss her trauma, if she wanted to, and to let her know that therapy after withdrawal would be very important, and to discuss referral pathways with her.

Trauma-focused treatment for PTSD and AOD use disorders

Some practitioners maintain the view that where trauma symptoms are accompanied by an AOD use disorder, the client's substance use must be treated first, and a significant period of abstinence achieved, prior to the commencement of trauma-focused treatment. In practice, however, this approach can lead to clients being moved between services, with little coordination of care, and the real possibility of clients "falling between the cracks" of the health system. It is important to recognise that although ongoing AOD use may impede therapy, it is not necessary to achieve abstinence before the commencement of PTSD treatment, and improvements can be obtained even in the presence of continued AOD use (Mills et al., 2012).

A growing number of psychotherapeutic interventions have been developed for the treatment of comorbid PTSD and AOD use over the last few decades. Existing approaches may be divided into either "past-focused" or "present-focused" therapies. Past-focused therapies include the use of exposure techniques in which the client is re-introduced to memories of previous traumas and are delivered individually. Present-focused therapies involve teaching clients coping skills to help them better manage their trauma symptoms in the present without revisiting the traumatic memory and may be delivered in either individual or group format. It is important to note that any treatment offered should come from a non-judgmental, sensitive and understanding perspective, regardless of focus.

A recent Cochrane review concluded that individual past-focused psychological interventions delivered alongside AOD treatment can reduce PTSD severity and AOD use, but that there is very little evidence to support the use of present-focused individual or group-based interventions (Roberts et al., 2015). Exposure-based treatments have long been considered the "gold standard" in treating PTSD, but these treatments were historically considered to be inappropriate for people with AOD use disorders, based on the belief that the emotions experienced may be overwhelming, and could lead to increased substance use. Evidence suggests that this is not the case: exposure therapy does not lead to an exacerbation of AOD use or the associated harms (Van Minnen et al., 2012, 2015), and has been shown to be protective with regards to relapse among people with Alcohol Use Disorders six months post-treatment (Foa et al., 2013).

Clinical researchers have also begun investigating the efficacy of integrated exposure-based programs that address PTSD and AOD use simultaneously. Typically, this involves psychoeducation regarding each disorder and their interrelatedness, coping skills training, relapse prevention work, and imaginal and/or in vivo exposure (that is, exposure to memories and physical reminders of the trauma, respectively). Support for these programs is growing, with an increasing number of studies providing evidence for their safety and efficacy. Participants in these studies have not demonstrated a worsening of symptoms or high rates of relapse. On the contrary, they demonstrated improvements in relation to both AOD use and PTSD outcomes.

Two of these studies, both randomised controlled trials, have been conducted in Australia. Mills and colleagues examined the efficacy of an integrated therapy called, "Concurrent Treatment of PTSD and Substance Use Disorders Using Prolonged Exposure" (COPE) among individuals with a range of AOD use disorders (Mills et al., 2012). Individuals randomised to receive COPE alongside treatment as usual for their AOD use demonstrated significantly greater reductions in PTSD severity compared with those randomised to receive treatment as usual for their AOD use alone (a 16.09 difference in change scores on the Clinician Administered PTSD Scale, with 49 per cent demonstrating a reliable and clinically significant reduction in PTSD symptoms), and this reduction in PTSD symptoms was accompanied by significant reductions in AOD use and severity of dependence. Also studying concurrent PTSD and Alcohol Use, Sannibale and colleagues compared the efficacy of Cognitive Behavioural Therapy (CBT) targeted at both PTSD and Alcohol Use with CBT targeted at Alcohol Use alone, in conjunction with supportive counselling (Sannibale et al., 2013). Participants who had received one or more sessions of Exposure Therapy for the PTSD component exhibited a two-fold greater rate of clinically significant change in PTSD severity compared with those who did not receive exposure therapy.

Conclusion

There is a clear need for AOD services to adopt a trauma-informed approach to the provision of treatment. A history of trauma exposure is more common than not among clients of these services, and, for many, this exposure is integrally linked to their AOD use. The reluctance of services to address trauma in their clients stems from valid concerns regarding client and practitioner safety, and a previous lack of evidence-based treatments to guide best practice. However, research in this area has grown substantially in recent years, highlighting the importance of addressing trauma among AOD clients and demonstrating the efficacy of trauma-focused treatments. It is the opinion of the authors that, by providing a supportive, trauma-informed model of care, and trauma-specific treatments, the outcomes for clients, and the health of the AOD workforce, may be substantially improved.

References

Anda RF, Felitti VJ, Bremner JD, et al. (2006) The enduring effects of abuse and related adverse experiences in childhood. *European Archives of Psychiatry and Clinical Neuroscience* 256: 174–186.

Barrett EL, Teesson M, Chapman C, et al. (2015) Substance use and mental health consequences of childhood trauma: An epidemiological investigation. *Drug and Alcohol Dependence* 146: e217–e218.

Brady KT and Sinha R (2005) Co-occurring mental and substance use disorders: The neurobiological effects of chronic stress. *American Journal of Psychiatry* 162: 1483–1493.

Chapman C, Mills K, Slade T, et al. (2012) Remission from posttraumatic stress disorder in the general population. *Psychological Medicine* 42: 1695–1703.

Cloitre M, Courtois CA, Charuvastra A, et al. (2011) Treatment of complex PTSD: Results of the ISTSS expert clinician survey on best practices. *Journal of Traumatic Stress* 24: 615–627.

Coffey SF, Read JP and Norberg MM (2008) Posttraumatic stress disorder and substance use disorder: Neuroimaging, neuroendocrine, and psychophysiological findings. In: Stewart SH and Conrod PJ (eds) *Anxiety and Substance Use Disorders*. Boston, MA: Springer, pp.37–57.

Darke S (2013) Pathways to heroin dependence: Time to re-appraise self-medication. *Addiction* 108: 659–667.

De Bellis MD (2002) Developmental traumatology: A contributory mechanism for alcohol and substance use disorders. *Psychoneuroendocrinology* 27: 155–170.

Dore G, Mills K, Murray R, et al. (2012) Posttraumatic stress disorder, depression and suicidality in inpatients with substance use disorders. *Drug and Alcohol Review* 31: 294–302.

Dube SR, Anda RF, Felitti VJ, et al. (2002) Adverse childhood experiences and personal alcohol abuse as an adult. *Addictive Behaviors* 27: 713–725.

Dube SR, Felitti VJ, Dong M, et al. (2003) Childhood abuse, neglect, and household dysfunction and the risk of illicit drug use: The Adverse Childhood Experiences study. *Pediatrics* 111: 564–572.

Dube SR, Miller JW, Brown DW, et al. (2006) Adverse childhood experiences and the association with ever using alcohol and initiating alcohol use during adolescence. *Journal of Adolescent Health* 38(4): 444.e1–10.

Elliott DE, Bjelajac P, Fallot RD, et al. (2005) Trauma-informed or trauma-denied: Principles and implementation of trauma-informed services for women. *Journal of Community Psychology* 33: 461–477.

Ewer PL, Teesson M, Sannibale C, et al. (2015) The prevalence and correlates of secondary traumatic stress among alcohol and other drug workers in Australia. *Drug and Alcohol Review* 34: 252–258.

Foa EB, Yusko DA, McLean CP, et al. (2013) Concurrent naltrexone and prolonged exposure therapy for patients with comorbid alcohol dependence and PTSD: A randomized clinical trial. *JAMA* 310(5): 488–495. doi:10.1001/jama.2013.8268.

Gilmore A, Bountress K, Barrett E, et al. (under review) Drug and alcohol abuse. In: Nemeroff CB and Marmar CR (eds) *Posttraumatic Stress Disorder*. New York, NY: Oxford University Press.

Goldstein RZ and Volkow ND (2011) Dysfunction of the prefrontal cortex in addiction: Neuroimaging findings and clinical implications. *Nature Reviews Neuroscience* 12: 652–669.

Goodhew M, Salmon AM, Marel C, et al. (2016) Mental health among clients of the Sydney Medically Supervised Injecting Centre (MSIC). *Harm Reduction Journal* 13: 29.

Hien DA, Jiang H, Campbell AN, et al. (2010) Do treatment improvements in PTSD severity affect substance use outcomes? A secondary analysis from a randomized clinical trial in NIDA's Clinical Trials Network. *The American Journal of Psychiatry* 167: 95–101.

Jaffe AE, DiLillo D, Hoffman L, et al. (2015) Does it hurt to ask? A meta-analysis of participant reactions to trauma research. *Clinical Psychology Review* 40: 40–56.

Kelly J, Harrison R and Palmer A (2016) Trauma and youth alcohol and drug use: Findings from a youth outpatient treatment service. *Journal of Applied Youth Studies* 1: 58–76.

Kessler RC, McLaughlin KA, Green JG, et al. (2010) Childhood adversities and adult psychopathology in the WHO World Mental Health Surveys. *The British Journal of Psychiatry* 197: 378–385.

Killeen TK, Back SE and Brady KT (2015) Implementation of integrated therapies for comorbid posttraumatic stress disorder and substance use disorders in community substance abuse treatment programs. *Drug and Alcohol Review* 34: 234–241.

Kingston REF, Marel C and Mills KL (2017) A systematic review of the prevalence of comorbid mental health disorders in people presenting for substance use treatment in Australia. *Drug and Alcohol Review* 36(4): 527–539.

Lee K, Harrison K, Mills K, et al. (2014) Needs of Aboriginal Australian women with comorbid mental and alcohol and other drug use disorders. *Drug and Alcohol Review* 33: 473–481.

Marel C, Mills K, Kingston R, et al. (2016) *Guidelines on the Management of Co-occurring Alcohol and Other Drug and Mental Health Conditions in Alcohol and Other Drug Treatment Settings, Second Edition*. Sydney, Australia: National Drug and Alcohol Research Centre.

Marsh A, Towers T and O'Toole S (2012) *Trauma-informed Treatment Guide for Working with Women with Alcohol and Other Drug Issues, Second Edition*. Perth, Australia: Improving Services for Women with Drug and Alcohol and Mental Health Issues and their Children Project.

Marsh A, O'Toole S, Dale A, et al. (2013) *Counselling Guidelines: Alcohol and Other Drug Issues, Third Edition*. Perth, Australia: Western Australia Alcohol and Drug Authority.

Mersky J, Topitzes J and Reynolds A (2013) Impacts of adverse childhood experiences on health, mental health, and substance use in early adulthood: A cohort study of an urban, minority sample in the US. *Child Abuse and Neglect* 37: 917–925.

Mills K, Teesson M, Ross J, et al. (2008) Predictors of trauma and PTSD among heroin users: A prospective longitudinal investigation. *Journal of Drug Issues* 38: 585–600.

Mills KL (2015) The importance of providing trauma-informed care in alcohol and other drug services. *Drug and Alcohol Review* 34: 231–233.

Mills KL, Ewer P, Dore G, et al. (2014) The feasibility and acceptability of a brief intervention for clients of substance use services experiencing symptoms of post traumatic stress disorder. *Addictive Behaviors* 39: 1094–1099.

Mills KL, Lynskey M, Teesson M, et al. (2005) Post-traumatic stress disorder among people with heroin dependence in the Australian treatment outcome study (ATOS): Prevalence and correlates. *Drug and Alcohol Dependence* 77: 243–249.

Mills KL, Teesson M, Back SE, et al. (2012) Integrated exposure-based therapy for co-occurring posttraumatic stress disorder and substance dependence: A randomized controlled trial. *Journal of the American Medical Association* 308: 690–699.

Mills KL, Teesson M, Ross J, et al. (2007) The impact of posttraumatic stress disorder on treatment outcomes for heroin dependence. *Addiction* 102: 447–454.

Mills KL, Teesson M, Ross J, et al. (2006) Trauma, PTSD, and substance use disorders: Findings from the Australian National Survey of Mental Health and Well-Being. *American Journal of Psychiatry* 163: 652–658.

Nadew GT (2012) Exposure to traumatic events, prevalence of posttraumatic stress disorder and alcohol abuse in Aboriginal communities. *Rural and Remote Health* 12: 1667.

Najavits LM (2004) Assessment of trauma, PTSD, and substance use disorder. In: Wilson J and Keane TM (eds) *Assessing Psychological Trauma and PTSD, Second Edition*. New York, NY: Guilford Press, pp.466–491.

Norman RE, Byambaa M, De R, et al. (2012a) The long-term health consequences of child physical abuse, emotional abuse, and neglect: A systematic review and meta-analysis. *PLOS Medicine* 9: e1001349.

Norman SB, Myers US, Wilkins KC, et al. (2012b) Review of biological mechanisms and pharmacological treatments of comorbid PTSD and substance use disorder. *Neuropharmacology* 62: 542–551.

Pineles SL, Mostoufi SM, Ready CB, et al. (2011) Trauma reactivity, avoidant coping, and PTSD symptoms: A moderating relationship? *Journal of Abnormal Psychology* 120: 240–246.

Read JP, Brown PJ and Kahler CW (2004) Substance use and posttraumatic stress disorders: Symptom interplay and effects on outcome. *Addictive Behaviors* 29: 1665–1672.

Roberts NP, Roberts PA, Jones N, et al. (2015) Psychological interventions for post-traumatic stress disorder and comorbid substance use disorder: A systematic review and meta-analysis. *Clinical Psychology Review* 38: 25–38.

Sannibale C, Teesson M, Creamer M, et al. (2013) Randomized controlled trial of cognitive-behaviour therapy for comorbid posttraumatic stress disorder and alcohol use disorders. *Addiction* 108(80): 1397–1410.

Schlenger WE, Jordan BK, Caddell JM, et al. (2004) Epidemiological methods for assessing trauma and PTSD. In: Wilson J and Keane TM (eds) *Assessing Psychological Trauma and PTSD, Second Edition*. New York, NY: Guilford Press, pp. 226–261.

Stephens MAC and Wand G (2012) Stress and the HPA axis: Role of glucocorticoids in alcohol dependence. *Alcohol Research: Current Reviews* 34: 468–484.

Van Minnen A, Harned M, Zoellner L, et al. (2012) Examining potential contra-indications for prolonged exposure therapy for PTSD. *European Journal of Psychotraumatology* 3:18805, doi:10.3402/ejpt.v3403i3400.18805.

Van Minnen A, Zoellner LA, Harned MS, et al. (2015) Changes in comorbid conditions after prolonged exposure for PTSD: A literature review. *Current Psychiatry Reports* 17: 1–16.

15 Biology and experience intertwined – trauma, neglect and physical health

Johanna Lynch and Anna Luise Kirkengen

While they treat the body as something that is alive, they persist in ignoring the body as something that is lived.

Gary Kielhofner, 1995, p.36

Introduction

The physical body can no longer be considered separate to the mind. Transdisciplinary research into physiological responses to threat and the impact of life experiences and relationships on brain structure and function, psychology and behaviour, reveals the intertwined nature of biology and lived-experience.

Modern biomedical scientific method is however still impacted by classical Greek notions of the mind–body divide. This has led to reductionistic specialised fields of study that often ignore salient information such as context, relationships, memories, meaning and sense of self. This dualist scientific philosophy has so impacted biomedical approaches to care that key aspects of the whole person often remain unacknowledged in everyday clinical practice. Even Descartes – famous for his theory of "mind–body dualism", the notion that the mind and body are quite separate – acknowledged the link between mind and body in a more intentional way than much of modern day biomedical science (Duncan, 2000). Recent research in attachment and interpersonal neurobiology, psychophysiology and psychoneuroimmunology clearly demonstrate how biology and experience can be integrated and understood.

This chapter aims to demonstrate that experiences, whether relational, cultural, spiritual or physical, influence each person's bodily health. Physiological stress can be evoked by real or perceived threat to integrity (McEwen, 1998), or by toxic stress, "associated with excessive, persistent, and/or uncontrollable adversity, without the buffering protection of stable adult support" (Shonkoff et al., 2009: p.2255). Building on extensive transdisciplinary knowledge, this chapter seeks to redirect the medical gaze towards the impact of lifetime adversity and social disadvantage on physical health (Reeve, 2010).

Adverse Childhood Experiences study

Paradigm-shifting research that has become known as the Adverse Childhood Experiences (ACE) study has identified a dose-dependent impact of childhood adversity on physical health (Felitti et al., 1998; Anda et al., 2006). This large epidemiological study grew out of the observation that a subset of people who regained weight after successfully losing weight had significant childhood maltreatment histories. This led to the inclusion of retrospective questions about eight and later ten categories of childhood adversity in a preventative health survey of 17,000 insured, middle-class respondents from San Diego in the USA. These categories included physical, emotional and sexual abuse, physical and emotional neglect, divorce or loss of a biological parent, alcoholism or drug use in the home, incarceration of a household member, depression or mental illness in the home and mother being treated violently. The respondents were assigned an ACE score – the number of different types of ACEs they had experienced – and monitored prospectively from 1995 using health outcome data from hospital discharges, doctor office visits, emergency room visits and the National Death Index. The results revealed an equal impact of each type of ACE, and higher than expected prevalence of each category: while one third of the population had no ACEs, half the population had between one and three ACEs, and one sixth of the population had four or more ACEs (Felitti and Anda, 2015). Clinicians will, therefore, very frequently see patients who have been subject to multiple adverse experiences in childhood.

The ACE study further demonstrated direct links between childhood adversity and risks to adult health, independent of behavioural risk factors, including cardiovascular disease, chronic lung disease, stroke, diabetes and cancer. The number of medically unexplained symptoms also increased in a dose-dependent relationship with ACEs. Behaviours that influence health – that are often ways to manage affect dysregulation and provide short-term stress relief – also increased significantly with the ACE score. These behaviours include smoking, alcohol and drug use, suicidality, promiscuity, broken relationships, and workforce absenteeism. The incidence of Depression, suicide attempts, impaired memory of childhood, hallucinations, and use of anxiolytic and antidepressant medications were also increased, so much so that Felitti and Anda stated, "It appears inescapable that a major portion of Depression and attempted suicide can be traced back to 10 categories of traumatising life experiences in childhood" (2015: p.209). Premature mortality was also clearly documented in those who had adverse childhood experiences, for example, up to 20 years less in those who had six or more ACEs (Felitti et al., 1998). These findings illustrate that clinicians need to be aware that life experiences and family environment, including neglect, impact significantly on health.

Australian studies confirm the prevalence of ACEs (Australian Institute of Health and Welfare, 2010), and the impact on physical health and behaviours. Reeve and Gool, using stringent measures of abuse, concluded that 15.5 per cent of those surveyed aged 16–85 were either physically or sexually abused in childhood (Reeve and Gool, 2013). They confirmed that abuse directly and indirectly increases rates of physical and mental illness, attempted suicide, alcoholism, drug use and overall health care costs. This study also confirmed the compounding effect of abuse, finding that those who had been both physically and sexually abused suffered the most with respect to both health conditions and health care costs. It should be noted that rates of emotional abuse and neglect were not measured in this study.

Research in this field has dramatically increased over the last 20 years, resulting in important shifts in understanding across many disciplines, requiring clinicians to acknowledge the link between adverse early experience and physical health (Charney et al., 1998; Perry and Pollard, 1998; Schore, 2001, 2006; Bremner, 2006; Van der Kolk, 2014).

Attachment research and interpersonal neurobiology

Cozolino (2006) has referred to the body's intricate interconnections with others through relationships as the "social synapse". From the existence of mirror neurones to evidence of failure to thrive in the face of emotional neglect, extensive research in this area has established that the quality of caregiving relationships in both childhood and adulthood affect the development, structure and function of the brain, immune function, autonomic nervous system, neuroendocrinological systems, procedural memory, sensory awareness of the self, and cortical capacity to down-regulate or soothe emotion. The experience of toxic stress in childhood contributes to a loss of synaptic connectivity and neuronal survival, causing significant disorganisation and loss of function (Perry et al., 1995). These changes impair affect regulation, and access to language and reason in day-to-day decision making (Teicher et al., 2016).

Attachment research and interpersonal neurobiology, enhanced by functional neuroimaging, have further established the effect of relationships on the body, especially in childhood. There are direct links between the experience of relationships and multiple physical health outcomes. This includes the impact of attachment on the experience of pain (Meredith et al., 2008), wound healing (Gouin and Kiecolt-Glaser, 2011), Depression (Burnette et al., 2009), Ischaemic Heart Disease (Anda et al., 1993) and experience-dependent brain maturation (Schore, 1996, 2001). Shonkoff and colleagues have extended this concept, viewing many adult diseases as developmental disorders that began in the context of toxic stress in childhood, and call for an "ecobiodevelopmental" framework that would encourage clinicians to be aware of the impact of childhood experiences on health (Shonkoff et al., 2012).

Van der Kolk summarises the impact of these attachment effects, "If you feel safe and loved, your brain becomes specialised in exploration, play and cooperation. If you are frightened and unwanted, it specialises in managing feelings of fear and abandonment" (Van der Kolk, 2014: p.56). This specialisation of function affects the capacity for an individual to adapt, access memory, integrate information, self-regulate and respond appropriately in day-to-day functioning. It also affects the capacity to trust – including health care professionals.

Psychophysiology

Each person uses their senses and autonomic nervous system to monitor the internal and external environment for danger and safety and to respond appropriately, the concept of neuroception (Porges, 2011). This monitoring feeds back to the hypothalamic–pituitary–adrenal (HPA) axis, sympathetic–adrenal–medullary (SAM) axis, and the immune system, impacting neurological, endocrine and metabolic systems. Sensory awareness can be dysregulated and disorganised by experiences of trauma and neglect. Sensation can be heightened and reactivated, or numbed and disconnected (Van der Kolk, 2014). Heightened sensation increases somatic awareness, and symptomatic and often unexplained presentations to medical care (Kirkengen et al., 1993; Maunder and Hunter, 2009). Numbness and experiences of emptiness and bodily inattention can alternately cause late presentation for medical care, loss of sense of agency and purpose (Van der Kolk, 2014), risk-taking, self-harming and often unnoticed physiological stress.

Toxic stress can also dysregulate homeostasis of the sympathetic and parasympathetic autonomic nervous systems. The sympathetic nervous system increases focused attention, movement and energy production, while the parasympathetic system encourages sleep, digestion, recuperation, cortical integration and social communication (Porges, 2011). Without parasympathetic modulation, the sympathetic system remains, "primed for threat and reacting to danger long since over" (Ogden et al., 2006: p.21). The parasympathetic system can be mobilised to "brake" the sympathetic system. In overwhelming situations, this brake can also cause "freeze" states, as explained by Porges' Polyvagal Theory. Although these states do have acute survival value, their interruption of neurological connections, sensations, memories, and the sense of self can cause long-term impacts on a person's life. Finally, the parasympathetic "social engagement system", involving the cranial nerves and the ventral vagus, is a vital part of the autonomic system response to threat (Porges, 2011). This system tunes into potential risk in the social environment, noticing the unconscious and nonverbal social cues of phonation and prosody, eye gaze, facial expression, neck orientation and tilting gestures of others. Disruption of this social engagement system may also have significant long-term impacts (Scaer, 2014).

When a person experiences toxic stress, their sympathetic nervous system can be intensely or chronically activated without the mediation of the parasympathetic system. This loss of autonomic nervous system modulation and sensory awareness can cause people to remain chronically alarmed, to find it difficult to accurately assess safety, to develop trauma-related altered states of consciousness (Frewen et al., 2015) and sensory fragments (including flashbacks and somatic experiences), and to have reduced expectation of reward (Teicher and Samson, 2016). This loss of awareness diminishes the capacity for self-soothing and the ability to soothe dependents. Other forms of soothing may be used, such as disconnection and distraction in its various forms, in a behavioural and often addictive attempt to cope with inner experience. Autonomic dysregulation may also underlie vascular, digestive, fatigue and musculoskeletal pain syndromes (Scaer, 2014).

Psychoneuroimmunology and metabolism

In a healthy person, glucocorticoids influence neurogenesis, myelination and neuronal synapse formation and maturation. Adaptive release of glucose gives energy for fight or flight responses, increases vigilance, attention and learning (Lupien et al., 2009), and buffers mitochondria against early apoptosis (Picard et al., 2014). When under stress, this system becomes dysregulated both directly, and indirectly through coping behaviours such as abuse of substances and medications. Researchers in this area use the term "allostatic load" to measure anything that affects the stability of the organism through change (Kirkengen and Lygre, 2015). Allostatic overload causes "multisystem physiological dysregulation" (Wiley et al., 2016) and disrupts the exquisitely balanced interactions between metabolic, endocrine, neurological and immune systems. The experience of chronic threat overwhelms these usually adaptive regulatory allostatic systems of the body causing physiological wear and tear, "weathering" (Geronimus et al., 2006), that silently impacts morbidity and mortality over a person's lifetime (Juster et al., 2011).

Experiences that disrupt homeostasis also affect the immune system (Fagundes et al., 2013; Straub, 2015), impacting inflammatory, infectious, mitotic (cancer) and autoimmune processes, including pro- and anti-inflammatory cytokines. The impact on the HPA and SAM axes disrupts metabolic function, cortisol levels and circulating glucose levels, directly increasing metabolic diseases such as Diabetes, Hypertension and Obesity. Prolonged elevation of glucocorticoids can cause metabolic oversupply, oxidative stress, systemic inflammation, telomere shortening, changes in "mitochondrial energetics" (Shaughnessy et al., 2014), epigenetic changes and premature cell death (Picard et al., 2014). Prolonged exposure to glucocorticoids has also been found to be neurotoxic (Gilbertson et al., 2002) and to contribute to aging (Sapolsky et al., 1986). Monoamine neurotransmitter regulation is affected (Cicchetti et al., 2007), impacting mood and dopaminergic responses to reward and to drugs of abuse (Anda et al., 2006; Lupien et al., 2009). Stress researchers from Selye (1956) to those working in the field of psychoneuroimmunology (Fleshner and Laudenslager, 2004) and other transdisciplinary fields (Juster et al., 2010) have confirmed the dysregulating impact of stressful experience on physiology and, therefore, health.

A vignette – "Carly"

Carly, a 42-year-old woman, presented to a new General Practitioner (GP) for a repeat prescription of her antidepressant. She said she had changed GPs because she thought her last GP was "sick of her coming" with pains for which no cause could be found, and she was hoping a new GP might help her find out what was "actually wrong" with her. She had already had multiple investigations for chest pain, muscle aches and pains, and dermatitis. Carly had been on a Selective Serotonin Reuptake Inhibitor form of antidepressant for 20 years for "Generalised Anxiety Disorder", and said it worked most of the time, but she felt it had increased her weight by 20 kilograms. She also said that all of the different medications she had been prescribed in the past had given her side effects. She gave a history of abdominal pain and intermittent diarrhoea since childhood, which had worsened at the time of her divorce 10 years ago when she was diagnosed with "Irritable Bowel Syndrome". Carly has several obsessive rituals that have annoyed other people who have lived with her over the years, and she now lives alone. She also has limited contact with her parents or younger brother as she gets very distressed when she sees them.

After building a relationship with Carly, her new GP asked her gently about her abdominal symptoms, and she described experiencing pain and tightness in her abdomen, even as a child, especially when she heard her father's unsteady alcoholic steps in the hallway, or when she felt she had let her mother or brother down when she couldn't protect them from her father's rages. She remembered being able to lessen her fear if she hid under the bed, or if she counted in sevens, and checked that her door was locked repeatedly. At present she finds living alone, her predictable job as an accountant, and comfort eating help to ease her distress.

Comprehensive assessment and family intervention as best practice

Traditional division of medical care into physical and psychological systems has not served patients well, especially those who have experienced the trauma of abuse and neglect. The terms "psychological" or "somatoform" should not in fact apply, since trauma is experienced concurrently in the whole person. As experts in this field have concluded, the divide between psychological and physical trauma is an illusion (Fleshner and Laudenslager, 2004). Human beings are organisms that embody and organise meaning-filled life stories, not just machines needing technical repair, and they cannot be reduced to organ-centric care without significantly decreasing the quality of the care provided. As such, there is an evidence-based ethical duty for medical professionals to regard the body as embedded in context, experience, relationships, emotions, thoughts and beliefs, and to attend to the whole person (Kirkengen and Thornquist, 2012). This approach needs to become best practice in all medical encounters, and if implemented has the potential to increase the person's understanding of their intuitive responses to their experiences and the subsequent impact of those experiences on their health. A thoughtful, trauma-aware approach also has the potential to assist in the coordination of care and to reduce health costs overall.

Because the mind and the body are so closely connected, and because trauma and forms of neglect are so common, all general health assessments need to be comprehensive and should be carried out under circumstances that allow for such complexity. This must involve creating an environment that helps reduce vigilance and facilitates disclosure, while offering the time and the safety required to do so. Approaches to the person should aim at listening intently and appraising a person's life story, their inner experience of threat and their relationships as part of the health care process. Understanding the link between life experience, bodily sensations and health may help those who minimise and ignore their physical experiences, and often avoid medical care, as well as those who are hypersensitive and vigilant about each physical sensation and seek medical attention and reassurance more often. Childhood maltreatment does increase adult multimorbidity, and therefore the clinician needs to educate and care for the whole person (England-Mason et al., 2018).

Assessment of those with a known trauma history, especially those who have experienced multigenerational trauma, dispossession or dislocation, such as Indigenous peoples and refugees, should also always include a full physical assessment. This should include vigilance for metabolic dysregulation, including awareness of blood pressure, weight, lipids, blood glucose and endocrine markers. Renal, cardiac and liver function also need to be considered, along with the potential for increased allergic, infectious or autoimmune processes. This involves paying attention to skin, teeth and hair, as well as musculoskeletal symptoms. It is additionally important to screen for and raise awareness of the physical impact of addiction to nicotine, alcohol, drugs (both pharmaceutical and illicit), exercise, eating compulsions, risk-taking, promiscuity and other coping behaviours.

A comprehensive assessment for Carly may have decreased the need for numerous investigations of her abdominal pain and may have helped her understand her life story and its impact on her body. An increased awareness of the risk of autoimmune disease, infection, cancer, endocrine and metabolic dysregulation should also have been maintained. This would involve education about the link between her childhood experiences of chronic hypervigilance and allostatic overload, cortisol and glucose dysregulation, and even the "behavioural allostasis" of her overeating (Garner, 2013). This may in turn motivate her to manage her weight and exercise, and to learn the importance of self-soothing and regulating without using food (Ismail et al., 2004). She would also be more informed about her lifelong risk for end organ damage including Diabetes, cardiac and renal damage. It may also be appropriate, once a good therapeutic relationship is established, to normalise Carly's hypersensitivity to medications, and her musculoskeletal and abdominal symptoms as normal sensory and neurological responses to trauma.

Visible or hidden evidence of trauma and neglect

The health practitioner also needs to be aware of the risk to each person they care for of direct physical injury at the time of trauma in the form of head injuries, fractures, bruising, cuts, burns, anal prolapse, vaginal tears and even genital mutilation, including ritual mutilation in some ethnic groups. Direct impacts can also include sexually transmitted diseases, pelvic pain, infertility, pregnancy and coerced abortion. Neglect can also cause direct physical impacts in the form of malnutrition, failure to thrive, obesity, infections, tooth decay, and delayed presentation for medical help. Another direct form of neglect involves injury to the infant from drug and alcohol abuse, including the risk of preterm birth, perinatal complications, including withdrawal, the impact on infant mental health of chronic maternal distress, through to Foetal Alcohol Syndrome (Hillis et al., 2004).

Carly did not reveal any physical trauma or substance-induced trauma to her body, however clinicians need to maintain an awareness that the patient may have life experiences they are not yet feeling safe enough to disclose, and they may also have sensory flashbacks to past physical pain.

Awareness of the meaning and impact of coping mechanisms

In those unable to achieve physiological and relational respite from dysregulated emotions, compelling strategies for relief – addictions – can become dominant. These "tension reduction behaviours" (Briere et al., 2010: p.772), or strategies to decrease inner experiences of threat can include an intuitive physiological craving for forgetting, distracting, altered mood, risk-taking, relational closeness or distance, disconnection or dissociation from self, and driven behaviours, including self-analysis, perfectionism, and workaholism. Awareness of the impact of threat on coping behaviours could increase understanding between patient and clinician of underlying reasons for addictions and decrease the diagnosis of "comorbid" conditions. Practitioners also need to be aware that trauma and neglect can lead to use of psychoactive drugs that cause "pharmaceutical allostatic load" (Juster et al., 2011) and impact on attention, memory, executive function, energy, weight and quality of life (De Jonghe and Swinkels, 1992; Reynolds and Kirk, 2010). This may lead to more informed discussions with patients about risks and benefits of long-term pharmaceutical treatments.

Carly uses routine, social withdrawal, obsessive rituals and food to modulate her mood. She has also been on antidepressants for many years that may not be effective. An open discussion with her about the way her life story has impacted her capacity to manage her affect, psychoeducation about grounding and other sensorimotor approaches to manage distress, and referral for ongoing trauma-focused therapy with an appropriate clinician may all help Carly decrease her maladaptive ways of coping.

Family and intergenerational approaches to assessment, treatment and prevention of toxic stress

Understanding the role of the intergenerational transmission of adversity is an important element of trauma-informed care of families. As well as epigenetic influences of trauma, environmental and relational adversity can be transmitted within families. It helps to be aware that, "The family literally embodies the fear-filled experiences its members have also shared" (Karr-Morse, 2012: p.15).

This means that awareness of family context, the capacity of adults to offer safe relational soothing (including the role of grandparents), and parenting capacity is an essential part of any health assessment. This also includes screening of children, parenting training, family therapy, and support for the relational and sensorimotor needs of each person. Trauma-informed interventions in schools to decrease bullying (Scott et al., 2014) and education that is designed to protect brain function through kindness (Shonkoff, 2011) are also key population-based interventions. Trauma-informed public health surveillance (Anda et al., 2010) is also required. These early interventions, if implemented at a population level, will have an impact on adult health care utilisation, health and productivity. In fact, a number of authors have determined that no society can afford economically to ignore childhood adversity (Heckman, 2006; Knudsen et al., 2006). Family and school-based interventions may have offered hope, prevention and strategic early intervention to Carly, improving both her life story and her lifelong health.

Conclusion

Moving toward a trauma-informed clinical care paradigm with respect to physical health will require changes to health care policy, clinical training, funding models, and processes of assessment and treatment. A shift in the understanding of how biology and experience are intertwined would bring about radical changes in the approach to whole person care, towards more comprehensive assessments, and relational, sensorimotor, metabolic, and family-focused treatments. The importance of community-wide awareness and prevention programs that decrease adverse childhood experiences by providing intensive family support to those families in distress, and prioritising stable adoptive homes for foster children, cannot be overstated.

Rather than identifying a subset of people requiring trauma-informed care, this chapter suggests a shift in awareness of the impact of each person's life experiences on their physical health. Experiences of trauma and neglect are so highly prevalent in the community (Felitti et al., 1998), and contribute so much to multi-morbidity (Tomasdottir et al., 2015). Integration of trauma-informed care needs to be implemented across the community, impacting the whole health system (Anda et al., 2010).

At present, an understanding of the physiological importance of whole person care is not embedded in medical, nursing or allied health undergraduate or postgraduate training. Training will be required across disciplines and at multiple levels. Change will also require new approaches to remuneration that do not discourage time spent with the patient, and the development of systems that highly prioritise the care of families, parents and couples.

This focus on trauma-informed care is inspired by the new knowledge that embodied humans can heal through positive experiences and relationships, and the restoration of hope, and agency. Positive neuroplastic changes can be facilitated by restoration of a "visceral sense of control and safety" (Van der

Kolk, 2014: p.31), and the rehabilitation of personal integrity and selfhood that is central to health.

Some areas of health care already offer a holistic storied understanding of health, notably those arising from an Indigenous worldview where it has long been understood that a person's body cannot be separated from his or her life story. This holistic wisdom could inform best practice care for the traumatised. The unique privilege of every clinician is to acknowledge their patients as people who embody their own story within their families and community.

References

Australian Institute of Health and Welfare (2010) *Child Protection Australia 2008–2009, Child Welfare Series*. Canberra, Australia: Australian Institute of Health and Welfare.

Anda RF, Butchart A, Felitti VJ, et al. (2010) Building a framework for global surveillance of the public health implications of adverse childhood experiences. *American Journal of Preventive Medicine* 39(1): 93–98.

Anda RF, Felitti VJ, Bremner JD, et al. (2006) The enduring effects of abuse and related adverse experiences in childhood. *European Archives of Psychiatry and Clinical Neuroscience* 256(3): 174–186.

Anda RF, Williamson D, Jones D, et al. (1993) Depressed affect, hopelessness, and the risk of ischemic heart disease in a cohort of US adults. *Epidemiology* 4(4): 285–294.

Bremner JD (2006) Traumatic stress: Effects on the brain. *Dialogues in Clinical Neuroscience* 8(4): 445–461.

Briere J, Hodges N and Godbout N (2010) Traumatic stress, affect dysregulation, and dysfunctional avoidance. A structural equation model. *Journal of Traumatic Stress* 23(6): 767–774.

Burnette JL, Davis DE, Green JD, et al. (2009) Insecure attachment and depressive symptoms: The mediating role of rumination, empathy, and forgiveness. *Personality and Individual Differences* 46(3): 276–280.

Charney DS, Grillon C and Bremner JD (1998) Review: The neurobiological basis of anxiety and fear: Circuits, mechanisms, and neurochemical interactions. *The Neuroscientist* 4(1): 35–44.

Cicchetti D, Rogosch FA and Sturge-Apple ML (2007) Interactions of child maltreatment and serotonin transporter and monoamine oxidase A polymorphisms: Depressive symptomatology among adolescents from low socioeconomic status backgrounds. *Development and Psychopathology* 19(4): 1161–1180.

Cozolino L (2006) *The Neuroscience of Human Relationships. Attachment and the Developing Social Brain.* New York, NY: WW Norton and Company.

De Jonghe F and Swinkels J (1992) The safety of antidepressants. *Drugs* 43(2): 40–47.

Duncan G (2000) Mind-body dualism and the biopsychosocial model of pain: What did Descartes really say? *The Journal of Medicine and Philosophy* 25(4): 485–513.

England-Mason G, Casey R, Ferro M, et al. (2018) Child maltreatment and adult multimorbidity: Results from the Canadian Community Health Survey. *Canadian Journal of Public Health.* https://doi.org/10.17269/s41997-018-0069-y.

Fagundes CP, Glaser R and Kiecolt-Glaser JK (2013) Stressful early life experiences and immune dysregulation across the lifespan. *Brain, Behavior, and Immunity* 27: 8–12.

Felitti VJ, Anda RF, Nordenberg D, et al. (1998) Relationship of childhood abuse and household dysfunction to many of the leading causes of death in adults: The Adverse

Childhood Experiences (ACE) Study. *American Journal of Preventive Medicine* 14(4): 245–258.

Felitti VJ and Anda RF (2015) The lifelong effects of Adverse Childhood Experiences. In: Chadwick DL, Alexander R, Giardino AP, et al. (eds) *Chadwick's Childhood Maltreatment: Sexual Abuse and Psychological Maltreatment.* Saint Louis, MO: STM Learning Inc.

Fleshner M and Laudenslager ML (2004) Psychoneuroimmunology: Then and now. *Behavioral and Cognitive Neuroscience Reviews* 3(2): 114–130.

Frewen P, Hegadoren K, Coupland NJ, et al. (2015) Trauma related altered states of consciousness (TRASC) and functional Impairment I: Prospective study in acutely traumatized persons. *Journal of Trauma and Dissociation* 16(5): 500–519.

Garner AS (2013) Home visiting and the biology of toxic stress: Opportunities to address early childhood adversity. *Pediatrics* 132(Suppl 2): S65–73.

Geronimus AT, Hicken M, Keene D, et al. (2006) "Weathering" and age patterns of allostatic load scores among blacks and whites in the United States. *American Journal of Public Health* 96(5): 826–833.

Gilbertson MW, Shenton ME, Ciszewski A, et al. (2002) Smaller hippocampal volume predicts pathologic vulnerability to psychological trauma. *Nature Neuroscience* 5(11): 1242–1247.

Gouin J-P and Kiecolt-Glaser JK (2011) The impact of psychological stress on wound healing: Methods and mechanisms. *Immunology and Allergy Clinics of North America* 31 (1): 81–93.

Heckman JJ (2006) Skill formation and the economics of investing in disadvantaged children. *Science* 312(5782): 1900–1902.

Hillis SD, Anda RF, Dube SR, et al. (2004) The association between adverse childhood experiences and adolescent pregnancy, long-term psychosocial consequences, and fetal death. *Pediatrics* 113(2): 320–327.

Ismail K, Winkley K and Rabe-Hesketh S (2004) Systematic review and meta-analysis of randomised controlled trials of psychological interventions to improve glycaemic control in patients with type 2 diabetes. *The Lancet* 363(9421): 1589–1597.

Juster R-P, Bizik G, Picard M, et al. (2011) A transdisciplinary perspective of chronic stress in relation to psychopathology throughout life span development. *Development and Psychopathology* 23(03): 725–776.

Juster R-P, McEwen BS and Lupien SJ (2010) Allostatic load biomarkers of chronic stress and impact on health and cognition. *Neuroscience and Biobehavioral Reviews* 35(1): 2–16.

Karr-Morse R (2012) *Scared Sick – the Role of Childhood Trauma in Adult Disease.* New York, NY: Basic Books.

Kielhofner G (1995) A meditation on the use of hands. *Scandinavian Journal of Occupational Therapy* 2(3–4): 153–166.

Kirkengen AL and Lygre H (2015) Exploring the relationship between childhood adversity and oral health: An anecdotal approach and integrative view. *Medical Hypotheses* 85(2): 134–140.

Kirkengen AL, Schei B and Steine S (1993) Indicators of childhood sexual abuse in gynaecological patients in a general practice. *Scandinavian Journal of Primary Health Care* 11(4): 276–280.

Kirkengen AL and Thornquist E (2012) The lived body as a medical topic: An argument for an ethically informed epistemology. *Journal of Evaluation in Clinical Practice* 18 (5): 1095–1101.

Knudsen EI, Heckman JJ, Cameron JL, et al. (2006) Economic, neurobiological, and behavioral perspectives on building America's future workforce. *Proceedings of the National Academy of Sciences* 103(27): 10155–10162.

Lupien SJ, McEwen BS, Gunnar MR, et al. (2009) Effects of stress throughout the lifespan on the brain, behaviour and cognition. *Nature Reviews Neuroscience* 10(6): 434–445.

McEwen BS (1998) Protective and damaging effects of stress mediators. *New England Journal of Medicine* 338(3): 171–179.

Maunder RG and Hunter JJ (2009) Assessing patterns of attachment in medical patients. *General Hospital Psychiatry* 31: 123–130.

Meredith P, Ownsworth T and Strong J (2008) A review of the evidence linking adult attachment theory and chronic pain: Presenting a conceptual model. *Clinical Psychology Review* 28(3): 407–429.

Ogden P, Minton K and Pain C (2006) *Trauma and the Body: A Sensorimotor Approach to Psychotherapy*. New York, NY: WW Norton and Co.

Perry BD, Pollard RA, Blakley TL, et al. (1995) Childhood trauma, the neurobiology of adaptation, and use dependent development of the brain: How states become traits. *Infant Mental Health Journal* 16(4): 271–291.

Perry BD and Pollard R (1998) Homeostasis, stress, trauma, and adaptation: A neurodevelopmental view of childhood trauma. *Child and Adolescent Psychiatric Clinics of North America* 7: 33–51.

Picard M, Juster R-P and McEwen BS (2014) Mitochondrial allostatic load puts the 'gluc' back in glucocorticoids. *Nature Reviews Endocrinology* 10(5): 303–310.

Porges SW (2011) *The Polyvagal Theory: Neurophysiological Foundations of Emotions, Attachment, Communication, and Self-regulation*. New York, NY: WW Norton and Co.

Reeve J (2010) Interpretive medicine: Supporting generalism in a changing primary care world. *Occasional Paper Royal College of General Practitioners* 88: 1–20.

Reeve R and Gool K (2013) Modelling the relationship between child abuse and long-term health care costs and wellbeing: Results from an Australian community-based survey. *Economic Record* 89(286): 300–318.

Reynolds GP and Kirk SL (2010) Metabolic side effects of antipsychotic drug treatment – pharmacological mechanisms. *Pharmacology and Therapeutics* 125(1): 169–179.

Sapolsky RM, Krey LC and McEwen BS (1986) The neuroendocrinology of stress and aging: The glucocorticoid cascade hypothesis. *Endocrine Reviews* 7(3): 284–301.

Scaer R (2014) *The Body Bears the Burden: Trauma, Dissociation, and Disease*. New York, NY: Routledge.

Schore AN (1996) The experience-dependent maturation of a regulatory system in the orbital prefrontal cortex and the origin of developmental psychopathology. *Development and Psychopathology* 8: 59–88.

Schore AN (2001) Effects of a secure attachment relationship on right brain development, affect regulation, and infant mental health. *Infant Mental Health Journal* 22(1–2): 7–66.

Scott JG, Moore SE, Sly PD, et al. (2014) Bullying in children and adolescents: A modifiable risk factor for mental illness. *Australian and New Zealand Journal of Psychiatry* 48(3): 209–212.

Selye H (1956) *The Stress of Life*. New York, NY: McGraw Hill.

Shaughnessy DT, McAllister K, Worth L, et al. (2014) Mitochondria, energetics, epigenetics, and cellular responses to stress. *Environmental Health Perspectives* 122(12): 1271.

Shonkoff JP (2011) Protecting brains, not simply stimulating minds. *Science* 333(6045): 982–983.

Shonkoff JP, Boyce WT and McEwen BS (2009) Neuroscience, molecular biology, and the childhood roots of health disparities: Building a new framework for health promotion and disease prevention. *Journal of the American Medical Association* 301(21): 2252–2259.

Shonkoff JP, Garner AS, Siegel BS, et al. (2012) The lifelong effects of early childhood adversity and toxic stress. *Pediatrics* 129(1): e232–e246.

Straub R (2015) *The Origin of Chronic Inflammatory Systemic Diseases and their Sequelae*. Waltham, MA: Academic Press.

Teicher MH and Samson JA (2016) Annual research review: Enduring neurobiological effects of childhood abuse and neglect. *Journal of Child Psychology and Psychiatry* 57(3): 241–266.

Teicher MH, Samson JA, Anderson CM, et al. (2016) The effects of childhood maltreatment on brain structure, function and connectivity. *Nature Reviews Neuroscience* 17(10): 652–666.

Tomasdottir MO, Sigurdsson JA, Petursson H, et al. (2015) Self reported childhood difficulties, adult multimorbidity and allostatic load. A cross-sectional analysis of the Norwegian HUNT study. *PLOS One* 10(6): e0130591.

Van der Kolk B (2014) *The Body Keeps the Score*. New York, NY: Viking.

Wiley JF, Gruenewald TL, Karlamangla AS, et al. (2016) Modeling multisystem physiological dysregulation. *Psychosomatic Medicine* 78(3): 290–301.

Part III

Individual treatment approaches

16 Sequenced relationship-based treatment for Complex Traumatic Stress Disorders

Christine A Courtois and Julian D Ford

Introduction

Complex Trauma refers to traumatic stressors that are complicated by a number of factors that differentiate them from single event or short-term exposures (Cook et al., 2005; Ford, 2017a). This statement should not be taken to minimise single event trauma as it is recognised that its occurrence and impact can be at extreme levels of severity, danger, and life threat. Traumatic events may have particularly complex sequelae, however, when they involve interpersonal causation with deliberate and often premeditated acts of physical and emotional intrusion and coercion, exploitation, assault, and when violence is perpetrated on the victim by another person, group of people, or organisation. A younger age of onset of victimisation, greater difference in age between victim and perpetrator, and closer degree of relatedness between them (for example, perpetration of harm or a failure to protect from harm by parents and others known to or related to the victim, and by those from whom he or she would normally expect safety and protection) add the dimension of interpersonal betrayal and predict greater severity of traumatic impact (Becker-Blease and Freyd, 2005).

Complex Trauma involves forms of assault and ongoing threats of danger that are chronic, ever-present, and usually inescapable. They may also escalate in severity over time. For example, sexual abuse that begins with grooming and fondling may escalate to physical penetration. Moreover, idiosyncratic and immutable characteristics of the individual, such as gender, physical size and strength, immaturity, sexual identity, sexual orientation, race, ethnicity, physical infirmity and disability, or illness, may lead people to be targeted for victimisation and associated forms of identity-based violence (Pole et al., 2008; Kira et al., 2011). Other factors such as membership of a particular group (family, ethnic group, tribe, religion, political party) can also be cause for traumatic levels of intergroup persecution and conflict that, in many cases, continues unabated over the course of generations. This is now referred to as intergenerational or historical trauma (Kirmayer et al., 2014; Mohatt et al., 2014), and includes colonialist oppression and domination by one group that is more powerful over another that is viewed as inferior in some way and has less power and resources available.

Complex developmentally-adverse interpersonal trauma (Ford, 2005) can result in symptoms that meet criteria for both Posttraumatic Stress Disorder (PTSD) and Complex Post-Traumatic Stress Disorder (C-PTSD), along with a large number of comorbidities, and are referred to here as Complex Traumatic Stress Disorders (Ford, 2017a). This chapter describes a treatment model that is carefully sequenced and incremental, designed to attend to the symptoms of PTSD and C-PTSD, as well as any associated physical, mental health, and relational issues. While the sequenced and phase-based treatment continues to be the standard of care for Complex Trauma treatment and is endorsed by clinical consensus (Cloitre et al., 2011; Schnyder et al., 2015), a recent critique (De Jongh et al., 2016) suggesting it is unnecessary and encouraging the use of evidence-based trauma-focused treatments applied very early in treatment will also be discussed. It is clearly acknowledged that "one size does not fit all" in terms of treatment (Cloitre, 2015) and therefore the sequenced model of trauma-focused psychotherapy is considered a meta-model within which different approaches and algorithms are embedded, according to client status and needs. Finally, it is important to note that addressing attachment and relational difficulties for those suffering with Complex Traumatic Stress Disorders is a central principle for all clinicians working with this client group and necessitates an emphasis on empathic attunement and the therapeutic relationship, regardless of the background, training, and inclinations of the clinician.

A vignette of C-PTSD – "Tina"

Tina was a 31-year-old Asian-American woman who was hospitalised twice over a six-month period for Depression and suicidality, complicated by bursts of energy and hearing voices telling her to kill herself, thought to be consistent with Bipolar II Disorder (a version of Bipolar I Disorder, without severe manic episodes) and a dissociative condition. She was a successful lawyer with five years' experience. She had been married for eight years to a journalist. The couple had two children, a seven-year-old boy and a two-year-old girl. Tina grew up in an intact upper-middle class family with parents she described as detached and demanding, with two older brothers she was close to. Tina was a star student and athlete, devoted to gymnastics until she had a serious accident in high school, when her plans for an athletic scholarship to college were derailed. During her recovery, she revealed that her coach had sexually molested her since she was six years old. Her parents filed charges and the coach was dismissed, and was then sentenced to probation, after a very public trial in which Tina testified against him. Other girls on the team defended him, however, and accused her of making up the story for attention and to gain compensation for her injury. After the sentencing, Tina and her family were ostracised in their community, leaving Tina isolated, stigmatised, and bereft.

Tina viewed this experience as the catalyst for her career as a family lawyer and an advocate for victims. She prided herself in taking on some of the most difficult cases of abuse and neglect. Apart from several months of family therapy at the time of the trial and brief experimentation with marijuana during her teenage years, Tina did not have any psychiatric or substance abuse history, until she experienced Postpartum Depression following the birth of her daughter, something that had not occurred after her son was born. In the intervening two years, Tina had experienced escalating symptoms of dysphoria, culminating in the severe recent affective and potentially psychotic and/or dissociative symptoms and ongoing suicidal ideation. Tina had also suffered with medically unexplained exhaustion, and blackouts in which her husband said she seemed to become another person.

Treatment for Complex Trauma – sequenced and relationship-based meta-model

The advent of the first comprehensive clinical framework for the diagnosis and treatment of psychiatric symptoms explicitly related to exposure to traumatic stressors was the PTSD diagnosis introduced in the Third Edition of the Diagnostic and Statistical Manual of Mental Disorders in 1980 (American Psychiatric Association, 1980). This coincided with the emergence of Cognitive Behavioural Therapy (CBT) as the dominant research-based approach to psychotherapy for Anxiety and Mood Disorders (Ford et al., 2015). Clinical research studies of these and related approaches, including Prolonged Exposure (PE/EX), Cognitive Therapy (CT), Cognitive Processing Therapy (CPT), and later Eye Movement Desensitisation and Reprocessing Therapy (EMDR), and Narrative Exposure Therapy (NET), demonstrated efficacy in diminishing the classic and debilitating symptoms of PTSD. Yet these techniques were not effective or sufficient for a sizable subgroup of recipients, even in studies that excluded individuals with the most pernicious symptoms and severe psychosocial impairment (for example, Acute Psychosis, Mania, Substance Abuse, suicidality, or self-harm) (Spinazzola et al., 2005; Bisson et al., 2013).

After studying the often widely differing clinical presentations associated with diverse types of exposure to traumatic stressors, Herman delineated the syndrome of Complex PTSD and proposed a relationally-focused sequenced approach to psychotherapy rather than the trauma memory-focused approach of the CBT models (Herman, 1992). This approach to psychotherapy for C-PTSD involved three defined though arbitrary phases of treatment, elaborating a model devised nearly a century earlier by the French psychiatrist Pierre Janet (Van der Hart and Friedman, 1989) for women who were designated as "Hysteric" at that time, a condition akin to the current Borderline Personality Disorder (Ford and Courtois, 2014). Phase 1 focused on client stabilisation, education, and skills training; Phase 2 on resolution of traumatic stress symptoms; and Phase 3 on life reconsolidation.

The three phases look simple and logical but are deceptively so because there are many variations and complications, both in the cohort requiring treatment and in the treatment process itself. Even when psychotherapy progresses smoothly, the three phases are not neatly sub-divided but tend to overlap, and treatment tasks may need to be frequently repeated before issues are sufficiently resolved and changes internalised. Although the model is linear, it is not designed, nor should it be applied, in a lock-step fashion, but according to the client's needs, personal and social assets, and personal goals and preferences. The sequenced model might better be visualised as a recursive spiral, with fluid movement across the three phases as clinically indicated, for example, due to periodic expectable relapses, especially during times of stress or change. Psychotherapy usually only progresses deliberately through the sequence in the prescribed manner when the client has a secure attachment style and a robust array of personal and social resources; unfortunately, this is not usually the case. In addition, C-PTSD places a severe strain not only on mental health but also on physical health and relationships. Loved ones, friends and colleagues, community, cultural, and religious influences, therapists and others who are highly supportive may be seriously tested by the clients themselves in terms of their needs, stories, and styles of interaction, and because of the secondary or vicarious trauma that they may experience. Members of the client's support systems may also have difficulty adapting to changes in their relationship when the client's symptoms improve, at times becoming defensive and "pushing back" to maintain the status quo if they find the changes emerging from therapy too discomforting or challenging.

In addition, individuals who have experienced Complex Trauma often bring issues into therapy that were not evident or reported during the initial assessment. These may become apparent as a result of the treatment itself, and in response to ongoing or unexpected life events and developmental transitions. Newly appearing issues and symptoms can either set back or accelerate the treatment and may mean that treatment plan and goals need to be revised, often several times. A very common example is the identification of dissociative symptoms that the client initially denied or obscured, which range in severity from occasionally "zoning out" or losing periods of time, to the more serious Dissociative Identity Disorder (DID), where entirely different personality states alternately make their appearance in the individual. Dissociation can be understood as a form of survival coping that, when identified and treated within a secure relationship and with skills for emotion regulation (Ford, 2017b), often emerges in Phase 2 as a crisis that requires a return to Phase 1 stabilisation work. Although this may appear to be "backtracking" or a loss of gains made in treatment, it is better understood as a way to begin moving into Phase 3 by enabling the client to process trauma symptoms or memories with enhanced self-awareness and skills for self-regulation (Ford, 2013), and thus to increase the durability of therapeutic gains. See Courtois and Ford (2013) for a more detailed discussion of what they term the sequenced, relationship-based model of treatment for Complex Trauma.

Phase 1

Therapy for C-PTSD begins with a wide-ranging psychosocial assessment that considers the whole person, all past and present life circumstances relevant to current safety and biopsychosocial health, functioning, and stability. Assessment should be viewed as the beginning of treatment, as an integral part of treatment, and not only as a precursor. The client's symptoms are not only enumerated but acknowledged nonjudgmentally and validated as understandable survival adaptations necessitated by past exposure to Complex Trauma. In addition to formulating a chronology of the client's psychiatric symptoms, drug and alcohol use and abuse, risky or harmful behaviours and relationships, major illnesses or injuries, involvement with healthcare, child and family services, and legal systems, it is also essential to assess personal strengths, resources, and accomplishments that demonstrate the client's self-capacities and sources of personal support. A thorough and empathic assessment is the basis of a strong therapeutic alliance, assists in the development of an individualised treatment plan, and begins the process of enhancing motivation by explaining that therapy is a vehicle for the achievement of goals, specifically those that relate to the client's personal values and hopes, in addition to helping them overcome the impairments caused by symptoms.

Creating a base for the remainder of the treatment is a major endeavour that involves helping the client to acquire or strengthen psychological and life skills and to make shifts in attitude, affect, and behaviour that underlie subsequent therapeutic activities and gains. Although many clients and some therapists would prefer to simply "make it all to go away" and "want this done yesterday", careful pacing and dosing of therapeutic work inevitably is the best way to "make haste slowly". This is accomplished by mirroring the client and challenging him or her to engage in rigorous and thorough self-reflection in a manner that is at times uncomfortable but always tolerable and informative rather than overwhelming. This enables clients to progressively expand their self-awareness, self-identification, and emotional "window of tolerance", while not precipitating iatrogenic crises, terminations, or "regressions".

Phase 1 is designed to assist the client in developing personal and developmental resources that they may have only partially or never learned, in lives interrupted or held hostage by Complex Trauma (Ford, 2017b). Skills building or strengthening starts with emotion identification (including both affective and somatosensory foci and regulation) and moves on to self-reflection as an adaptive alternative to unhelpful ongoing survival reactions. The client's safety from risky or self-harming behaviours as well as from external sources of harm needs routine and repeated assessment, including attention to ongoing relationships to ensure as much as possible that they are not violent, abusive, coercive, or otherwise destabilising. Similarly, the client's current and historical behavioural choices should be assessed for potential dangers or crises, to develop strategies for gaining control over impulsive behaviour, self-destructive thoughts and behaviours, dangerous interpersonal situations, addictions, ongoing dissociation, and affect discharges that lead to risk and re-traumatisation.

Although the first phase does not specifically focus on trauma processing and resolution, much of the work relates, either directly or indirectly, to traumatic antecedents and posttraumatic reactions and their secondary elaborations. The major difference between Phases 1 and 2 is that trauma memories and trauma-related symptoms are addressed mainly from an exploratory and cognitive-educational perspective in Phase 1. Exploration is done in a context of getting to know each client and helping him or her self-examine through attunement and reflection, as a preparation for formulating customised treatment goals and for moving into deeper self-reflection with a strengthened foundation of safety, stability, and trust in the therapist, the therapeutic process, and themselves.

However, an important caveat applies. When clients have intense acute traumatic re-experiencing symptoms, for example, overwhelming flashbacks or nightmares, some processing of trauma may need to occur first, "out of order". These clients are unable to stop reliving traumas and cannot stabilise from their posttraumatic symptoms and achieve a modicum of safety without immediate assistance. They may "spill" memories of trauma intentionally or involuntarily at the outset of therapy, in part to test whether the therapist can tolerate this intensity, but also in a primal attempt to unburden themselves from the painful "baggage" of their Complex Trauma experiences. If not provided with guidance in containing the emotion and finding meaning in the memories or symptoms, these clients may resort to risky (for example, drugs, alcohol, sex, violence) or explicitly self-harming behaviours, to cope with the unrelenting pressure of intrusive trauma re-experiencing. In these situations, it is advisable for the therapist to consider how best to help the client to gain some sense of control over these intense and heretofore apparently uncontrollable trauma-related memories and feelings, drawing on aspects of the CBT protocols for trauma memory/symptom processing or utilising a CBT or EMDR technique out of the usual order.

Despite the fact that trauma is the reason that the majority of clients seek mental health care, it is important to note that it is still the case that training in traumatic stress in the relevant disciplines is frequently inadequate. Therapists who treat trauma therefore have an obligation to gain knowledge and skills, often on their own initiative. It is particularly important to note that traumatised clients may have transference reactions (known as traumatic transference) based in their own history, that impact on their needs and modes of interacting with others. This includes their relationships with therapists, who, in return, may display strong emotional responses, or countertransference. It is therefore important for the therapist to seek the help of relevant educational material, supervision, and, as needed or on an ongoing basis, specialised consultation. It is also important for the therapist to attend to personal emotional and mental health, to have a support system, and to have ways to decompress and to restore themselves.

Phase 2

Some clients leave treatment after completing Phase 1, in some cases, prematurely or via a "flight into health" and, in others, after choosing not to undertake trauma processing work because they feel unready, unsafe, or insufficiently supported, or their current life status demands their full attention and energy. Alternatively, their life and symptoms may be sufficiently upgraded that they decide to take a break, planning to return later if symptoms persist or if life again becomes problematic. At times, the shift into Phase 2 is explicitly initiated by the therapist, based on their evaluation of the client's readiness to safely and productively examine the impact that Complex Trauma has had on his or her emotions, beliefs, relationships, health, and life pursuits. At other times, Phase 2 commences more seamlessly as clients spontaneously engage in self-reflection about the impact of the trauma over the life course, and how symptoms that began as survival adaptations became maladaptive. Trauma processing occurs in many ways, but with a focus on helping the client to think about the many formerly unacknowledged and unintegrated feelings, cognitions, and beliefs. Relapse planning is also an essential component in Phase 2. Clients are expected to relapse, that is, experience distress that triggers a resurgence of survival coping and associated symptoms. When this occurs, they are encouraged to view the "slip" as a problem to be solved, rather than as a deterioration or failure. They are further encouraged to apply the plans they made and the skills they learned in Phase 1 to regain self-regulation with respect to both emotion and behaviour.

Phase 2 starts with an explanation that the therapist will systematically encourage, but not pressure, the client to reflect carefully on critical memories – both current and from the distant past – while experiencing the emotional impact as fully as they can tolerate. The client is urged to apply the self-regulatory skills developed in Phase 1 to modulate emotional experiencing and to not just re-experience but actively find meaning and a sense of personal control that was not possible in the remembered experience. The client is further supported in separating past from present, and in understanding that the traumatic circumstances are in the past rather than continuing in the present. The therapist functions first as a stimulus, assisting the client to explore the feelings and to learn to regulate them to the point of manageability and resolution. Importantly, the therapist also acts as a "container", through close attunement and co-regulation with the client, and with the provision of emotional support and validation of the meaning that the experiences now have, validation the client may never have had previously. In this way, the emotions and anguish associated with traumas, including intense anger, shame, and grief, begin to make sense, feel manageable in the current moment and in the context of support, and are no longer experienced as uncontrollable and mystifying symptoms.

It is important that the therapist not become emotionally or physiologically overwhelmed in Phase 2, especially to the point of detachment/avoidance, as this may replicate previous experiences of abandonment. Nor is it helpful if the therapist becomes emotionally over-involved to the point of encouraging avoidance as a means of protecting the client, thereby inadvertently giving the message that the client is not strong enough to manage or that the trauma is too awful to face. As previously noted, clients suffering in the wake of Complex Trauma often engender such strong feelings in others, including therapists, and this must be understood, repeatedly recognised, and managed, and it is therefore imperative that the therapist determine his or her own capacity to stay emotionally engaged with the client during this emotional and working-through process. The therapist's own ability to self-regulate and stay closely attuned in response to the client's emotional state is a major part of the relational basis of treatment. The importance of supervision and consultation in this context cannot be over-emphasised.

Phase 3

Phase 3 can be seen as the culmination of the very difficult work of self-reflective trauma processing, and as a time of growth and renewal; it may also be a very challenging period. Clients may continue to feel like "misfits", or as though they were deprived of their lives and now need to play "catch-up". It is important that therapists do not assume that clients with Complex Trauma histories are only able to achieve marginal lives and minimal functioning, because this can unwittingly reinforce clients' own fears and sense of stigma. Some of the most inspiring success stories in the treatment of C-PTSD belong to those who have struggled for most, or even really all, of their lives with severe mental illness, addiction, learning disabilities, homelessness, conflicted or empty relationships, and other pervasive life challenges, but who have overcome them with treatment, perseverance, intention, and support. It should also be noted that some clients with C-PTSD are highly functional in their lives, their skills and strengths reinforced in treatment.

Phase 3 is designed to enable clients to fully shift from the survival coping mode by transforming their beliefs, aspirations, lifestyle, and relationships using the self-awareness and personal capacities and resources developed or strengthened in Phases 1 and 2. Identifying and grieving losses continues in Phase 3 and extends to additional losses that occur in the present when clients recognise that they must make new choices that may profoundly change or end key relationships and activities. On a more positive note, Phase 3 can include using and fine-tuning the self-regulatory and other life skills developed earlier, to apply to yet unresolved developmental deficits and fixations. Some of the issues that receive focus in this phase are the development of trustworthy relationships and intimacy, improved and healthy sexual functioning, improved ability to parent, self-oriented career and other life decisions, ongoing discussions with or confrontations of abusive or neglectful others, determining courses of action for ongoing self-protection, and so on. In this phase, as in the others, the therapist continues to provide a source of emotional support and encouragement.

A vignette of treatment – "Tina" continued

During her two admissions, Tina was assessed with respect to her symptoms and her history. Although she was diagnosed with Bipolar II Disorder during her first admission, for which she was primarily treated with a mood-stabiliser medication, she did not improve. During her second stay in a hospital that operated from a trauma-informed philosophy of practice, the diagnoses were revised to PTSD, Dissociative Subtype with delayed expression, C-PTSD, and Major Depressive Disorder (MDD). She was prescribed an antidepressant, of the Selective Serotonin Reuptake Inhibitor class suggested for PTSD in relevant treatment guidelines, to which she had a good response. Her Depression also lessened in response to the intensive efforts that were made by staff to her ongoing suicidality. She was helped to understand that the birth of a daughter had been one of several precipitants related to the emergence of her symptoms and their intensity. She both loved and feared for her daughter and her future welfare, feelings that touched on her own vulnerability and prior history of abuse. Tina was provided education about the role of her past trauma in her present-day symptoms. Once the association was made, she felt relieved and less hopeless about her ability to adequately parent her children, especially her daughter.

After a short hospital stay, Tina was referred to outpatient therapy, where the initial focus was on supporting the gains she had made in the hospital and improving her functioning at home and at work. Her therapist assessed her degree of dissociation and taught her skills to identify when she "spaced out" and strategies for staying present and for coping more effectively. Tina and her therapist also discussed how the coach abuse, the trial, and her social and athletic losses had impacted her, and how she had tried to cope by "getting beyond it" and largely avoiding her own history. Tina stabilised over the course of approximately six months during which she began to tell her story in more detail and to express her long-avoided memories and emotions. Her husband attended several sessions to provide her with emotional support.

At this point, the therapist introduced Tina to various evidence-based methods for a more directed focus on the trauma, Phase 2. After hearing about each approach, Tina decided on a course of EMDR. She initially found it very helpful, but at one point felt overwhelmed to the point of again becoming suicidal. The EMDR was suspended for several sessions as she and her therapist discussed and processed what had come up for her and her suicidal ideation subsided. Eventually, Tina processed her years of sexual abuse and arrived at a point of emotional resolution. She told her therapist she now had a better understanding of herself and her life choices. During Phase 2, her husband again attended several sessions to support Tina, and to discuss the impact of the trauma on him, their marriage, and on parenting their children.

In Phase 3, Tina decided to research her former coach and found that he had been accused of molesting other girls. He had lost his job but remained out of gaol. She decided to take further legal action by filing a civil lawsuit against him. When her lawsuit became public, other victims came forward and a criminal case was reopened. This time, the coach was found guilty and imprisoned, to Tina's great relief. Her civil lawsuit was settled in her favour before trial but included a non-disclosure clause. During this period, Tina also made the decision to move from her full-time position to work half-time, so she could be exposed to less work-related stress and so she could have more time for both herself and for her children. She also began to describe her satisfaction at being a good and attentive parent to both. She was very careful about their safety, especially when they began to engage in organised sports. Tina eventually reported that she felt like she got her life back again. She continued in therapy for several years because she felt the need for her therapist's ongoing support and validation.

Status of sequenced treatment for C-PTSD

Sequenced treatment is recommended by clinical consensus in all the professional practice guidelines for C-PTSD, based on research evidence and the experience and consensus opinion of practicing clinicians (Cloitre et al., 2011). However, the sequenced model for C-PTSD has a more limited research evidence base to support its efficacy than CBT therapies for PTSD (Bisson et al., 2013; Ford, 2017b). Research on treatments for C-PTSD is particularly challenging because many different strategies have been developed to address the wide range of symptoms and comorbidities that extend well beyond those of traditional PTSD. The absence of a universally accepted and formally codified C-PTSD syndrome or diagnosis further impedes a clinical or scientific consensus.

Recently, the sequenced approach to the treatment of C-PTSD has been criticised for these scientific limitations (De Jongh et al., 2016). Critics have particularly challenged the legitimacy of a stabilisation phase preceding trauma processing, asserting that this may unduly delay, or lead to a failure to provide, that central component of treatment. The critics are correct in pointing out that trauma-focused CBT therapies have demonstrated efficacy with recipients who have Complex Trauma histories and for symptoms that extend beyond PTSD, for example, depression, dissociation, grief, and shame. However, there is no approach to PTSD psychotherapy, including all CBT models, that requires or recommends commencing trauma processing without the assessment, education, safety planning, and engagement/therapeutic alliance activities specified in Phase 1. The issue is not whether to prepare clients sufficiently for trauma processing, but exactly how the preparation is best done, for how long, and for whom. No research study has addressed these key questions, and the wide variability in symptoms, circumstances, histories, and self- and relational-capacities of survivors of Complex Trauma strongly suggests that they must be addressed on a client-by-client basis, and not using a "one size fits all" approach (Courtois and Ford, 2013; Cloitre, 2015). Client-centred outcome research on treatment for survivors of Complex Trauma therefore should not be limited to studies comparing static interventions but instead should be designed to develop systematic algorithms for deploying, sequencing, and evaluating the effectiveness of strategies for assessing and ensuring adequate client safety and stability, engagement and motivation, readiness and preparedness, skills for self-regulation and trauma processing, relapse anticipation and prevention, and generalisation of gains to daily living.

It should finally be emphasised that for those clients who have been abused by others, by far the majority of those presenting with Complex Traumatic Stress Disorders, there are always issues with personal safety and trust, and a focus on the relational via attention to the therapeutic relationship is paramount, and it is not advisable for trauma processing can proceed without this fundamental principle in place.

Conclusion

This chapter has described Complex Trauma and C-PTSD and a clinically-endorsed sequenced approach to its treatment. C-PTSD is differentiated from classic PTSD based on deficits in self and relational capacity, ability to self-regulate, dissociation, and somatosensory and other medical indicators. As a result of the myriad of symptoms of C-PTSD, and the presenting problems that are often in evidence when a client seeks treatment, a multi-focused, systemic, and hierarchical application of treatment tasks is recommended. It is suggested that trauma-focused treatments, that is, those with the strongest evidence-base to date, are very important in the treatment of PTSD symptoms but are not always therapeutic as a first line treatment for C-PTSD. It is recommended that multi-modal and integrative treatment approaches be used that incorporate evidence-based and other treatments according to a variety of factors in a client's presentation.

References

American Psychiatric Association (1980) *Diagnostic and Statistical Manual of Mental Disorders, Third Edition*. Washington, DC: American Psychiatric Publishing.

Becker-Blease KA and Freyd JJ (2005) Beyond PTSD: An evolving relationship between trauma theory and family violence research. *Journal of Interpersonal Violence* 20(4): 403–411.

Bisson JI, Roberts NP, Andrew M, et al. (2013) Psychological therapies for chronic post-traumatic stress disorder (PTSD) in adults. *Cochrane Database Systematic Reviews* 13 December (12): CD003388.

Cloitre M (2015) The "one size fits all" approach to trauma treatment: should we be satisfied? *European Journal of Psychotraumatology* 6: doi:10.3402/ejpt.v6.27344.

Cloitre M, Courtois CA, Charuvastra A, et al. (2011) Treatment of complex PTSD: Results of the ISTSS expert clinician survey on best practices. *Journal of Traumatic Stress* 24(6): 615–627.

Cook A, Spinazzola J, Ford JD, et al. (2005) Complex Trauma in children and adolescents. *Psychiatric Annals* 35(5): 390–398.

Courtois CA and Ford JD (2013) *Treating Complex Trauma: A Sequenced Relationship-Based Approach*. New York, NY: Guilford.

De Jongh A, Resick PA, Zoellner LA, et al. (2016) Critical analysis of the current treatment guidelines for complex PTSD in adults. Review. *Depression and Anxiety* 33(5): 359–369.

Ford JD (2005) Treatment implications of altered neurobiology, affect regulation and information processing following child maltreatment. *Psychiatric Annals* 35: 410–419.

Ford JD (2013) How can self-regulation enhance our understanding of trauma and dissociation? *Journal of Trauma and Dissociation* 14(3): 237–250.

Ford JD (2017a) Complex Trauma and complex PTSD. In: Cook J, Gold S and Dalenberg C (eds) *Handbook of Trauma Psychology, Volume One*. Washington, DC: American Psychological Association, pp.281–306.

Ford JD (2017b) Emotion regulation and skills-based interventions. In: Cook J, Gold S and Dalenberg C (eds) *Handbook of Trauma Psychology, Volume Two*. Washington, DC: American Psychological Association, pp.227–252.

Ford JD and Courtois CA (2014) Complex PTSD, affect dysregulation, and borderline personality disorder. *Borderline Personal Disorder and Emotion Dysregulation* 9: 1–9.

Ford JD, Grasso DG, Elhai JD, et al. (2015) *Posttraumatic Stress Disorder: Scientific and Professional Dimensions, Second Edition*. New York, NY: Academic Press.

Herman JL (1992) Complex PTSD: A syndrome in survivors of prolonged and repeated trauma. *Journal of Traumatic Stress* 5(3): 377–391.

Kira I, Templin T, Lewandowski L, et al. (2011) Cumulative tertiary appraisal of traumatic events across cultures: Two studies. *Journal of Loss and Trauma* 16(1): 43–66.

Kirmayer LJ, Gone JP, Moses J, et al. (2014) Rethinking historical trauma. *Transcultural Psychiatry* 51(3): 299–319.

Mohatt NV, Thompson AB, Thai ND, et al. (2014) Historical trauma as public narrative: A conceptual review of how history impacts present-day health. *Social Science and Medicine* 106: 128–136.

Pole N, Gone JP, Kulkarni M, et al. (2008) Posttraumatic stress disorder among ethnoracial minorities in the United States. *Clinical Psychology: Science and Practice* 15(1): 35–61.

Schnyder U, Ehlers A, Elbert T, et al. (2015) Psychotherapies for PTSD: What do they have in common? *European Journal of Psychotraumatology* 6(1): doi:10.3402/ejpt.v6.28186.

Spinazzola J, Blaustein M and Van der Kolk BA (2005) Posttraumatic stress disorder treatment outcome research: The study of unrepresentative samples? *Journal of Traumatic Stress* 18(5): 425–436.

Van der Hart O and Friedman B (1989) A reader's guide to Pierre Janet on dissociation: A neglected intellectual heritage. *Dissociation: Progress in the Dissociative Disorders* 2(1): 3–16.

17 Treating Posttraumatic Stress Disorder with evidence-based psychological treatments

Carla J Walton and Christopher W Lee

Introduction

Posttraumatic Stress Disorder (PTSD) is one of the most common mental health disorders in Australia, with a 12-month prevalence of between 3 per cent and 7 per cent, depending on the diagnostic criteria used (Peters et al., 1999), and a lifetime prevalence of approximately 8.3 per cent (Kilpatrick et al., 2013). PTSD develops after direct or indirect exposure to potentially traumatic events. The core symptoms of the disorder involve re-experiencing the trauma, alterations in arousal and reactivity, avoidance and numbing, and negative changes in mood and cognition (Friedman et al., 2007). Exposure to traumatic events confronts the individual's basic beliefs about safety and personal control, and responses often involve fear and helplessness. For approximately two-thirds of individuals exposed to a significantly traumatic event, any sequelae resolve spontaneously with time, however, one third will go on to develop PTSD (Cusack et al., 2016). In approximately 10–20 per cent of those who develop PTSD, the course of the disorder is chronic, with debilitating symptoms that impact on quality of life, relationships, work and physical health (Fletcher et al., 2010).

Several factors influence the prevalence and severity of PTSD. The prevalence increases as the number of traumatic events increase (Brewin et al., 2000; Ozer et al., 2008). PTSD is also more likely to occur after more severe types of trauma, such as childhood sexual abuse, adult rape or military combat (Friedman et al., 2007). In addition, the prevalence increases in situations where harm was deliberately inflicted (Santiago et al., 2013).

Although there is evidence for the use of pharmacotherapy in reducing the symptoms of PTSD (Phoenix Australia – Centre for Posttraumatic Mental Health, 2013), research shows that most people prefer non-pharmacological approaches (Simiola et al., 2015). Most guidelines recommend that trauma-focused psychological interventions are used as the first line of treatment for PTSD (Phoenix Australia – Centre for Posttraumatic Mental Health, 2013), and outcome studies show that the majority of individuals no longer meet the criteria for PTSD following treatment. Specifically, there are more than 80 randomised controlled trials (RCTs) showing that trauma-focused Cognitive Behavioural Therapy is effective in the treatment of PTSD (Bisson et al., 2013).

Most of these RCTs have been for single-incident or adult-onset trauma. There is also research on effective interventions for adults who have PTSD arising from childhood events. Ehring et al. (2014) conducted a meta-analysis of 16 RCTs evaluating psychological interventions for PTSD as a result of childhood abuse. They found that overall there is good evidence for these interventions and that trauma-focused treatments had better outcomes than interventions that were not trauma-focused.

Early development of structured therapies

Ivan Pavlov, a Russian physiologist, initially studied the digestive system of dogs. Through these observations he developed a theory known as "classical conditioning", and he later became pivotal in behaviour modification approaches. He observed that external phenomenon that occurred at the time that dogs produced salivation in anticipation of food could also elicit salivation, even when food was not present. He subsequently trained dogs to salivate in response to non-food stimuli. John B Watson became interested in Pavlov's work, and extended the study to humans. In 1913, he called for psychology to focus on observable behaviour, that is, the prediction and control of behaviour, rather than on internal mental processes, which he regarded as unverifiable. He carried out one of the most controversial experiments in psychology when he conditioned a nine-month-old orphan, "Little Albert", to be scared of a white rat by banging on an iron rod when the rat was presented. Whilst Albert had not initially been afraid of the rat, he later showed fear around it. The study demonstrated that emotions could become conditioned, and "behaviourism" – the theory that behaviour can be explained in terms of conditioning without regard to thought or feeling – became the dominant paradigm of the early twentieth century. Watson was followed by BF Skinner, who, rather than focusing on the events or stimuli that triggered behavioural responses, focused on what happened after the behaviour. He observed that the strength of a behaviour is modified by reward or punishment, a concept known as "operant conditioning". This work contributed significantly to the understanding that the consequences of a behaviour directly influence the likelihood of a recurrence of this behaviour. Skinner is often considered to be the most influential psychologist of the twentieth century. Joseph Wolpe, a South African Psychiatrist who had treated soldiers diagnosed with what is now considered PTSD, studied both Pavlov and Watson's work, and developed the form of treatment now known as Systematic Desensitisation, or Graded Exposure Therapy. Useful for Phobias and Anxiety Disorders, a hierarchy of fears is established, and once a relaxation technique has been learned, individuals gradually face and overcome their feared stimuli. In their focus on behaviour, Pavlov, Watson, Skinner and Wolpe have all had a profound impact on the range of psychological treatments available today.

Alongside the behaviourists, in the 1960s, Aaron Beck began to develop Cognitive Therapy (Beck, 1979). Beck had begun his career as a psychoanalyst, but, in carrying out a series of studies to test the psychodynamic theory of

Depression, his experimental findings contradicted the generally accepted hypothesis that depressed patients have "a need to suffer". He also noted that many of his students and colleagues, in analysis for years, did not improve, and that his own patients reacted adversely to psychodynamic interventions. Instead he began studying internal thoughts, beliefs and attitudes, and their role in influencing individuals. He developed his theory through the observation of his patients. If the theory was validated by several individuals, he developed interventions consistent with the theory. He eventually determined that negative views about oneself, the world and the future are important in the development of depressive states, and he called this the "cognitive triad". This led to interventions aimed at challenging negative or distorted thoughts. Cognitive Behavioural Therapy, usually referred to as "CBT", a mixture of both types of interventions, was originally developed for the treatment of Depression, but over time expanded to other conditions.

From Beck's perspective, traumatic incidents in childhood may create the potential for later distress by generating dysfunctional underlying beliefs (Beck et al., 1985). In relation to PTSD, the key beliefs involved are related to personal safety or vulnerability, lessened trust in others, dangerousness of the world, self-blame and guilt, and the "unfairness" of events. From a behavioural perspective, trauma is also seen to be associated with other material that can later evoke responses, similar to those evoked by the trauma itself; the brain "pairs" the two. For example, if an abuser wore a distinctive aftershave, the smell of this aftershave in unassociated circumstances could trigger flashbacks of the original abuse, even though the individual is currently safe. This may lead to avoidant behaviour.

In the context of PTSD, trauma, and CBT, it is relevant to note that there are now several structured psychotherapies that are primarily "trauma-focused". This means that the treatment centres on either the memory of the traumatic event or its meaning. This chapter will focus on the three trauma-focused therapies with the strongest research evidence base: Prolonged Exposure Therapy, Cognitive Processing Therapy, and Eye Movement Desensitisation and Reprocessing. Each of these therapies has been found to be superior to no treatment and superior to supportive counselling (Bisson et al., 2013).

Prolonged Exposure Therapy (PE)

Although there are several CBT treatments for PTSD, Prolonged Exposure Therapy (PE), developed by Edna Foa, is the most researched (Foa and Rothbaum, 2001). In a recent meta-analysis of PTSD, the average effect size for PE was 1.27 (Cusack et al., 2016). Effect sizes are a standardised metric that measure the size of the difference between two groups. An effect size of 1.27 means that the score of the average person receiving PE is 1.27 standard deviations above the average person in the control group. This effect size would be considered a very large effect for any treatment given that 0.5 is described as a medium effect and 0.8 as a large effect.

The theoretical basis for PE relies upon a learning model, such that the individual's response to the trauma did not reduce sufficiently, and the association between the memory of the event and the message of danger had not been extinguished, even though the danger had passed. As a result, people with PTSD usually try to avoid the things that remind them of the trauma. Though this helps people feel better in the short term, in the long term it sustains the trauma symptoms. The goal is to facilitate emotional processing of the memory that incorporates corrective information about the experience and the actual amount of danger. PE aims to help people to gain control by facing the triggers that they have been avoiding.

In PE, the therapist helps the person to confront their trauma memories in the session and schedules a series of structured homework assignments to confront the triggers of their PTSD symptoms between sessions. In both situations, the person is required to do this for an extended period to allow habituation to occur, such that physiological and emotional responses substantially diminish. Typically, the therapist will ask that experiences be described in the first person and in the present tense. At the session, the person retells their experience of the trauma several times. As they repeatedly focus on the details of the memory in the safety of the therapist's office, the arousal associated with the memory is expected to decrease. Over the course of treatment, the therapist encourages the person to increasingly focus on the worst aspects of their memory, so that eventually the person can recall even the most difficult details and not experience distress. Habituation to memories in the session facilitates the ability to confront triggers of distress outside of the session.

Harned et al. (2012) have adapted PE for the treatment of PTSD in people with a diagnosis of Borderline Personality Disorder who are suicidal and self-harming by integrating PE into another form of CBT designed specifically for those with this condition, Dialectical Behaviour Therapy (DBT). This approach involves helping people develop the necessary self-regulation skills to cease their self-harming or suicidal behaviour prior to commencing PE, and then using PE concurrently with DBT.

Cognitive Processing Therapy

Cognitive Processing Therapy (CPT) is another CBT treatment that, rather than focusing on the retelling of trauma experiences, emphasises the person's cognitions about their traumatic experiences. The evidence for the effectiveness of CPT is substantial and the treatment effect size is also very large at 1.40 (Cusack et al., 2016).

In contrast to PE, CPT emphasises reappraisal of the meaning of the trauma memory. It was originally developed by Patricia Resick for survivors of rape (Resick and Schnicke, 1992), but has now also been developed for military populations and people with a history of childhood trauma (Chard, 2005). The underlying assumption is that avoidance of thinking about traumatic events contributes to people not recovering. In CPT, there is a focus on identifying and changing negative thoughts that develop in response to the trauma, for example, what happened was the fault of the sufferer, or that the world is dangerous. The therapist uses "Socratic questioning", the practice of asking probing questions, to facilitate reflection and explore erroneous conclusions embedded in the appraisal. The person then talks with their therapist about cognitions related to the trauma, with emphasis on specific themes of shame, self-blame, intimacy, trust, and anger. The element of exposure in CPT involves the person writing down their trauma memory, and reading it out aloud, although evidence shows that the written element is optional, that is, the act of verbally recounting any memories is sufficient.

Eye Movement Desensitisation and Reprocessing

Eye Movement Desensitisation and Reprocessing (EMDR) was developed by Francine Shapiro after she experienced some disturbing thoughts and found that they reduced when moving her eyes rapidly back and forth (Shapiro and Forrest, 2001). She studied the phenomenon further and developed procedural guidelines so that EMDR would help people process memories, thoughts and feelings utilising a "dual processing" model.

The efficacy of EMDR has been demonstrated in comparison with both standard care and waitlist groups, as well as to a range of psychological and pharmacological interventions including CBT, PE, stress management, fluoxetine and placebo (Marcus et al., 1997; Lee et al., 2002; Rothbaum et al., 2005; Van der Kolk et al., 2007; Van den Berg et al., 2015). EMDR has been shown to be effective in treating PTSD when delivered as a stand-alone treatment or as an adjunct to other psychological or pharmacological therapies (Marcus et al., 1997; Carlson et al., 1998). In the most recent meta-analysis on EMDR, the effect size was found to be 1.28 (Dominguez and Lee, 2017). This is comparable to the effect sizes for Prolonged Exposure and Cognitive Processing Therapy. In RCTs that have directly compared EMDR with CBT, EMDR had been found to be equivalent or superior (Chen et al., 2015).

Common to other trauma-focused structured therapies, a history is taken, and the person is orientated to the treatment. The person is encouraged to recollect the traumatic memory, and is then asked to describe what occurred, the feelings associated with the event, and the negative cognitions associated with the worst part of the experience. Information sought about the event includes what the person remembers seeing, hearing or smelling. The person is also assisted to develop a positive cognition that will replace the negative themes associated with the event.

The next stage of the treatment is a desensitisation stage, where the therapist again asks the person to recollect the traumatic event, associated negative beliefs, and somatic sensations connected to this memory. The person is then instructed to focus on these three aspects of the memory, and to follow the therapist's finger as it moves backwards and forwards, resulting in side-to-side eye movements. During this dual attention task, the therapist instructs the person to simply observe what is happening, without making any judgement. After each set, the person is asked to take a break, and then to describe whatever they are experiencing at that time. The process is continued with subsequent sets until positive material emerges. Once the positive material is stable, the level of distress associated with the traumatic memory is then reassessed on a, "Subjective Units of Distress Scale", or "SUDS" scale (Wolpe, 1969), where zero represents no distress, and 10 is as uncomfortable as feelings can get. When the distress level is less than two, the therapy moves to the next phase, where the therapist pairs the memory of the trauma with a positive belief and continues the dual attention task. This phase continues until the positive belief is strongly felt to be true. The final check of the procedure is for the person to imagine their old memory and to repeat the positive phrase, while the therapist ensures that there is either a positive somatic experience, or if any negative somatic sensations are present, that they are minimal.

The mechanism of action underlying EMDR is still uncertain. One of the most common theories involves a working memory model, in which it is hypothesised that the traumatic images of the event are held in a system that has very limited capacity, specifically the "visuospatial sketchpad", a component of working memory (Jeffries and Davis, 2013). It is proposed that performing the dual attention task while focusing on the unpleasant memory disrupts the already limited capacity of working memory, and this results in less vivid recall of the images (Andrade et al., 1997). This subsequently decreases the intensity of the emotions associated with the image. Though there is empirical support for this hypothesis, more research is needed to confirm what aspects of the dual task are critical, and what the ideal level of complexity is to produce this effect (Jeffries and Davis, 2013).

There has also been controversy around whether the effectiveness of EMDR is due to the exposure to the trauma memory, or whether there is added benefit from the dual stimulation. The most recent meta-analysis of studies that looked at this issue found that adding an eye movement task resulted in significant improvements to symptom reduction and reduced vividness and emotionality of the trauma memory, compared with no eye movement control conditions (Lee and Cuijpers, 2013).

A vignette – "Karina"

Karina was a 44-year-old married woman with a 13-year-old daughter. She worked part-time in a craft shop. She was referred to a private psychologist by her General Practitioner, with a long history of PTSD and depressive symptoms. In the first session she stated that she had seen psychologists and psychiatrists, "all my life". She added that her Depression began in high school, and she described currently experiencing a poor opinion of herself, low mood, little enjoyment, and sleep difficulties. She said that when she was depressed she had thoughts like, "I am bad", "I am worthless" and that, "I have tricked people into thinking that I am good, but one day they will find out the truth".

In addition to the depressive symptoms, she also had flashbacks, hyperarousal, and avoidance symptoms associated with several traumatic memories. These included emotional and physical abuse from her father, including threats to her life. She reported that he would often say that he was going to kill the entire family, and sometimes he held a knife in his hand when he said this. She also reported that she was sexually abused for a year when she was 13 by a family friend. She stated that her PTSD symptoms had increased since her daughter's last birthday. She appeared unaware of the connection between the exacerbation of her symptoms, her daughter's age, and the age when she was abused.

Karina stated at the start of therapy that she could only afford to come for 10 sessions as part of a government subsidised scheme. Given this limitation, there would not be any opportunity to facilitate stabilisation strategies, and, given that none of her previous therapies had involved a trauma-focused approach, it was decided to treat her PTSD with EMDR. Prior to treatment commencing, in the first session, the clinician completed a general psychological assessment which included a symptom history, a developmental, attachment and trauma history, and an evaluation of client strengths and weaknesses. Importantly, it was noted that Karina was not suicidal, she appeared to have a good relationship with her daughter, and she had held her current job for six months. Her level of PTSD symptomatology was however assessed with the "Impact of Events" scale at 54, the average score for people presenting with PTSD in Australian treatment centres (Vaughan et al., 1994; Lee et al., 2002).

In the second session, the initial target memory for EMDR treatment was identified as the first incident of sexual abuse, in which she was wearing bathers at the perpetrator's house. She stated that she remembered feeling scared, and that something bad was happening. She said that she could still see the staircase below her, and she had an accompanying sense that she needed to run away. She then said that she remembered the perpetrator coming up from behind, putting his hand under her bathers, and penetrating her with his fingers. She rated her distress associated with this memory at nine on the SUDS scale. She remembered having a tight feeling in her chest and the thought that, "I am bad, and it must have been my fault".

In the subsequent session the desensitisation phase of EMDR was administered. After 10 minutes of treatment she reported that the initial memory had begun to fade. During the following 20 minutes she described that she no longer saw the staircase, rather she remembered other aspects of that day, including leaving the building and putting on her clothes. After 50 minutes, she reported that her SUDS score had dropped to five. In the next 20 minutes she expressed anger that her father had not protected her from this situation, and anger that, because of his own issues, no one in the family could feel safe. At the end of this 90-minute session, her SUDS score had dropped to two. Subsequent sessions involved strengthening of the positive beliefs like, "I am good", and, "It wasn't my fault". Other childhood memory events, involving her father threatening to kill the family, were also desensitised. At the end of the 10 sessions, Karina's score on the Impact of Event Scale had reduced to 27, similar to the scores obtained when PTSD has been successfully treated in Australian clinics (Vaughan et al., 1994; Lee et al., 2002).

Key components of all trauma-focused structured therapies

Different trauma-focused therapies have different treatment components. Therapists might ask which treatment to use, or which components are necessary for a successful outcome. In a seminal paper on what the psychotherapies for trauma have in common, pioneers in the development and evaluation of these interventions identified the mutual elements across the treatments (Schnyder et al., 2015). These included: psychoeducation about the nature and course of posttraumatic stress reactions; teaching of emotion regulation and coping skills; exposure to the person's memory of their traumatic experience in a safe environment; cognitive processing or meaning-making of the experience; and reorganisation of memory functions to create a coherent trauma narrative. The goals of all trauma-focused structured therapies are: to help the person develop a more realistic appraisal of threat; to address the traumatic memories to develop mastery over them; to promote the capacity to regulate emotions and reduce shifting between states of numbing and hyperarousal; and to establish or re-establish healthy relationships.

A thorough history must be taken first to develop an individualised case formulation. This approach identifies the key maintaining factors, including trauma cues and avoidance of emotions, as well as any negative core beliefs, any emotional dysregulation, and the state of interpersonal relationships. Such an individualised approach will include an assessment of any areas that may need to be addressed before using a structured trauma approach. Individuals with PTSD often present with other comorbid psychiatric disorders and these may need to be considered. The extent to which the comorbid issues should be focused on prior to treating PTSD will depend upon which difficulty is primary. In the case of PTSD and Substance Abuse, there is some evidence favouring a combined approach (Phoenix Australia – Centre for Posttraumatic Mental Health, 2013).

It is also important to note that all the trauma-focused therapies require the person to disclose information about what occurred to them during the trauma. Sharing this information is likely to evoke memories, emotions, and thoughts that may increase vulnerability. In many cases, particularly sexual assault, shame is often associated with the event and/or the person's reaction. Attentive listening, sensitivity, and empathy are all required by therapists who treat people with PTSD. Where the trauma is interpersonal, the ability to trust others is likely to have been significantly impacted, and work must be done towards building a safe, therapeutic relationship. Consistent with evidence for other psychological disorders, the establishment of a good therapeutic relationship has been shown to improve the outcomes for PTSD (Phoenix Australia – Centre for Posttraumatic Mental Health, 2013).

As with the non-structured therapies for the treatment of trauma, in structured therapies, clinicians need to be aware of transference and countertransference responses arising in the therapeutic relationship. People with extensive trauma histories, particularly, can evoke strong emotional reactions, and secondary or vicarious traumatisation in the treating clinician. Clinical supervision is extremely important so that therapists can be supported and assisted to process and understand their emotional reactions to the person.

Sessions of up to 90 minutes are usually required in trauma-focused therapies to ensure there is adequate time to complete the necessary work and to return the person to a safe baseline. The number of sessions required is highly variable, but twelve sessions may be sufficient when the trauma is not complex. When there have been multiple traumas, significantly more sessions may be required.

Factors to consider that may influence treatment outcome

While therapists can be confident that PTSD symptoms will often improve with one or more of the trauma-focused structured treatments, trauma processing may be insufficient for people whose PTSD developed following repeated or chronic interpersonal trauma, such as sexual or physical abuse in childhood. Complex PTSD is a term used to describe the core symptoms of PTSD in conjunction with symptoms that occur in addition to those well-recognised in PTSD, such as decreased attention and consciousness, including dissociation, disturbances in emotion regulation, somatic distress or disorganisation, poor relational capacities, and changed belief systems (Cloitre et al., 2012). The condition can follow lengthy abuse in adulthood, but most commonly refers to the sequelae of trauma in childhood, which is a developmentally vulnerable time, and a period in which the effects of trauma may impact significantly on a child's biopsychosocial development. Developmental trauma affects multiple brain structures, including the hippocampus, anterior cingulate cortex, amygdala and corpus callosum (Teicher and Samson, 2016).

The International Society for Traumatic Stress Studies (ISTSS) Guidelines for the Treatment of Complex Trauma (Cloitre et al., 2012) recommends a phase-based approach that begins with a focus on the reduction of psychiatric symptoms, increasing key functional capacities for self-regulation, and strengthening psychosocial and environmental factors. It has been proposed that this early stabilisation phase is necessary before any trauma-focused structured treatment is attempted. However, other researchers have disputed these guidelines and the need for such a phased approach (De Jongh et al., 2016). Though the ISTSS guidelines purport that the failure to address emotion regulation skills and stabilisation may lead to drop-out from interventions such as PE or EMDR, a recent meta-analysis failed to find evidence that this occurs in the treatment of adults with PTSD resulting from childhood events (Ehring et al., 2014). The case described above provides an example of an adult with childhood trauma who was treated with EMDR without a stabilisation phase. In those cases where chronic self-harm and suicidal ideation are present, more time and attention to stabilisation and engagement may however be required in preparation for trauma-focused structured therapy, as suggested by Cloitre and colleagues (2012). Issues of chronic self-harm and suicidal ideation are particularly more likely in those with Complex PTSD (Krysinska and Lester, 2010), so that individuals should be carefully assessed and only those identified as low risk should be offered trauma-focused treatment, as the emotional activation inherent in the process may elevate suicide risk. It is however worth noting potential exceptions here, for example, that some individuals with PTSD may have ongoing suicidality until the traumatic experience is addressed, in which case any delay in trauma-focused therapy should be avoided as much as possible (Harned et al., 2012).

It is also important to note that the majority of traumatic experiences can be well integrated into coherent internal narratives with therapy. In highly traumatic situations, however, people may dissociate to remove themselves from an inescapable situation, so as not to be present or connected to the trauma. If the trauma is ongoing, dissociation can become habitual, and, if severe, may even constitute a disorder in itself. In the field of trauma-focused therapies, significant dissociation is generally a contra-indication, as the problem needs to be addressed in its own right before other work can begin, and this process may be lengthy. Any of the structured trauma therapies also involve some level of emotional activation, and individuals with significant difficulties regulating affect may also require more stabilisation before commencing trauma work.

Despite evidence of the effectiveness of specialised trauma treatments, research suggests that many therapists are fearful to utilise them, or even talk about trauma with those they treat, out of concern that symptoms may worsen or that there will be drop-outs (Becker et al., 2004). There is no empirical evidence that this is the case. Whilst it is understandable that therapists may be apprehensive about exacerbating symptoms, it is also lacking in compassion and unethical to leave people suffering with a disorder that can be effectively treated. Therapists should also not deliver interventions beyond their level of expertise but should seek appropriate training and supervision to do so.

It is finally important to note that in the Australian healthcare system treatment for people with PTSD is likely to be provided by private therapists or by those in federal and state government funded services. There is a wide variation in the availability of treatment in different states and territories, and between urban and rural areas. Sessions are however generally only funded on an hourly basis, contrary to the 90-minute sessions recommended, and, currently, treatment is often limited to 10 sessions in a calendar year, which may be sufficient to treat some with trauma, but is insufficient for many.

Conclusion

The prevalence of PTSD in people with a history of trauma is high, and people with this disorder commonly present to mental health settings in Australia. If left undiagnosed and untreated, the disorder can become chronic, and can significantly impact multiple areas of a person's life. It is critical to note though that there is extensive evidence that PTSD can be successfully treated using trauma-focused structured approaches, so there is good reason to be hopeful about outcomes, when specific training in one of the trauma-focused therapies has been obtained, and therapy is delivered in a humane and compassionate way.

References

Andrade J, Kavanagh D and Baddeley A (1997) Eye-movements and visual imagery: A working memory approach to the treatment of post-traumatic stress disorder. *British Journal of Clinical Psychology* 36: 209–223.

Beck AT (1979) *Cognitive Therapy of Depression*. New York, NY: Guilford Press.

Beck A, Emery G and Greenberg R (1985) *Anxiety Disorders and Phobias: A Cognitive Approach*. New York, NY: Basic Books.

Becker CB, Zayfert C and Andersen D (2004) A survey of psychologists' attitudes towards and utilization of exposure therapy for PTSD. *Behaviour Research and Therapy* 42: 277–292.

Bisson JI, Roberts NP, Andrew M, et al. (2013) Psychological therapies for chronic post-traumatic stress disorder (PTSD) in adults. *Cochrane Database of Systematic Reviews* Issue 12 Art. No.: CD003388. DOI: 10.1002/14651858.CD003388.pub4.

Brewin CR, Andrews B and Valentine JD (2000) Meta-analysis of risk factors for post-traumatic stress disorder in trauma-exposed adults. *Journal of Consulting and Clinical Psychology* 68: 748–766.

Carlson JG, Chemtob CM, Rusnak K, et al. (1998) Eye movement desensitization and reprocessing (EDMR) treatment for combat-related posttraumatic stress disorder. *Journal of Traumatic Stress* 11: 3–24.

Chard KM (2005) An evaluation of cognitive processing therapy for the treatment of posttraumatic stress disorder related to childhood sexual abuse. *Journal of Consulting and Clinical Psychology* 73: 965–971.

Chen L, Zhang G, Hu M, et al. (2015) Eye Movement Desensitization and Reprocessing versus Cognitive-Behavioral Therapy for adult Posttraumatic Stress Disorder: Systematic review and meta-analysis. *The Journal of Nervous and Mental Disease* 203: 443–451.

Cloitre M, Courtosis CA, Ford JD, et al. (2012) *ISTSS expert consensus treatment for complex PTSD in adults*. Available at: istss.org/treating-trauma/istss-complex-ptsd-treatment-guidelines.aspx.

Cusack K, Jonas DE, Forneris CA, et al. (2016) Psychological treatments for adults with posttraumatic stress disorder: A systematic review and meta-analysis. *Clinical Psychology Review* 43: 128–141.

De Jongh A, Resick PA, Zoellner LA, et al. (2016) Critical analysis of the current treatment guidelines for Complex PTSD in adults. *Depression and Anxiety* 33: 359–369.

Dominguez SK and Lee CW (2017) Errors in the 2017 APA Clinical Practice Guideline for the Treatment of PTSD: What the data actually says. *Frontiers in Psychology* 8: 1–7.

Ehring T, Welboren R, Morina N, et al. (2014) Meta-analysis of psychological treatments for posttraumatic stress disorder in adult survivors of childhood abuse. *Clinical Psychology Review* 34: 645–657.

Foa EB and Rothbaum BO (2001) *Treating the Trauma of Rape: Cognitive-Behavioral Therapy for PTSD*. New York, NY: Guilford Press.

Fletcher S, Creamer M and Forbes D (2010) Preventing post traumatic stress disorder: Are drugs the answer? Review. *Australian and New Zealand Journal of Psychiatry* 44: 1064–1071.

Friedman MJ, Resick PA and Keane TM (2007) *Handbook of PTSD: Science and Practice*. New York, NY: Guilford Press.

Harned MS, Korslund KE, Foa EB, et al. (2012) Treating PTSD in suicidal and self-injuring women with borderline personality disorder: Development and preliminary evaluation of a Dialectical Behavior Therapy Prolonged Exposure Protocol. *Behaviour Research and Therapy* 50: 381–386.

Jeffries FW and Davis P (2013) What is the role of eye movements in eye movement desensitization and reprocessing (EMDR) for post-traumatic stress disorder (PTSD)? A review. *Behavioral and Cognitive Psychotherapy* 41: 290–300.

Kilpatrick D, Resnick H, Milanak M, et al. (2013) National estimates of exposure to traumatic events and PTSD prevalence using DSM-IV and DSM-5 criteria. *Journal of Traumatic Stress* 26: 537–547.

Krysinska K and Lester D (2010) Posttraumatic stress disorder and suicide risk: A systematic review. *Archives of Suicide Research* 14: 1–23.

Lee CW, Gavriel H, Drummond P, et al. (2002) Treatment of PTSD: Stress inoculation training with prolonged exposure compared to EMDR. *Journal of Clinical Psychology* 58: 1071–1089.

Lee CW and Cuijpers P (2013) A meta-analysis of the contribution of eye movements in processing emotional memories. *Behavioural Therapy and Experimental Psychiatry* 44: 231–239.

Marcus SV, Marquis P and Sakai C (1997) Controlled study of treatment of PTSD using EMDR in an HMO setting. *Psychotherapy* 34: 307–315.

Ozer EJ, Best SR, Lipsey TL, et al. (2008) Predictors of posttraumatic stress disorder and symptoms in adults: A meta-analysis. *Psychological Trauma: Theory, Research, Practice and Policy* 1: 3–36.

Peters L, Slade T and Andrews G (1999) A comparison of ICD-10 and DSM-IV criteria for posttraumatic stress disorder. *Journal of Traumatic Stress* 12(2): 335–343.

Phoenix Australia – Centre for Posttraumatic Mental Health (2013) *Australian Guidelines for the Treatment of Acute Stress Disorder and Posttraumatic Stress Disorder*. Melbourne, Australia: Phoenix Australia.

Resick PA and Schnicke MK (1992) Cognitive processing therapy for sexual assault victims. *Journal of Consulting and Clinical Psychology* 60: 748–756.

Rothbaum BO, Astin MC and Marsteller F (2005) Prolonged exposure versus eye movement desensitization and reprocessing (EMDR) for PTSD rape victims. *Journal of Traumatic Stress* 18: 607–616.

Santiago PN, Ursano RJ, Gray CL, et al. (2013) A systematic review of PTSD prevalence and trajectories in DSM-5 defined trauma exposed populations: Intentional and non-intentional traumatic events. *PLOS One* 8: e59236.

Schnyder U, Ehlers A, Elbert T, et al. (2015) Psychotherapies for PTSD: What do they have in common? *European Journal of Psychotraumatology* 6: 1–10.

Shapiro F and Forrest M (2001) *EMDR: Eye Movement Desensitization and Reprocessing*. New York, NY: Guilford Press.

Simiola V, Neilson EC, Thompson R, et al. (2015) Preferences for trauma treatment: A systematic review of the empirical literature. *Psychological Trauma: Theory, Research, Practice and Policy* 7: 516–524.

Teicher MH and Samson JA (2016) Annual research review: enduring neurobiological effects of childhood abuse and neglect. *Journal of Child Psychology and Psychiatry* 57: 241–266.

Van den Berg DP, de Bont PA, van der Vleugel BM, et al. (2015) Prolonged exposure vs eye movement desensitization and reprocessing vs waiting list for posttraumatic stress disorder in patients with a psychotic disorder: a randomized clinical trial. *JAMA Psychiatry* 72: 259–267.

Van der Kolk BA, Spinazzola J, Blaustein ME, et al. (2007) A randomized clinical trial of eye movement desensitization and reprocessing (EMDR), fluoxetine, and pill placebo in the treatment of posttraumatic stress disorder: Treatment effects and long-term maintenance. *Journal of Clinical Psychiatry* 68: 37–46.

Vaughan K, Armstrong M, Gold R, et al. (1994) A trial of eye movement desensitization compared to image habituation training and applied muscle relaxation in post-traumatic stress disorder. *Journal of Behavior Therapy* 25: 283–291.

Wolpe J (1969) *The Practice of Behavior Therapy*. New York, NY: Pergamon Press.

18 Trauma-informed Psychodynamic Psychotherapy – a brief history and contemporary application

Joan Haliburn

> Experiencing is the sense of my state of being … the psychotherapist must stay with the immediate experience.
>
> Robert Hobson, 1985, p.34

Introduction

Psychodynamic Psychotherapy has its roots in Classical Psychoanalysis. A short history is provided in this chapter, with emphasis on the role of trauma and traumatic memories in shaping psychoanalysis and psychotherapy. This is followed by a brief summary of the Conversational Model (CM), a contemporary, trauma-informed, relational model of therapy. The case of "Lilly", a young patient who was treated in the early 1980s in a psychiatric ward of a general hospital, demonstrates the use of the model. The need to look beyond symptoms and signs is emphasised, because the current diagnostic classification system generally in use does not take into account aetiology, and thereby inadvertently negates individual experiences. The necessity for a humanistic approach to patients cannot be overstated.

A short history of Trauma Theory

Jean-Martin Charcot, a leading physician in Paris, was the first to make the link between the condition then known as "Hysteria" and early trauma. Hysteria at the time encompassed a broad range of symptoms including conversion, somatisation and dissociation, and conditions that would now be known as Borderline Personality Disorder and Posttraumatic Stress Disorder (Van der Hart and Friedman, 1989). Charcot's work on Hysteria was then taken up by Pierre Janet, a French psychologist, who proposed that "vehement emotions" were aroused as a result of traumatic events, and when difficulty was experienced integrating the event it would be split off or dissociated, laying the foundations of a psychodynamic understanding of trauma. Two of Charcot's other pupils, Georges Gilles de la Tourette and Joseph Babinski, focused their research on the topic of "suggestibility", which initially held sway as a reason for the "problem of Hysteria". This led to sufferers of trauma in World War I being exposed to ineffective and questionable treatments to "boost their desire for health", and, after Charcot's death, Janet became a "lone voice" in the psychoanalytic field in the area of trauma (Van der Kolk et al., 1996: p.67). Just before the turn of the twentieth century, however, Sigmund Freud, an Austrian neurologist and the eventual founder of psychoanalysis, had also begun to recognise trauma and the relevance of traumatic memories.

Freud worked with Josef Breuer, a respected Viennese physician, well known for his case of "Anna O", a woman with a multitude of hysterical symptoms. Both Freud and Breuer realised that their patients, who mainly presented with hysterical symptoms, "suffered from reminiscences" (Breuer and Freud, 1893: p.7). Freud initially attributed these symptoms to the effects of childhood sexual abuse, ranging from sexual advances to actual sexual activity by elders. Known as the "Seduction Theory", Freud quickly abandoned these ideas involving the disturbing area of pathology in families, favouring instead a "fantasy model", believing that the recollections of these patients were not tied to real events, but to regressed infantile wish-fantasies (Hanly, 1986).

Freud, like Breuer, initially used hypnosis as a method of treatment, but he abandoned this as well, thinking that the benefit of hypnosis was unreliable, its therapeutic effect being too closely related to the personality of the hypnotist and the relationship with the patient. Instead, he started to use the technique of "free association" in which the patient is encouraged to say whatever comes to mind, so that patient and analyst may access unconscious material which could help with understanding and therefore the development of awareness. Free association was regarded as the real birth of psychoanalysis, along with the development of the concept of the unconscious. Freud also wrote at length about other matters, and developed what has been described as a "one-person" or intrapsychic theory of psychopathology, involving instinctual drives, psychological defence mechanisms, particularly repression, and the production of symptoms when an appropriate balance of energy cannot be achieved. The seminal work of Ellenberger (1970) provides details of this history.

Karl Jung, a Swiss psychiatrist and psychoanalyst, and the developer of concepts including archetypes and the collective unconscious, demonstrated the presence of what he referred to as "feeling-toned complexes". He linked these to splinter elements of the psyche, which were unacceptable and disturbing to the conscious mind, and which conflicted with the individual's conscious attitudes. He wrote, "it [trauma] behaves like an animated foreign body in the sphere of consciousness" (Jung, 1934/1970: p.7).

Sandor Ferenczi, a Hungarian psychoanalyst, reiterated that the sexual abuse of his female patients actually occurred when they were children, leading to fragmentation and dissociation (Ferenczi, 1932a). He described these experiences as "shocks", and opposed Freud's fantasy model. Ferenczi also believed that empathy on the part of the analyst was central to the therapy. Balint, who had been Ferenczi's patient, however, commented on Ferenczi's literal responses towards his patients' regressions (Ferenczi, 1932b) and his failure to preserve boundaries, for both of which he was ostracised by the psychoanalytic community.

It was Abram Kardiner's 1941 conceptualisation of the effects of war in returned soldiers as a "physioneurosis", suggesting that direct physiological changes resulted in chronic irritability, startle reactions and explosive aggression (Brett, 1996), that finally led to a different perspective being taken. From this work emerged the recognition of the distinct condition Posttraumatic Stress Disorder (PTSD), which eventually also included the suffering of sexually abused women (Herman, 1981; Miller, 1981). The American Psychiatric Association first included PTSD in the Third Edition of its Diagnostic and Statistical Manual of Mental Disorders, the DSM-III (American Psychiatric Association, 1980), and continued to refine it in later editions. Trauma-based treatments evolved outside of psychoanalysis following these developments in classification as a result of the work with veterans and because of the work of feminists, for example Herman (1992), and inside psychoanalysis via others, like Davies and Frawley, who wrote about approaches to those who have been sexually abused (1992).

A number of other psychoanalytic schools developed in parallel to and after Freud. These are important to note as all have made contributions to the understanding of the mind, the practice of psychodynamic psychotherapy, and the relevance of trauma to symptoms, understanding and treatment.

The emergence of the Object Relations Schools

Melanie Klein was a major influence in the British Psychoanalytic Institute, where there were three groups – one aligned with Freud, one with Klein, and a third sided with neither. Klein held that children's emotional problems were almost entirely due to fantasies derived from internal conflict, rather than as a result of real events in the external world (Klein, 1932). Klein is best known for her emphasis on the "internal object", which meant the taking in, or metaphorically internalising, of the significant other, the mother, and placed little or no significance on the environment. Klein introduced the complex concept of projective identification, referring to a state in which one forces unwanted parts of oneself into a significant other with the unconscious aim of controlling them. Klein saw her patient's self-destructive behaviour as an expression of their drives and repression, much like Freud (Knox, 2003).

The British Object Relations school, which included Ronald Fairbairn, Harry Guntrip, Michael Balint and Donald Winnicott, maintained that man's primary motivation is to seek relationship with others, and that early relational trauma boded dire consequences (West, 2016). Harry Stack Sullivan, who similarly believed in the power of early relationships, developed Interpersonal Psychoanalysis (Sullivan, 1953), dismissing the Freudian one-person model and placing emphasis on the interaction between the child and significant others.

Attachment Theory

Attachment Theory is the joint work of John Bowlby and Mary Ainsworth (Ainsworth and Bowlby, 1991). Bowlby wrote about the mother–child relationship, particularly the effects of an emotionally deficient environment on later infant development, and three papers contain the first formal statements of Attachment Theory (Bowlby, 1958, 1959, 1960). Drawing on ethology, cybernetics, information processing, developmental psychology, and psychoanalysis, Bowlby revolutionised the way in which the mother–child relationship and the effects of deprivation, separation and loss are considered. The main concept that a young child needs to develop a close relationship with at least one caregiver for social and emotional development to occur normally is now widely accepted. His concept of the "internal working model" of early mother–infant relationship as a template of the first relationship on which other relationships are patterned upon, and direct a person's manner of relating, and the subsequent intergenerational transmission of patterns of attachment, has been influential. Ainsworth expanded the theory, contributing to the concept of the attachment figure as a secure base from which the infant could explore the world in safety. She designed the "strange situation" procedure to determine the health of the early mother–child relationship, and to categorise the attachment as either secure, anxious-resistant or anxious-avoidant. A colleague of Ainsworth's, Mary Main, added a fourth group, the disorganised/disoriented attachment style, in which the child reacted unpredictably (Main and Solomon, 1986).

Attachment Theory was initially criticised as mechanistic, non-dynamic, and a total misunderstanding of psychoanalytic theory (Freud, 1960; Schur, 1960; Spitz, 1960), "renouncing drives, conflicts, the Oedipal complex and unconscious fantasy" (Fonagy, 2001: p.2). For the next several decades Bowlby was an outcast in the field. Research in Attachment Theory has however made a significant impact in the field of developmental psychopathology and, today, Attachment Theory is seen to be pivotal to the way in which both mother–infant dyads and the therapeutic relationship are understood (Holmes, 2001).

Self Psychology

In his school of Self Psychology, Heinz Kohut deviated markedly from traditional psychoanalysis and began the shift to a more relational way of working. He felt that internal instincts and motivations were insufficient to explain normal emotional life and the development of psychopathology, and that the patient's sense of well-being was directly related to their sense of self. Kohut reasoned that one needed to be emotionally connected to others, and to both idealise one's carers and to be validated by them, to develop a healthy sense of narcissism and to promote a sense of self-agency, as opposed to the development of pathological narcissism (Kohut, 1971). Kohut felt that others must be understood in treatment via the process of "vicarious introspection", or empathy, the ability to emotionally understand another. Kohut addressed the core needs of individuals whom he described as suffering from a disturbance of self-esteem, feelings of inner emptiness, lack of motivation and social and sexual problems, which he felt were ill-recognised and he referred to as a Narcissistic Personality Disturbance, or a defect in the sense of cohesion and continuity of the self. Strenuous attempts were later made to integrate Self Psychology with Object Relations Theory (Kernberg, 1975; Bacal, 1991) as relationships were considered pivotal.

The Relational School of Psychoanalysis

Further attempts to move away from Freud's internal drive and defense model and to place relationships, both early infant–caregiver and later therapist–patient, at the forefront, resulted in the development of the Relational School (Mitchell, 1986). Philip Bromberg (2011) has contributed significantly to the development of relational theory, particularly the relevance of trauma to early relationships, self-organisation and states of consciousness. He believes that a wave of dysregulated affect, a "tsunami", hits the infantile mind and if not processed by a carer leaves a "shadow" that may have a significant impact on future affect regulation capacity and upon relationships. He felt that it is important to not only recognise the inescapable effects of relational trauma, such as fragmentation and dissociation, but focus on the need for therapists to develop techniques to address fragmentation and to help to integrate dissociative states of mind.

Psychodynamic Psychotherapy

Psychodynamic Psychotherapy is a talking therapy which aims to help patients become aware of their own emotional states in order to help them with their problems. It has arisen and developed in the context of the schools of psychotherapy previously discussed. The primary focus in this form of therapy is on feelings and relationships, in contrast to thoughts, which form the basis of cognitive types of therapy. These problems include anxious and depressive symptoms, often described as "worries", relationship difficulties, lack of achievement and struggles with living, which are all traumatic in one way or other. Solid evidence supports its value (Holmes and Bateman, 2002). Traditional Psychoanalytic Psychotherapy, practiced now for over a century, was originally scheduled for four to five times a week, however, more contemporary Psychodynamic Psychotherapy usually involves only one or two sessions each week. Therapy may often extend over months and sometimes years. Research into the manner in which psychotherapy works is still in its early stages and is incomplete. Neuroscience studies however show that psychotherapy follows the principles of evolutionary adaptation, and is consonant with genetics, changing brain function and structure (Glass, 2008). Such studies Glass adds "have shown that psychotherapy affects regional cerebral blood flow, neurotransmitter metabolism, gene expression, and persistent modification in synaptic plasticity" (p.1589).

Short Term Psychodynamic Psychotherapy

The need to develop more time-effective psychotherapy was seen as urgent, both by patients and by third parties, even though a role for long-term dynamic psychotherapy was seen as necessary for some patients (Malan, 1976; Sifneos, 1979; Davanloo, 1980). Early forms like those of Malan and Davanloo, who worked together, involved active interpretation; the therapy was labelled as Intensive Short Term Dynamic Therapy. Later, Klerman et al. (1996) developed Interpersonal Psychotherapy for the treatment of Depression. Four areas involving grief, role disputes, role transitions and interpersonal deficits were looked at over 12 to 16 sessions. This therapy was psychodynamically informed but also utilised more structured principles from Cognitive Behaviour Therapy. Two types of short term therapy have been based on the Conversational Model of Psychotherapy, Short Term Dynamic Interpersonal Psychotherapy (STDIP), which has been manualised in Australia (Haliburn, 2017), and Psychodynamic Interpersonal Therapy, which is practiced in the UK (Guthrie, 1999). The difference between STDIP and other models of short term therapy is that it is trauma-informed, a distinct manner of assessment is advocated, assuming that all patients who present for help have experienced trauma. The following example helps to illustrate the process of psychotherapy in general, but in a shorter form.

A vignette – "Mr X"

Mr X saw his family doctor for increasingly depressed feelings, preceded by several months of anxiety and panic attacks for which he could find no reason. He reported feeling no better after several trials of antidepressant medication, and he was worried that he would lose his job, which would create further problems for his family. He was referred for psychotherapy.

During the assessment phase, Mr X outlined the history of his problems, as well as his personal and relationship history. It soon became clear to both the therapist and to Mr X that the onset of his difficulties coincided with his eldest daughter announcing that she planned to travel and live overseas for a period of time. He disagreed with her plans, but could not effect any change in her decision. Mr X was seen to have a number of strengths and no significant comorbid difficulties. As a result, it was decided that Mr X could undergo a trial of short term psychodynamic psychotherapy, on a weekly basis.

Exploring the difficulties with his daughter, it was clear that Mr X felt helpless and at a loss to know what to do. Further discussion of his situation revealed that two years earlier his mother had died. Mr X had had a difficult relationship with her since his adolescence. He had not resolved this relationship, and as his eldest daughter with whom he had a special relationship with was now leaving the family to live overseas, he found himself in turmoil. He said he had never felt "angry" towards her before, but did now. He felt that he could not come to terms with her decision, and at the same time he could not speak his mind, and said that he had gradually felt worse as the time of her departure got closer. The impending loss of his daughter had brought up for Mr X hitherto unacknowledged feelings towards his mother and her death which he was not consciously aware of, and which had resulted in his symptoms. Allowed to uncover and process these feelings, Mr X was able to recognise that his daughter was separating from the family in a way that was developmentally normal, and that he needed to allow her to separate. He also needed to work through the tumultuous relationship he had with his own mother, because of his own desire to be a separate individual as opposed to his mother's requirement to have him dependent on her. After 15 weeks of therapy it was clear that Mr X's symptoms had resolved, and he was able to move on. Contact at six months verified that his gains had been maintained.

The Conversational Model

The Conversational Model (CM) is one of several contemporary models of Psychodynamic Psychotherapy (Meares, 2004). Grounded in psychoanalytic theory, it was pioneered in the late 1960s by Robert Hobson and Russell Meares in the UK, and it has continued to evolve since the 1980s in Sydney, Australia with Meares and colleagues. Briefly aligned with Self Psychology, the CM returned to its original path in a more systematic way to potentiate the development of self that had been derailed by trauma, primarily in childhood and primarily in relationship. It has continued to evolve as it incorporates the latest findings in infant research, developmental theory, neurophysiology, brain dynamics and linguistics.

In the CM, traumatised patients are seen to be suffering a primary and fundamental disturbance: a disruption of the core of their being, or "self" (James, 1890). Types of trauma are wide-ranging and may include chronic early emotional deprivation, serious difficulties with attachment, emotional abuse in the form of chronic criticism, devaluation and shaming, and physical and/or sexual abuse. Ongoing trauma causes cumulative effects (Khan, 1963), and subsequent difficulties may be myriad and occur across multiple domains including affect, consciousness, self-perception, and relationship (Herman, 1992). The stage of development at which abuse occurs, the severity of the abuse and the relationship of the abuser to the abused are important factors. Sexual abuse by an entrusted care-giver, for example, may lead to severe fragmentation of the personality, and to the development of a Dissociative Disorder. This type of abuse also gives rise to symptoms like flashbacks, hypervigilance, and exaggerated startle reflexes, similar to those seen in Post-traumatic Stress Disorder (PTSD), and, with other symptoms, is referred to as Complex Post-Traumatic Stress Disorder (Steele et al., 2017).

The CM is primarily relational in its mode of action, and the type of dialogue used is characterised by an emphasis on feeling tones (Hobson, 1985). The CM approach to trauma is unique in that it suggests that the language of the therapist should fit with the capacity of the patient and his or her general functioning, and not to the patient's psychopathology (Meares, 1999a, 1999b). Efforts are particularly made to attempt to enter the patient's world and their pain by gently speculating with the patient about how they are feeling and what they might be struggling with. The CM is also a phasic model, much like all others for trauma treatment. Three arbitrary but inter-related phases can be described: an initial phase of stabilisation, a middle phase of identifying and processing traumatic memories, and a later phase of integrating trauma into the sense of self.

Applications of the CM

Applicable in day-to-day mental health care, the CM is taught to trainees through close supervision of audio-recorded sessions of patients (Meares et al., 2012). Originally pioneered in the treatment of patients diagnosed with Borderline Personality Disorder (BPD), and for whom Classical Psychoanalysis failed to be of help, it was found that at the end of one year of intensive twice-weekly therapy that 30 per cent of patients no longer met the DSM criteria for BPD (Stevenson and Meares, 1992). It has since been routinely used for the treatment of Personality Disorders (Haliburn et al., 2017), for Treatment Resistant Depression (Stevenson et al., 2015) and for Somatisation Disorders (Meares et al., 2008; Haliburn, 2011). It is applicable to adolescents, in parent–child psychotherapy (Haliburn, 2017), and is currently being trialled in group therapy. It has been adapted to short term therapy (Haliburn and Baker, 2014) and for single session crisis care whether in the emergency room or other setting (Haliburn, 2017).

A vignette – "Lilly"

Lilly was aged 16 when first seen in the 1980s by the author, who was then in both psychiatry and psychotherapy training. She was initially assessed in an emergency department. A waif of a girl, with a far-away look, Lilly was merely skin and bone as a result of total self-starvation, and covered with bruises and contusions. Remaining mute, her mother provided the history, while Lilly clung to her.

An anxious child who startled easily, she had become suddenly ill at the age of 12 years, when she stopped eating and drinking and refused to go to school. She also began to seriously self-harm, as a result of which she had multiple hospitalisations and outpatient attendances. Over the years she had been diagnosed with Major Depression, Eating Disorder, and Obsessive Compulsive Disorder, and treated accordingly with medication, Cognitive and Behaviour Therapy, including Exposure Therapy, all to no avail. She was last discharged from an adolescent unit where she was said to be non-compliant with therapy; she had been asked to confront her fear of looking at herself.

On assessment, using the classification system in use at the time, the DSM-III (American Psychiatric Association, 1980), Lilly fulfilled the diagnostic criteria for the following:

Axis I

1 Major Depressive Disorder
2 Obsessive Compulsive Disorder
3 Anorexia Nervosa
4 Separation Anxiety Disorder with School Phobia

Axis II

1 Borderline Personality Disorder

A dynamic formulation in the context of her presenting problems and her history was also developed. Her mother was found to be quite rejecting of her, and there were concerns that Lilly had not found her home life sufficiently safe or nurturing. Lilly's self-depriving behaviour, her failure to eat and drink, and to care for herself, were seen as a response to distressing internal stimuli and possibly to feelings of guilt. She also seemed to respond to internal stimuli by harming herself. Lilly's obsessive-compulsive behaviours were regarded as a way of engaging herself, namely, coping in order to prevent distressing thoughts from entering her mind.

Lilly's immense fear and her lack of insight caused her to cling to her mother and to avoid leaving her mother or go to school. What appeared to be Separation Anxiety and School Phobia was thought to reflect the avoidance behaviour characteristic of post-trauma syndromes. It was additionally thought that Lilly had in fact been subjected to further re-traumatisation by the systems of care that had previously misunderstood her presentation, particularly being forced to look at herself naked in a mirror in order to overcome her distress with her own body.

The Diagnostic and Statistical Manual of Mental Disorders

In response to the lack of diagnostic accuracy used in psychoanalysis, the American Psychiatric Association Task Force on Nomenclature and Statistics attempted to make the DSM-III a mainly descriptive document that was atheoretical in regard to aetiology, primarily for scientific rigour and to assist with communication and research. Most importantly, descriptive data can be framed in relatively clear statements which achieve diagnostic reliability, which offer certainty that clinicians and researchers are looking at the same entity. The Task Force also compared and contrasted the descriptive orientation in psychiatry with the psychodynamic orientation, and concluded that the two approaches overlap, are complementary and necessary to each other, and that there was a descriptive data base underlying dynamic psychiatry which could also be usefully included in future nomenclatures (Frances and Cooper, 1981). At the time, the aetiology of most psychiatric disorders was unknown, controversial, and thought to be the sum of multiple interacting causes. Reliability of diagnosis came to be seen as most important. However, over subsequent years, it has become increasingly clear that the aetiology of most psychiatric disorders remains uncertain, and that the DSM has done little more than to delineate symptom clusters, while not diagnosing actual disorders or diseases. In the process, the stories of individual patients have come to be seen as less and less significant. As a result, a focus on assessment in terms of the DSM system using the symptom clusters has frequently dictated contemporary "diagnosis" and "management". However, what is required of a competent psychiatrist or other mental health worker is the ability to gather data by structuring the interaction while also listening to the flow of a patient's conversation, so that a psychiatric and psychodynamic diagnosis or formulation are both possible within a reasonable time-frame. The previous approach to Lilly, in contrast, epitomises the difference.

Lilly – continued

Lilly was admitted to an adult psychiatry ward where she was treated by the author. She saw Lilly briefly every day, during the first week, and gradually reduced the frequency thereafter. Stabilisation of her mental state was the first aim, and this was achieved via the containing functions of the therapist, limited use of medication, and via the ward staff who were encouraged to help to understand Lilly and to validate both her distress and her personal story.

Another psychiatry trainee was allocated as case manager to Lilly. Simple and flexible behavioural techniques were used on a daily basis to encourage food and fluid intake, and to restrict ritualistic behaviour. The treatment team, so important in day-to-day management, was supported with frequent case discussions, and background relevant reading to help understand Lilly's situation. It cannot be overemphasised that acceptance of the patient and her problems, a general empathic and non-punitive attitude, provision of a validating and containing milieu, use of appropriate and timely limit-setting, and respect for one another in the treatment team, are vitally necessary in units who care for patients like Lilly.

During her inpatient stay, her mother gave a history of Lilly's older sister having been sexually abused by her father, who was charged accordingly and excluded from the family home. He was a returned soldier who consumed large amounts of alcohol, and appears to have suffered with PTSD. The possibility that Lilly herself might have been abused was raised by her mother, however whether or not this occurred was not verified.

Psychotherapy with Lilly

After two weeks of difficult, largely silent sessions, marked mostly by the therapist's speculations and reflective observations, Lilly began to respond and engage, allowing twice-weekly therapy to become the mainstay of her treatment in hospital. She was discharged after four months, having reached her optimum weight, with almost total reduction of ritualistic and self-harming behaviour. Continuity of care was seen to be an important factor in Lilly's treatment, and the author continued to see her in twice-weekly therapy as an outpatient for a further three years.

As the work progressed, Lilly began to experience safety within the confines of the therapeutic relationship, and she began to talk about herself and her family. She first expressed bewilderment about the removal of her father from the family home. She missed him and referred to him as, "the only one who loved me". Her pining for him brought forth scornful remarks from her mother and older sister and Lilly said, "they always put me down and compare my looks to those of my father". In the first six months, Lilly required brief re-admissions on three different occasions: the first due to escalating self-harm, the second on account of an increase in suicidal ideation, and the third as a result of a serious overdose of her antidepressants.

Traumatic memories

As she talked about her friends, Lilly began to remember that her illness started when she was in grade six, when she saw her best friend and boyfriend "making out" at her best friend's birthday party, when "I rushed home and began to bash my head against the wall, until the blood was running". With this memory came further fragments of memories of repeated sexual molestation by her father, and with it, recollections of there being "nobody at home" except her father, because her mother worked. She thought she might have been less than five years of age when this occurred, as she had not as yet started school.

Traumatic memories are experienced differently from narrative memories, because they are not integrated into the autobiographical history of the patient (Van der Hart et al., 1993) and therefore do not emerge in narrative form, but rather as partial or unformed memories, activated by internal or external triggers and sometimes, by no obvious trigger at all. Lilly also disclosed being physically beaten by her father when she "did not do as he asked". She could not understand this, "because he loved me so much". She rubbed her arms up and down, as if she remembered or perhaps was trying to erase some memory. Early traumatic memories are frequently only stored in implicit or unconscious and procedural memory systems, and arise as a collage of sensations, emotions, and behaviours (Levine, 2015). When activated, memories become labile again, and can be destabilising with associated disturbing thoughts, feelings and behaviours, very often of a self-punishing nature.

Self-harming and eating behaviours

Lilly saw herself as "bad". She described her need to punish herself by hitting, scratching and cutting herself, whenever she had memories of the abuse, and if she as much as saw her reflection in a mirror or a window pane she would become hyperaroused and harm herself. She experienced an inordinate amount of guilt and shame, and viewed herself as undeserving, and, when punishment was deemed by her to be insufficient, she began to deprive herself of food and then refused to drink water. She could not touch her own body, which resulted in deteriorating, and then absent, self-care. She also did not want to look like her father, "big and strong", which was a comparison her mother and sister often made. At one point, she remembered her mother holding her for the first time, after she became seriously ill, and added, "I always thought she didn't like me". Lilly had been diagnosed in earlier presentations as having primarily Anorexia Nervosa, and treated unsuccessfully with behavioural techniques.

Progress and betrayal trauma

Psychotherapy using the CM, with regular supervision, gradually brought about substantial change, and Lilly was able to return to school and complete her education, a dramatic turnaround. She did not socialise initially as she was afraid "that people could see what had happened to me", such was her experience of shame, which caused her to avoid the pain of exposure. She began to feel very guilty for loving her father, when in fact he had betrayed her, and it was at first difficult for her to recognise that she was left in the care of her father while her mother worked, while his role was to take care of her and protect her. Herman (1981) argues that the horror of incest is not in the sexual act but in the corruption of parental love. Indeed, child sexual abuse by an attachment figure creates mixed feelings of affection, love, anger and pain, and along with it, feelings of betrayal (Freyd and Birrell, 2013). These failures led to Lilly being robbed of any opportunity to develop a sense of self of any kind, because of the guilt. She had to come to terms with the fact that she was not to know that her father would indeed abuse her, and that she was very young when the abuse occurred. Lilly was eventually able to clearly express this, "How could he have done this to me? I loved him, and he was supposed to take care of me", showing remarkable self-awareness.

Conclusion

Responses to trauma have been many and varied, but the process of classification within psychiatry and mental health, and too few psychotherapeutic options for those suffering with mental illness and trauma-related conditions over the last several decades, have tended to obscure personal trauma histories. The fact that trauma results in pain and suffering to individuals and families, and an economic burden to society, is well known, but is only just having an impact. Being a psychiatrist, psychotherapist or other mental health worker who sees patients with varying dimensions of trauma is not just a matter of acquiring skills or techniques, as in the CM or in any other model. It takes a lifetime of learning, of attempting to understand others, and, even then, the work is incomplete. However, every moment spent with a patient can leave an indelible mark on a psychotherapist that can only assist others going forward. The case of Lilly is not an isolated one. Every psychiatrist and mental health worker will come across many such patients, if only the relevance of trauma is understood and the signs looked for.

That psychotherapy is costly is a myth that has for so long prevented appropriate resources being invested in the care of those who have experienced serious trauma. This myth has also prevented the growth of clinicians, and deprived them of an appropriate training experience. Psychodynamic psychotherapy has been ostracised for too long, and by too many, in positions of authority and of power. The demise of psychodynamically oriented ward milieus, the downgrading or eliminating of training programs in psychodynamic psychotherapy, the failure to support the provision of psychotherapy, because all are seen as non-essential, are changes to be resisted at all cost; psychotherapy is worth the effort (Lazar, 2010).

References

Ainsworth M and Bowlby J (1991) An ethological approach to personality development. *American Psychologist* 46: 331–341.

American Psychiatric Association (1980) *Diagnostic and Statistical Manual of Mental Disorders, Third Edition*. Washington, DC: American Psychiatric Publishing.

Bacal HA (1991) Notes on the relationship between Object Relations Theory and Self Psychology. *Progress in Self Psychology* 7: 36–44.

Bowlby J (1958) The nature of the child's tie to his mother. *International Journal of Psychoanalysis* 39: 350–373.

Bowlby J (1959) Separation anxiety. *International Journal of Psychoanalysis* 41: 1–25.

Bowlby J (1960) Grief and mourning in infancy and early childhood. *The Psychoanalytic Study of the Child* 15: 9–52.

Brett EA (1996) The classification of Posttraumatic Stress Disorder. In: Van der Kolk BA, McFarlane AC and Weisaeth L (eds) *Traumatic Stress: The Effects of Overwhelming Experiences on Mind, Body, and Society*. New York, NY: The Guilford Press, pp.117–128.

Breuer J and Freud S (1893) On the psychical mechanisms of hysterical phenomena: In: Strachey J (ed and trans) *The Standard Edition of the Complete Psychological Works of Sigmund Freud*. London, UK: The Hogarth Press and the Institute of Psychoanalysis.

Bromberg P (2011) *The Shadow of the Tsunami and the Growth of the Relational Mind*. New York, NY: Routledge.

Davanloo H (1980) *Short Term Psychodynamic Psychotherapy*. New York, NY: Jason Aronson.

Davies JM and Frawley MG (1992) Dissociative processes and transference-countertransference paradigms in the psychoanalytically oriented treatment of adult survivors of childhood sexual abuse. *Psychoanalytic Dialogues* 2: 5–36.

Ellenberger H (1970) *The Discovery of the Unconscious*. London, UK: Allen Lane.

Ferenczi S (1932a) Confusion of tongues between adults and the child. In: Balint M (ed), Mosbacher E (trans) (1955) *Final Contributions to the Problems and Methods of Psychoanalysis: The Selected Papers of Sandor Ferenczi, MD, Volume III*. London, UK: The Hogarth Press, pp.156–167.

Ferenczi S (1932b) On shock. In: Balint M (ed), Mosbacher E (trans) (1955) *Final Contributions to the Problems and Methods of Psychoanalysis: The Selected Papers of Sandor Ferenczi, MD, Volume III*. London, UK: The Hogarth Press, pp.253–284.

Fonagy P (2001) *Attachment Theory and Psychoanalysis*. New York, NY: Other Press.

Frances A and Cooper AM (1981) Descriptive and dynamic psychiatry: A perspective on DSM-III. *American Journal of Psychiatry* 139(9): 1198–1202.

Freud A (1960) Discussion of Dr Bowlby's paper, "Grief and Mourning in infancy and early childhood". In: Freud A (author) *The Writings of Anna Freud, Volume Five*. New York, NY: International Universities Press, pp.167–186.

Freyd J and Birrell P (2013) *Blind to Betrayal: Why We Fool Ourselves We Aren't Being Fooled*. New York, NY: Wiley and Sons.

Glass RM (2008) Psychodynamic Psychotherapy and the research evidence: Bambi survives Godzilla? *The Journal of the American Medical Association* 300: 1587–1589.

Guthrie E (1999) Psychodynamic Interpersonal Psychotherapy. *Advances in Psychiatric Treatment* 5: 135–145.

Haliburn J (2011) From traumatic attachment to somatisation disorder. *Australasian Psychiatry* 19: 401–405.

Haliburn J (2017) *An Integrated Approach to Short Term Dynamic Interpersonal Psychotherapy*. London, UK: Karnac.

Haliburn J and Baker A (2014) What has happened to the practice of short term dynamic psychotherapy in Australian mental health services? A multidisciplinary training program in Western Sydney. *Australasian Psychiatry* 22(5): 443–446.

Haliburn J, Stevenson J and Halovic S (2017) Integration in the psychodynamic psychotherapy of severe personality disorders: The Conversational Model. *Journal of Personality Disorders* 31: 1–17.

Hanly C (1986) The assault on truth: Freud's suppression of the seduction theory. *International Journal of Psychoanalysis* 67: 517–519.

Herman J (1981) *Father Daughter Incest*. Cambridge, MA: Harvard University Press.

Herman J (1992) *Trauma and Recovery*. New York, NY: Basic Books.

Hobson R (1985) *Forms of Feeling: The Heart of Psychotherapy*. London, UK: Tavistock.

Holmes J (2001) *The Search for the Secure Base: Attachment Theory and Psychotherapy*. Hove, UK: Brunner-Routledge.

Holmes J and Bateman A (eds) (2002) *Integration in Psychotherapy: Models and Methods*. Oxford, UK: Oxford University Press.

James W (1890) *Principles of Psychotherapy, Volume I*. New York, NY: Holt.

Jung C (1934/1970) A review of the Complex Theory. In: Jung C (author) Adler G and Hull RFC (eds and trans) *Collected works of CG Jung, The Structure and Dynamics of the Psyche, Volume Eight, Edition Two*. Princeton, NJ: Princeton University Press.

Kernberg O (1975) *Borderline Conditions and Pathological Narcissism*. New York, NY: Aronson.

Khan MR (1963) The concept of cumulative trauma. *Psychoanalytic Study of the Child* 18: 286–306.

Klein M (1932) *The Psychoanalysis of Children*. London, UK: The Hogarth Press.

Klerman GL, Weissman MW, Rounsaville BJ, et al. (1996) *Interpersonal Psychotherapy of Depression*. Northvale, NJ: Aronson.

Knox J (2003) Trauma and defences. *Journal of Analytic Psychology* 48: 207–233.

Kohut H (1971) *The Analysis of the Self*. New York, NY: International Universities Press.

Lazar SG (ed) (2010) *Psychotherapy Is Worth It: A Comprehensive Review of Its Cost-Effectiveness*. Washington, DC and London, UK: American Psychiatric Publishing.

Levine PA (2015) *Trauma and Memory: Brain and Body in a Search for the Living Past.* Berkeley, CA: North Atlantic Books.

Main M and Solomon J (1986) Discovery of a new, insecure-disorganised/disoriented attachment pattern. In: Yogman M and Brazelton TB (eds) *Affective Development in Infancy*. Norwood, NJ: Ablex, pp.95–124.

Malan DH (1976) *The Frontiers of Brief Psychodynamic Psychotherapy*. New York, NY: Plenum Press.

Meares R (1999a) Value, trauma and personal reality. *Bulletin of the Menninger Clinic* 63: 443–465.

Meares R (1999b) The 'adualistic' representation of trauma: On malignant internalisation. *American Journal of Psychotherapy* 53: 392–402.

Meares R (2004) The Conversational Model: An outline. *American Journal of Psychotherapy* 58(1): 51–66.

Meares R, Gerrull F, Korner A, et al. (2008) Somatisation and stimulus entrapment. *Journal of the American Academy of Psychoanalysis and Dynamic Psychiatry* 36(1): 165–180.

Meares R, Bendit N, Haliburn J, et al. (2012) *Borderline Personality Disorder and the Conversational Model: A Clinician's Manual.* New York, NY: WW Norton.

Miller A (1981) *Prisoners of Childhood: The Drama of the Gifted Child and the Search for the True Self.* New York, NY: Basic Books.

Mitchell SA (1986) Roots and status. *Contemporary Psychoanalysis* 22: 458–466.

Schur M (1960) Discussion of Dr John Bowlby's paper. *Psychoanalytic Study of the Child* 15: 63–84.

Sifneos PE (1979) *Short Term Psychodynamic Psychotherapy*. New York, NY: Plenum Press.

Spitz R (1960) Discussion of Dr John Bowlby's paper. *Psychoanalytic Study of the Child* 15: 85–94.

Steele K, Boon S and Van Der Hart O (2017) *Treating Trauma-Related Dissociation: A Practical, Integrative Approach.* New York, NY: WW Norton.

Stevenson J and Meares R (1992) An outcome study of psychotherapy for borderline personality disorder. *American Journal of Psychiatry* 149: 358–362.

Stevenson J, Haliburn J and Halovic S (2015) Trauma, personality disorder and chronic depression: The role of the Conversational Model in the treatment of resistant depression. *Psychoanalytic Psychotherapy* 2: 135–148.

Sullivan HS (1953) *The Interpersonal Theory of Psychiatry*. New York, NY: Norton.

Van der Hart O and Friedman B (1989) A reader's guide to Pierre Janet: A neglected intellectual heritage. *Dissociation* 2: 3–16.

Van der Hart O, Steele K, Boon S, et al. (1993) The treatment of traumatic memories: Synthesis, realization and integration. *Dissociation* 6: 162–180.

Van der Kolk BA, Weisaeth L and Van der Hart O (1996) The history of trauma in psychiatry. In: Van der Kolk B, McFarlane A and Weisaeth L (eds) *The Effects of Overwhelming Experience on Mind, Body, and Society*. New York, NY: Guilford Press, pp.47–76.

West M (2016) *Into the Darkest Places: Early Relational Trauma and Borderline States of Mind.* London, UK: Karnac.

19 Working with body and mind – trauma-informed somatic psychotherapy

Marianne Kennedy and Narelle McKenzie

> Our most refined thoughts and best actions, our greatest joys and deepest sorrows, use the body as a yardstick … and suffering, whether it starts in the skin or in a mental image, happens in the flesh.
>
> Antonio Damasio, 1994, p.xviii

Introduction

An enduring core concept in Psychoanalysis and traditional therapy has been the recognition that "Words and other forms of emotional communication have the power to interact with biological systems to bring about change in bodily systems, not only in ideas" (Bucci, 2008: p.51). What has equally been a central principle in body psychotherapy is that the reverse is also true, that intervention at a bodily level changes ideas and feelings, not just bodily systems.

All somatic psychotherapeutic approaches are grounded in a belief in the functional unity of body and mind: the soma, or lived body, and the psyche, form a single holistic entity, often called the "bodymind". Thought, emotion and somatic experience are understood as inextricably linked. Within both the mental health and broader community there is now a growing understanding and acceptance of this fundamental idea, which has led to increasing interest in exploring somatic psychotherapies and other body-based approaches, particularly in relation to the effects of both acute and developmental trauma. In Australia, somatic psychotherapy is also referred to as body psychotherapy, body-oriented or body-centred psychotherapy.

Historical background

Wilhelm Reich (1897–1957), a psychoanalyst and a student of Freud, is generally acknowledged to be the father of body psychotherapy, although its roots go back further, to Pierre Janet and others. Following a split between Freud and Reich in the 1930s, due to Reich's radical political and social views and his increasing attention to the body, psychoanalysis and body-oriented approaches took different paths into exploring and working with the psyche. However, it is now becoming evident that Reichian theory foreshadowed a contemporary understanding of the centrality of limbic and autonomic regulatory processes in affective and mental life (Sletvold, 2014). Somatic psychotherapy has always been based in an understanding that, in a myriad of subtle and cumulative ways, early developmental experiences shape and form not only our minds but our very embodiment.

Reich's theory of the development of character structure described ways in which emotional and physical disruptions, inhibitions, blockages, invasions and abuse are experienced, expressed and maintained somatically. He argued that the effects of historical traumas are carried in the body, in behavioural holding patterns, in deep muscle structures (called "muscular armouring"), in visceral tensions, and even in the shape and morphology of the body. These effects are also evident in patterns of emotional perception, organisation, and relationship (Reich, 1945/1983; Young, 2006). A fundamental tenet has therefore been the therapeutic value of establishing, or re-establishing, the free "flow" of psychic and physical energy, which Reich termed the "life force", necessary for psychological health.

In the USA, UK and Europe, a range of body-oriented models of theory and practice developed out of the work of Reich and his early students, including Fritz Perls (Gestalt Therapy), Alexander Lowen (Bioenergetic Analysis), Charles Kelley (Radix), John Pierrakos (Core Energetics), Gerda Boyesen, (Biodynamic Psychotherapy) and Stanley Keleman (Formative Psychology).

During the latter part of the twentieth century, the body psychotherapy tradition became associated with and incorporated philosophy and practices from the humanistic and existential psychology traditions, and several new models were advanced. In the early years of this development, these influences led to an emphasis on supporting and encouraging the humanistic ideals of self-actualisation and free expression. In some models, therapeutic catharsis was used to achieve these ideals and, as a result, less careful attention was paid to safety, containment, and relational issues. It was in this context that "neo-Reichian" somatic psychotherapy was introduced to Australia through the personal growth movement in the 1970s and until relatively recently these approaches have continued to be regarded by many as "alternative" and outside mainstream psychology and psychotherapy.

However, both in Australia and internationally, body psychotherapy, like other models of psychotherapy, has been informed and deeply influenced by the significant expansion in neurobiological and developmental research that has occurred over the past three decades. Insights into the processes and neurobiology of early attachment, infant development and parent–infant communication (Beebe and Lachman, 2002; Tronick, 2007; Schore, 2012; Beebe, 2013), the processes of self and dyadic regulation (Schore, 2012), and the psychobiological impact of trauma (Van der Kolk, 1996, 2014; Levine, 1997, 2010; Ogden et al., 2006; Ogden and Fisher, 2015) have helped to explicate many aspects of body psychotherapy theory and have led to new treatment approaches. There is also now a growing body of contemporary theory, based on neurobiological research and more specifically on infant research, that demonstrates that movement and the registration of that movement is an essential aspect of embodiment and self-experience. Both the impulse to movement and the constriction of that movement shapes bodily structure, forms body schema and body image, and is instrumental in shaping self-structure (Gallagher, 2005).

Neuropsychological research now clearly demonstrates that traumatic experiences reach deeply into the affective and autonomic domains and are stored in the limbic system (Marlock and Weiss, 2015). When people have experienced trauma, whether single incident or complex developmental trauma (Complex Trauma), in many different ways, "the body keeps the score" (Van der Kolk, 1996, 2014). Trauma may be encoded in incomplete patterns of fight or flight sympathetic nervous system arousal, or in a behavioural freeze or shutdown, which is a parasympathetic nervous system vagal response (Levine, 2010; Porges, 2011). There can also be a thwarted fight/flight arousal response along with a freeze response (Levine, 2010; Schore, 2012). Research is also now starting to make clear the long-term impact of early childhood trauma on people's relationship to their own bodies (Price, 2007; Van der Kolk, 2014). Body awareness, body attitude and body satisfaction may all be negatively affected, for example, in dissociation from body experience or in feelings of deep shame, disgust or hatred towards their bodies or parts of their bodies that are associated with trauma, especially sexual trauma (Scheffers et al., 2017).

There is also growing recognition of the powerful parallels between early developmental processes, the profound psychobiological effects of traumatic experience, and the growth-facilitating processes of psychotherapy (Porges, 2011; Schore, 2012; Beebe, 2013; Van der Kolk, 2014). Before other therapeutic work can be done, it is often essential to help traumatised clients to strengthen their somatic and emotional regulatory capacities, to be able to tolerate arousal states and to stay present in the moment. "Psychotherapeutic methods that are primarily cognitive and verbally oriented are thus not particularly well equipped to meet the demands of [the] somatic reality at the root of subjective experience" (Marlock and Weiss, 2015: p.2). Engaging in a here-and-now, "bottom up" therapy approach (Ogden et al., 2006; Van der Kolk, 2014) represents a shift of focus from "top-down" attention to explicit, analytical, conscious, verbal and rational left hemisphere functioning, towards implicit, integrative, unconscious, non-verbal, bodily-based emotional right hemisphere functioning (Schore, 1994, 2012). Assisting clients to re-connect to their bodies, to learn to better modulate the intensity of their emotions and arousal levels and to begin to establish a greater sense of safety and agency in interpersonal relationships should now form a significant part of the initial phase of any trauma-informed treatment.

Somatic approaches to working with trauma

Somatic approaches can be used to treat those who have suffered single incident trauma, adult onset trauma or Complex Trauma. Several distinct body-oriented approaches to working with trauma can be identified and there are variations in the degree to which touch, movement and physical contact are used. Most trauma-informed somatic psychotherapies integrate verbal reflection and psychodynamic exploration with more direct work with embodied experience and patterns of expression, when appropriate. Some more recent models have been specifically developed for treating trauma, and therapists who are trained in these models frequently also combine the somatic work with other "talk" therapies. Body-focused work within all these approaches may be engaged to help clients develop greater body awareness, self and other contact, containment, boundaries, self-regulation capacity, flexibility and spontaneity, as well as in the exploration of traumatic experiences, including body memory. There is also an extensive range of other body therapies, such as massage, yoga and stress release therapies that may be valuable as adjunct treatments for some clients.

Regardless of the specific modality involved, a three-phase process is now generally considered most appropriate for the treatment of the severe, pervasive and long-term effects of Complex Trauma (International Society for the Study of Trauma and Dissociation, 2011). Phase one focusses on establishing safety, stabilisation, and symptom reduction; phase two involves confronting, working through, and integrating traumatic memories; and phase three involves identity integration and rehabilitation. Body-centred approaches to working with dysregulated psychobiological states are especially valuable in addressing issues in the first phase of treatment. They are also important in helping to stabilise and support integration when processing traumatic memories during phase two and to help build and strengthen somatic and relational resources and increase resilience in phase three.

Working in this way, somatic approaches can help address deep-seated difficulties with affect regulation, body image distortion, self-injury, shame, dissociation and somatisation, as well as the trust and relational difficulties commonly experienced. Clients with Complex Trauma, especially when resulting from ongoing childhood abuse and neglect, are likely to gain most benefit from a psychotherapeutic approach in which the somatic work is integrated within a therapy that provides an ongoing opportunity to experience a safe, holding relationship, an experience that was disrupted and/or was unavailable in early life. Much of what follows in the remainder of this chapter refers to this type of treatment.

Assessment

At the beginning of therapy, a thorough assessment is undertaken, including acute safety matters, somatic symptoms and a personal history. Attention is paid to the client's embodied presence and vitality; the intensity, strength and qualities of their engagement in the relationship; their regulation of emotions and their self-awareness. Embodied character patterns that may be reflected in physical posture and movement are carefully observed. Signs of dissociation and disconnection from the bodymind and any other indications of trauma responses are especially noted and will determine the pace and timing of somatic interventions used. When there is significant disconnection or dissociation, the therapist attends to the client's body signals while at the same time working verbally to establish rapport, to assess the client's capacity for self-regulation and to clarify goals and the current support system. Work with physical contact and movement in most cases is contra-indicated when significant dissociation is present because of the risk of further dysregulation or re-traumatisation. However, movement and emotional expression and even touch may at times be used to assist a client to feel contained and to help address dissociative behaviour. Any decision to work in this way is based on careful assessment and skillful tracking by the therapist. During the assessment phase a clear contract is negotiated and agreed to, as would be the case for any other form of psychotherapy. The boundaries or frame of the therapy are clearly outlined, particularly in regard to the possibility of work involving touch.

Fundamental principles

Attention to and work with bodily experience

Careful observation and tracking of embodied experience, through attention to sensation, impulse, movement and emotion, has always underpinned somatic psychotherapy. This engages a process of non-judgmental attention to experience akin to that used in "mindfulness" practice, although the meditative aspects are not typically present. To assist with this, somatic psychotherapists are also trained to become sensitively attuned observers of their own physiology and the associated bodily changes and emotions, as well as those of their clients, and to draw on these observations for information about moment-to-moment interactions.

Initially, a therapist will unobtrusively observe and "read" a client's body structure and patterns of physical organisation and relational engagement, including the intonation, inflection and modulation of the voice and their facial and gestural expressions. Habitual body postures that may reflect longstanding beliefs and self-regulation strategies are also noted, especially those that may indicate chronic trauma responses, such as extreme rigidity in the torso, lack of muscle tone in the limbs, or deadened, blank or lifeless eyes (Ogden et al., 2006). Gradually the client's attention may be drawn to noticing their own body sensations, including aspects such as body temperature, tension, pain, numbness or tingling, energy levels and distribution, vibrations and subtle movements. Through observation, tracking and exploration of such experiences in concert with the emotions, thoughts, images and memories that accompany them, clients gradually begin to recognise and experience them with more acceptance and to develop a greater sense of self-agency. When appropriate, structured body-focused activities may also be used to help a client explore the impact that a particular body position (Smith, 1985), stress position (Lowen, 1975), or other body posture or movement has on their emotional and energetic arousal and their capacity to stay regulated, and whether it functions to enhance or interrupt connection with themselves and with others.

Clients who have experienced significant early developmental trauma may particularly need to learn how to identify and connect to their own body sensations – both proprioceptive (awareness of where the body is in space) and interoceptive (awareness of internal sensations and emotions) – and to develop a vocabulary for naming and describing these sensations. In the early stages of the work, the trauma and accompanying symptoms are acknowledged but the events are not explored in detail. The focus at that point is on the relief of symptoms, the therapeutic relationship, and the development of a greater sense of awareness and control over bodily and cognitive functioning, including flashbacks.

Body-based interventions with those who have experienced trauma may also involve teaching techniques of "grounding", which broadly means being in touch with reality, having a grip on the world and being able to stand on your own two feet (Lowen, 1975). For example, improved reality testing through the experience of the reliability of the musculoskeletal system and the stability and solidity of the ground enables anxiety-provoking thoughts and memories to be tolerated from a position of greater self-awareness and safety (Röhricht, 2015). Grounding also supports the regulation of physiological and emotional responses like shaking, shivering, crying, anger and dissociation. Bringing dissociatively withdrawn and traumatically "frozen" energy back into the hands, arms, feet, legs and eyes (Lowen, 1975; McKenzie, 2015) may also promote a greater sense of presence (that is, maintaining awareness of both inner and external experience without dissociating) and agency.

A vignette – "Rodney"

Rodney was 35 years old and had a history of severe childhood abuse. A recent interpersonal conflict at his work had re-triggered some of his earlier trauma responses. He felt ambushed by these and found himself bursting into tears, feeling frightened and unsafe around work colleagues, and being startled by sudden unexpected noises. As he began to describe this to his therapist, it became apparent that he was disconnected from his experience. His gaze was fixed, his speech was rapid, his breathing shallow, his level of arousal was increased, and he was generally less embodied. His therapist asked him to pause, to slowly inhale and, as he exhaled, to gently push his feet into the floor. After a few repetitions, Rodney started to settle. The therapist then suggested that he blink a little, look around at objects in the room, and describe their texture and colour. This was initially difficult, and he took a little time, as he was anxious to return to the original story. There was a lot of emotion in his body, and it was clear to the therapist that he needed more grounding to be able to process it, so she suggested that Rodney stand up and feel his feet on the floor, and then bend his knees slightly. With each inhalation he was encouraged to curl over, letting his head gradually drop toward the floor as he felt his legs and hips supporting him. Then, after slowly returning to an upright position and staying aware of the rhythm of his breath, he was asked to slowly straighten his legs on inhaling, and to bend them a little on exhaling. After a few minutes, Rodney reported that he felt more aware of the strength in his legs and feet, more connected to himself, and more present in the room and with the therapist. He was then able to sit down and continue his story more calmly and without disembodiment or emotional dysregulation.

Working within the window of tolerance

Learning to differentiate between the body sensations of moderate physiological arousal (such as shaking, rapid heart rate) and significant emotional arousal, such as terror, is often necessary in working with the sequelae of trauma. Directly attending to the body sensations and learning to observe, name and gradually regulate them helps develop a safer base from which to process trauma-related emotion (Ogden et al., 2006). This will usually occur in phase one, during which time the therapist may need to function as an "interactive psychobiological regulator" for the client (Schore, 2012). For example, the therapist may use the tone and rhythm of their voice and the regulation of their own breath and presence to help the client calm and return to their "window of tolerance", that is, the zone within which a person is able to process stimuli and function effectively. At times, physical contact may be used if appropriate and negotiated. Schore argues that just as the psychobiologically attuned caregiver regulates the affective states of a child, so a therapist's attunement to both their own and the client's unconscious, non-verbal, bodily based functioning is fundamental to helping traumatised clients learn to regulate their arousal states (Schore, 2012).

Specific breathing patterns have been shown to serve important functions in both the conscious and unconscious regulation of emotional arousal (Moore et al., 2011; Ogden and Fisher, 2015). For example, deepening and extending the exhalation phase engages the ventral vagal nervous system necessary for calming hyperarousal and the flight/fight response and for moving out of a freeze response (Porges, 2011). Developing awareness and an ability to use the breath to modulate arousal can also help to modulate the intensity of spontaneous flashbacks and intrusive memories. Similarly, the breath may be used to bring enlivenment.

Working with touch

Touch communicates a vast range of meanings that are influenced by the relational context in which the touch occurs, as well as the type and intention of the touch. Emotional regulation in early life occurs through attuned and modulated attention and affect provided by the caregiver, communicated through gaze, prosody of voice and touch (Schore, 1994). A sense of self and self-and-other is also partially derived in early infancy from the presence and quality of the touch from important attachment figures (Brazelton and Cramer, 1991), whereas lack of touch, or inappropriate touch, can result in serious developmental disruption (Van der Kolk, 2014).

The use of physical touch within the psychotherapeutic setting remains controversial among mental health practitioners due to concerns about the risk of boundary crossings and violations, particularly of a sexual nature. If physical contact from therapist to client occurs at all, it is typically in the context of providing a holding, nurturing or comforting experience at a given time. However, within the body-centred tradition, the skilful use of touch and other physical contact may provide a much broader range of therapeutic functions, beyond the social communication of comfort.

Contactful touch is a multilayered, complex, intersubjective interaction that involves moment-by-moment, here-and-now mindful connection (Westland, 2011). Appropriate and carefully negotiated touch may help clients to focus and deepen self-awareness and emotional experience, enable experimentation with different patterns of contact and withdrawal, facilitate sensorimotor organisation and activation and support somatic structuring (Cornell, 2008, 2015; LaPierre, 2012), as well as developing the capacity for "play". The therapeutic use of touch may also help traumatised clients to regulate and contain their emotions, reducing their fear and helping them to reality test and build new somatic resources (Westland, 2015).

There are many variations in the ways and degrees to which somatic therapists from different modalities use direct physical contact, either between therapist and client or through guided use of self-touch by the client. For example, a client may explore various forms of touch and pressure to bring greater awareness and aliveness to their own arms. In any session, depending on what is emerging for the client, touch may be the main focus of a session, or there may be brief moments of touch, or none at all.

Training in the skills necessary for observing and evaluating the appropriateness of any physical intervention is essential for understanding the clinical and ethical considerations involved in this work. This is especially important when negotiating touch. Close attention to the congruence between the client's bodily and verbal communications is fundamental as, for example, a client may verbally agree to touch but subtly flinch or become still, indicating difficulty.

A vignette – "Sally"

Sally, a client with a history of sexual abuse, was working on her underdeveloped sense of physical and emotional boundaries. Her therapist suggested that she explore some self-touch to develop a sense of her body as a container. Guided by her therapist as both sat in their chairs, with each inhalation of her breath Sally applied gentle but firm pressure to her right arm, starting at her shoulder and moving slowly down, releasing the pressure on each exhale. Sally then applied this rhythm of pressure to her left arm, to the sides of her torso, her thighs and calves. At the end of the exercise, Sally sobbed. Prior to this session she had experienced her body, "like a balloon on a string, all head and no body". Now she shared that she had a sense of the substance of her body and its physical boundaries – a sense of a container. This reduced her fears considerably.

Confronting, working through and integrating traumatic memories

In phases two and three of work with clients with Complex Trauma, continued attention to the client's developing somatic awareness and capacity for emotional regulation provides a platform from which they can more safely explore traumatic memories. Differentiating between types of traumatic experience is especially important here, for example, medical trauma, prolonged combat or terrorism experiences and early developmental trauma, which may include abuse of a sexual, physical and/or emotional nature. Throughout the trauma work, interventions will emerge through the client's and the therapist's growing awareness of the nature of the ongoing therapeutic relationship and what may be helpful or needed. They may collaboratively agree that a client is ready to deepen the exploration of a memory or the impact of a traumatic event. However, not all clients will wish to work with traumatic memories, and some will not have strong and stable enough resources to do so without significant disruption.

Processing traumatic memory requires very careful attention to arousal levels and titration of exposure and focus. Somatic flashbacks and somatosensory intrusions and symptoms, along with body memories – those traumatic memories encoded in body sensations and experience – may emerge and be highly disturbing. "The therapist needs to elicit, carefully and slowly, fragments of the memory at a pace that enables the client to approach the edges of the window of tolerance but not remain in a hyper- or hypoaroused zone", accessing enough of the traumatic material to work with, without causing re-traumatisation or dissociation (Ogden et al., 2006: p.243). Usually the work will begin away from the specific area of trauma or discomfort, and the therapist will "pendulate" the experience by helping the client to move back and forth between an aroused and/or dysregulated state or traumatic memory and a more resourced and regulated state (Levine, 2010).

Some trauma-specific approaches work directly at a physiological level, paying careful attention to small spontaneous movements that reveal interrupted impulses and actions and bringing them to conscious attention. The focus here is on releasing bodily tensions safely within the context of the therapeutic relationship (Levine, 2010; Brom et al., 2017), allowing for the expression of meaningful actions that were not able to be completed at the time of the trauma. These may include protective orienting actions, fight/flight responses and coming out of freeze responses, with the intention of enabling healing without the need for a full or explicit telling of the traumatic events (Levine, 2010).

The somatic experiences and their implications need to be reflected on and, when possible, integrated into a coherent narrative memory. Employing both verbal and somatic approaches in the exploration of traumatic memories supports the development and/or the restoration of a subjective experience of a more "bounded, cohesive, continuous and agentic self" (Boulanger, 2007: p.74).

Encouraging emotional expression and expanding the window of tolerance

Siegel has written that "Our well-being depends on widening the window of tolerance so that we can hold the elements of our internal world in awareness – without being thrown into rigidity (depression, cut-offs, avoidance) or chaos (agitation, anxiety, rage)" (2012: p.139). In the later phases of therapy there is a shift in emphasis as the person's capacity for more flexible emotional regulation increases. Emotional regulation moves beyond the reduction of affective intensity or the dampening of negative emotions to also include more intense experiences of positive emotion, enabling more complex self-organisation (Schore, 2012). Stronger emotions, affective memories and bodily sensations can be experienced and integrated, further lessening the need for dissociative processes. Developing a greater capacity for "dual awareness" makes it possible to attend to both internal sensations and external cues simultaneously when evaluating the safety of a situation or environment (Rothschild, 2011).

In phase three, experiences of positive emotion, trust in the self, and in the felt sense of "going-on-being" – the ability to just "be" without intrusion – are sought and consolidated. Attention is also paid to building and restoring effective relationships as clients learn and practise actions and expressions that further promote integration and adaptation in normal life (Ogden et al., 2006). Though the need to alleviate symptoms may arise and require attention, the focus is increasingly on the person's growing sense of safety within themselves and in the world, their capacity for presence and aliveness in relationship, their capacity to be in contact with reality and their ability to express or contain emotions, thoughts and actions, and to establish and maintain appropriate emotional, cognitive and physical boundaries.

A client who has been subjected to abuse may at this stage feel able, for the first time, to express grief or rage at their abuser, having developed a greater capacity to express intense emotion without becoming destabilised and losing connection to themselves or the therapist. They are more able to stay present and integrate the experience within both body and mind and, when necessary, to use newly developed skills to regain self-regulation.

Training, supervision and personal therapy

It is important that therapists who work with traumatised clients have adequate training and supervision in trauma-informed therapy. This is equally true when working directly with the embodied aspects of traumatic experience. Accredited somatic psychotherapists in Australia have usually had prior training and experience in a relevant field, such as psychology, social work, medicine, nursing, counselling or psychotherapy. They are then typically required to undertake formal postgraduate level training of a minimum of two to three years, providing theoretical and clinical skills for both verbal and body-oriented psychotherapy, including professional and ethical standards of practice. In most models of somatic psychotherapy, therapists are required to have undertaken their own personal psychotherapy and are expected to engage in ongoing clinical supervision of their work to maintain accreditation.

Research

Somatic psychotherapy approaches for Complex Trauma and trauma-specific body-oriented treatments are still a relatively new, though growing area of practice in Australia, as indeed they are elsewhere. Although strong links are being made to the substantial body of evidence from studies in affective neuroscience, there has to date been little systematic investigation into the efficacy of body psychotherapy (Röhricht, 2009) and the need for more rigorous research involving comparative studies and clinical trials is now well recognised. Several recent studies and exploratory investigations of specific models of somatic treatment for trauma hold promise, and a number of larger research projects are currently being undertaken.

Some preliminary research evidence provided by small pilot studies has found empirical support for the use of bodywork, particularly focusing on body awareness, combined with psychotherapy, in reducing dissociation and assisting recovery from sexual abuse in women (Price, 2005, 2007). A recent study (Brom et al., 2017), the first randomised controlled study investigating the effectiveness of Somatic Experiencing, a neurobiologically based trauma-specific body-oriented therapy (Levine, 1997), showed significant effects for both depressive and posttraumatic symptom severity. Exploratory field studies using brief Somatic Experiencing as an early intervention treatment with tsunami survivors (Leitch, 2007; Parker et al., 2008), also found significant symptom improvement immediately post-treatment and at eight to 12 months follow-up.

Two recent pilot studies used techniques derived from Sensorimotor Psychotherapy (Ogden et al., 2006), a quasi-experimental pilot study with traumatised adolescents in residential treatment (Warner et al., 2014) and a 12 session Sensorimotor Psychotherapy group therapy treatment with a severely and chronically ill population in a trauma centre (Gene-Cos et al., 2016). Both found statistically significant changes on a range of measures and offer promising directions for use in the stabilisation and skills building phase of treatment for Complex Trauma. However, the authors of all of these studies caution that more systematic controlled outcome research with larger samples is needed.

Conclusion

A reduction in symptoms and distress, greater emotional regulation capacity and sense of agency, and improved relationships are among the central goals of all trauma treatment approaches. However,

> If there is one way in which body psychotherapy continues and will continue to distinguish itself from other psychotherapies, it will no doubt be through its continued attachment to a concept of vitality – more than acceptance, more than adjustment, more than self-confidence [and] more than a 'contract for living'.
>
> (Randolph, 2015: p.450)

Assisting traumatised clients to gain a stronger sense of aliveness and vitality remains an inherent vision for trauma work in somatic psychotherapy.

References

Beebe B and Lachman F (2002) *Infant Research and Adult Treatment: Co-constructing Interactions*. New York, NY: The Analytic Press.

Beebe B (2013) *The Origins of Attachment: Infant Research and Adult Treatment*. New York, NY: Routledge.

Boulanger G (2007) *Wounded by Reality: Understanding and Treating Adult Onset Trauma*. New York, NY: Psychology Press.

Brazelton TB and Cramer B (1991) *The Earliest Relationship: Parents, Infants and the Drama of Early Relationship*. London, UK: Karnac.

Brom D, Stokar Y, Lawi C, et al. (2017) Somatic Experiencing for Posttraumatic Stress Disorder: A randomized controlled outcome study. *Journal of Traumatic Stress* 30(3): 304–312.

Bucci W (2008) The role of bodily experience in emotional organization: new perspectives on the multiple code theory. In: Anderson FS (ed) *Bodies in Treatment: The Unspoken Dimension*. New York, NY: The Analytic Press, pp.51–76.

Cornell W (2008) *Explorations in Transactional Analysis: The Meech Lake Papers*. Pleasanton, CA: TA Press.

Cornell W (2015) *Somatic Experience in Psychoanalysis and Psychotherapy*. New York, NY: Routledge.

Damasio A (1994) *Descartes' Error: Emotion, Reason and the Human Brain*. New York, NY: Putnam.

Gallagher S (2005) *How the Body Shapes the Mind*. Oxford, UK: Clarendon Press.

Gene-Cos N, Fisher J, Ogden P, et al. (2016) Sensorimotor psychotherapy group therapy in the treatment of Complex PTSD. *Annals of Psychiatry and Mental Health* 4(6): 1080. 1–7.

International Society for the Study of Trauma and Dissociation (2011) Guidelines for treating dissociative identity disorder in adults, third revision. *Journal of Trauma and Dissociation* 12: 115–187.

LaPierre A (2012) *Healing Touch: Honoring the Somatic Dimension of Psyche*. eBook: cellula rbalance.com.

Leitch ML (2007) Somatic Experiencing treatment with tsunami survivors in Thailand: Broadening the scope of early intervention. *Traumatology* 13(11): 11–20.

Levine P (1997) *Waking the Tiger: Healing Trauma.* Berkeley, CA: North Atlantic Books.

Levine P (2010) *In an Unspoken Voice: How the Body Releases Trauma and Restores Goodness.* Berkeley, CA: North Atlantic Books.

Lowen A (1975) *Bioenergetics.* New York, NY: Coward, McCaan and Geoghegan.

Marlock G and Weiss H (2015) The field of body psychotherapy. In: Marlock G, Weiss H, Young C, et al. (eds) *The Handbook of Body Psychotherapy and Somatic Psychology.* Berkeley, CA: North Atlantic Books, pp.1–18.

McKenzie N (2015) Visual contact, facing, presence and expression: The ocular segment in body psychotherapy. In: Marlock G, Weiss H, Young C, et al. (eds) *The Handbook of Body Psychotherapy and Somatic Psychology.* Berkeley, CA: North Atlantic Books, pp.658–665.

Moore M, Brown D, Money N, et al. (2011) *Mind-body skills for regulating the autonomic nervous system, Version 2.* Arlington, VA: Defense Centers of Excellence for Psychological Health and Traumatic Brain Injury.

Ogden P, Minton K and Pain C (2006) *Trauma and the Body: A Sensorimotor Approach to Psychotherapy.* New York, NY: Norton and Co.

Ogden P and Fisher J (2015) *Sensorimotor Psychotherapy: Interventions for Trauma and Attachment.* New York, NY: Norton and Co.

Parker C, Doctor RM and Selvman R (2008) Somatic therapy treatment effects with tsunami survivors. *Traumatology* 14(3): 103–109.

Porges S (2011) *The Polyvagal Theory: Neurophysiological Foundations of Emotions, Attachment, Communication and Self-Regulation.* New York, NY: Norton and Co.

Price C (2005) Body-oriented therapy in recovery from child sexual abuse: An Efficacy Study. *Alternative Therapies in Health and Medicine* 11(5): 46–57.

Price C (2007) Dissociation reduction in body therapy during sexual abuse recovery. *Complementary Therapies in Clinical Practice* 13(2): 116–128.

Randolph M (2015) On vitality. In: Marlock G, Weiss H, Young C, et al. (eds) *The Handbook of Body Psychotherapy and Somatic Psychology.* Berkeley, CA: North Atlantic Books, pp.444–453.

Reich W (1945/1983) *Character Analysis, Third Edition.* New York, NY: Farrar, Straus and Giroux.

Röhricht F (2009) Body-oriented psychotherapy: The state of the art in empirical research and evidence-based practice: A clinical perspective. *Body, Movement and Dance in Psychotherapy* 4(2): 135–156.

Röhricht F (2015) Body psychotherapy for the treatment of severe mental disorders – an overview. *Body, Movement and Dance in Psychotherapy* 10(1): 51–67.

Rothschild B (2011) *Trauma Essentials: The Go-To Guide.* New York, NY: Norton and Co.

Scheffers M, Hoek M, Bosscher R, et al. (2017) Negative body experience in women with early childhood trauma: associations with trauma severity and dissociation. *European Journal of Psychotraumatology* 8(1): 1–9.

Schore A (1994) *Affect Regulation and the Origin of the Self: The Neurobiology of Emotional Development.* New York, NY: Psychology Press.

Schore A (2012) *The Science of the Art of Psychotherapy.* New York, NY: Norton and Co.

Siegel D (2012) *Mindsight: Change Your Brain and Your Life.* Melbourne, Australia: Scribe.

Sletvold J (2014) *The Embodied Analyst: From Freud and Reich to Relationality.* London, UK: Routledge.

Smith E (1985) *The Body in Psychotherapy.* Jefferson, NC: McFarland and Co.

Tronick E (2007) *The Neurobehavioural and Social-Emotional Development of Infants and Children.* New York, NY: Norton and Co.

Van der Kolk B (1996) The body keeps the score: Approaches to the psychobiology of Posttraumatic Stress Disorder. In: Van der Kolk B, McFarlane A and Weisbath L (eds) *Traumatic Stress: The Effects of Overwhelming Experience on Mind, Body and Society.* New York, NY: The Guilford Press, pp.214–241.

Van der Kolk B (2014) *The Body Keeps the Score: Brain, Mind and the Body in the Healing of Trauma.* New York, NY: Viking.

Warner E, Spinazzola J, Westcott A, et al. (2014) The body can change the score: Empirical support for somatic regulation in the treatment of traumatized adolescents. *Journal Child and Adolescent Trauma* 7(4): 237–246.

Westland G (2011) Relating through physical touch in contemporary body psychotherapy. *The Psychotherapist* 48: 17–19.

Westland G (2015) Touch in body psychotherapy. In: Marlock G, Weiss H, Young C, et al. (eds) *The Handbook of Body Psychotherapy and Somatic Psychology.* Berkeley, CA: North Atlantic Books, pp.494–508.

Young C (2006) One hundred and fifty years on: The history, significance and scope of body psychotherapy today. *Body, Movement and Dance in Psychotherapy* 1(1): 17–28.

20 Meditation and yoga for trauma

Timothea Goddard

Introduction

Meditation and yoga emerged from rich Eastern spiritual traditions which offer multifaceted pathways of training including practice, study, and ethics. Yoga arose from the Hindu Vedantic tradition more than 5000 years ago, and mindfulness meditation developed out of the Buddhist tradition more than 2,500 years ago. These practices have spread across many different continents and cultures and have recently become more mainstream, so that people suffering from trauma are now regularly seeking meditation courses and yoga classes. Interest in these approaches has been driven by clinicians and researchers who have become concerned that conventional treatments often fail to fully address the complexities of trauma. Some of these difficulties include loss of experiential awareness in the present moment, somatic disturbances, affect dysregulation, inability to experience satisfaction and pleasure in life, and an overall lack of integration between the sense of self and the body (West et al., 2016).

With a more nuanced understanding of the role of overwhelming stress on physiological, neurological and emotional development (Schore, 1994; Siegel, 2001) it can be seen that the balanced regulation of bodily systems, particularly that of the brain and autonomic nervous system (ANS), is a sign of psychological health. ANS dysregulation, brought about by trauma, often impedes the development of healthy cognitive, emotional and relational functioning (Cook et al., 2005). Within the field, attention to the whole human organism, including direct experience of the "body" as a site of possible healing and transformation, has grown substantially over the past 15 years (Van der Kolk, 2014). Drawing on the work of Damasio (2000), Van der Kolk (2014) points to the central role of the registration of bodily sensations, conveying the inner state of the body, that gives rise to a coherent and relatively stable sense of self.

Developmental neglect and abuse alter brain functioning in ways that shut down the capacity to access ordinary body-based experience, so that those who have suffered trauma become unable to accurately read their own physiological needs and emotional states, or to respond accordingly.

An important aspect of both meditation and yoga is the development of body awareness in ways that are psychologically salient and useful. These approaches can contribute to self-regulation skills, including enhanced interoception (the capacity to both feel and appraise body sensations); proprioception (awareness of where one's body is in space); affect differentiation and distress tolerance (the ability to accurately identify and manage one's emotions); increased sense of safety and self-agency; and the possibility of simply just enjoying being alive (Hölzel et al., 2011). These practices offer a strengths-based approach, fostering growth and empowerment. They may also have considerable relevance to the existential aspects of trauma as they may facilitate a greater sense of connection, and offer a fresh way of being and living, rather than simply being a "treatment" for problems. Today, these practices are offered in diverse ways with different emphases from fitness and strength, to self-regulation, resilience and self-knowledge, and finally to spiritual awakening.

In recent years, as specific approaches have become more carefully tailored to those who have been traumatised, it has become important to recognise that yoga and meditation now necessarily span two powerful yet quite different paradigms. The first is the Western scientific approach, with its emphasis on objectivity, evidence-based practice, cost-effectiveness and generalisabilty. The second is the paradigm of spiritual development, drawing on Vedantic and Buddhist psychologies, with their emphasis on experiential, embodied and phenomenological learning, and on values such as wholeness, integrity, ethics, wisdom and compassion.

Meditation

Although there are many forms of meditation, mindfulness meditation has been most rigorously researched in the field of mental and physical health. Mindfulness can be understood as the non-judgemental acceptance and "open-hearted" investigation of present moment experience, including body sensations, internal mental states, thoughts, emotions, impulses and memories (Kabat-Zinn, 2003). Mindfulness meditation is the method by which mindfulness is cultivated.

Mindfulness meditation involves training in where and how attention is placed, and the perspective brought to what is being attended to, in the interests of relieving suffering and developing insight and wisdom about the human condition, and how to live. It initially involves concentration practice, choosing to attend to one object, for example the breath, or sounds, which can calm the nervous system. It also involves "open monitoring practice" which tracks and observes the unfolding of experience over time, leading to insights about the nature of the mind and the experience of "self" and "self-in-relationship" (Kabat-Zinn, 1996).

A key contributor to the spread of mindfulness meditation in the West has been Jon Kabat-Zinn, a molecular biologist who has long held a passionate interest in the potential of Buddhist meditation practices and Hatha yoga to relieve human suffering. Over the past 35 years, his original mindfulness meditation training program, Mindfulness Based Stress Reduction (MBSR), has been adapted and translated into many Mindfulness Based Programs (MBPs) which are used to treat a wide range of mental and physical health issues, including those that may be trauma-related. Many different mindfulness approaches are now available, some of which use meditation as a central pillar (mindfulness-based programs), whereas others draw on it less intensively (mindfulness-informed approaches) (Crane et al., 2017). Mindfulness-integrated Cognitive-Behavioural Therapy is a mindfulness-based approach applicable to trauma which draws on a similar rationale but with a different pedagogical style from the MBPs described here, more strongly privileging Cognitive Behaviour Therapy principles in thinking about case formulation, symptom maintenance, exposure and behavioural change (Cayoun, 2011). Dialectical Behaviour Therapy (DBT) and Acceptance and Commitment Therapy (ACT) are mindfulness-informed approaches sharing some rationale with MBPs, which, however, do not use mindfulness meditation practice systematically.

Yoga

Hatha yoga is the basis of all modern forms of yoga and has been recognised as having many mental and physical health benefits (West et al., 2016). Although originally involving many different practices of self-development including ethics and meditation, yoga is most widely known as a practice of physical postures which emphasise fitness, strength and flexibility. The word "yoga" means to yoke together the body and mind and can be understood to cultivate mindfulness through careful attention to physical movement, breathing and deliberate relaxation.

Trauma Sensitive Yoga (TSY), a specific application of Hatha yoga for trauma, was developed by David Emerson and colleagues at the Trauma Centre in Boston (Emerson et al., 2009; Emerson and Hopper, 2011; Emerson, 2015). It was born out of a collaboration between Emerson, a social worker and an experienced yoga teacher, and Van de Kolk, a leading trauma researcher and clinician. TSY has five key elements that inform the teaching: a focus on interoception, shared authentic experience, invitational language, choice-making and non-coercion.

An overview of Mindfulness Based Programs (MBPs)

MBPs traditionally run over eight weeks, with the group meeting for between two to two and a half hours each week, with one silent practice day. Participants are encouraged to practice formal mindfulness meditation up to one hour each day and are given detailed audio instructions to guide the practice at home. These include exercises involving awareness of breath, body scan, movement practice (based on Hatha yoga, and walking), and paying attention to the sensations of emotion, and ultimately, to the processes involved in thinking. There is an emphasis on bringing curiosity-laden attention to all experience, whether it is pleasant, unpleasant or neutral, and therefore encouraging less reactivity to what would normally be avoided or held on to.

By paying attention, awareness is developed, of both immediate unfolding experience, as well as recognition of patterns arising in the body, posture, emotional and mental life, behaviour and relationships. This is explored in class through a process of interactive dialogue and inquiry. There is also an emphasis on exploring one's capacity to take responsibility in smaller and larger ways for one's own actions, and to discover how they increase or decrease one's suffering. The teaching style is experience-near, invitational and empowering of participants to honour and understand their own experience through investigation.

An overview of Trauma Sensitive Yoga

TSY is generally conducted in small groups, for an hour a week, for 10 to 12 weeks. An appropriately skilled teacher provides guidance so that participants can practice gentle exploratory movements in a safe, supportive context. This helps participants tune in to physical sensations, enhance their experience of rhythm, to make their own choices and to take effective action in response to what they are experiencing (Emerson and Hopper, 2011). All these human capacities are undermined by the experience of trauma, and TSY deliberately targets them to help build or renew a more strongly "felt" sense of the body through interoception, leading to self-agency and competence in responding to one's own signals. Ongoing practice after an initial program is ideal.

A key principle in TSY is that of non-coercion in the relationship between teacher and participants. Within a containing structure, participants are invited to make their own choices to move, or not to move, how they move, for how long and in what direction. Participants are free to choose more ease and comfort, or more challenging experiences, in any moment. There is no pressure to strive for attainment of any posture or state, and whatever experience the participant discovers, however they pay attention, and whatever choices they make are honoured as their authentic experience in the moment.

An experience of rhythm and flow in the body is facilitated in TSY by offering explorations of simple movements intra-personally. For example, by connecting the breath with a simple movement within one's own body or finding a pace and scope that is satisfying or interesting. Inter-personally, this could be explored by negotiating with another person to explore rhythms of movements between people.

An important aspect of trauma is that it often disrupts the sense of time; people can feel trapped in states that seem to never end. In TSY, there is a significant emphasis on noticing how experiences are constantly beginning and ending. Participants are particularly invited to notice the impermanence of sensations: how they arise, get more or less intense, and end, over and over again.

The TSY teacher engages participants in ways which may be very different from an ordinary yoga class. Language is invitational. Teachers do not offer physical touch to assist students with movements. Postures are called by the neutral word "form". Teachers speak throughout the class so that there is little silent time. Like other yoga classes, however, there is no time given to directly processing emotion or discussing immediate past or current life issues, even if these experiences arise in the class (Emerson, 2015). Participants are also free to self-regulate by leaving the class at any time.

How programs work

MBPs and TSY share much theoretical, pedagogical and philosophical ground, as well as being different in key respects. Emerson and other proponents of TSY have conceptualised MBSR alongside some mindfulness-informed psychotherapies such as DBT and ACT as a, "cognitively-oriented treatment without body work" (Emerson, 2015; West et al., 2016). This is a misunderstanding of the MBSR program which is grounded in embodied somatic exploration, including Hatha yoga-based movement practice.

Attention training

Most humans live on "auto-pilot", with attention being drawn in spontaneous ways to all manner of internal and external phenomena, often out of conscious awareness. Practice in MBPs involves the recognition of this and reinforces the capacity for attention: being able to sustain attention on an object (for example, the breath or the body), being able to notice mind-wandering ("What am I going to have for dinner?", "I am worthless"), one's response to it (for example, frustration or sadness), and to be able to switch attention back to a chosen object. This basic training strengthens the capacity in daily life for choosing where to place one's attention and being able to shift it to something salient and of value in the moment. Participants begin to purposefully recognise the difference between the experiencing mode of direct sensing and the conceptualising mode, including thinking of all kinds – memories, beliefs, preoccupations, plans – and to step out of conceptualising mode if one chooses.

In TSY, participants are invited to pay attention to the shifting sensations in their bodies as they explore movements, but there is no emphasis on returning to a particular object or cultivating the ability to pay attention in a sustained way. The rationale for this is so that participants do not feel coerced by the teacher to have certain experiences or to behave in certain ways. This is particularly important for those who have been traumatised by others over extended periods as may have experienced chronic coercion, and these power dynamics need to be reversed.

Body awareness and interoception

Simple awareness practices focusing on body-based experience are used in both meditation and yoga, often resulting in the regulation of physiological arousal by the activation of calming parasympathetic states which assist with emotional regulation (Hölzel et al., 2011), although in both MBPs and TSY it should be noted that physiological regulation is seen as a by-product of practice rather than a goal to be strived for. Focusing on the body, however, increases both interoception and proprioception and provides a pathway to ground attention in the present moment, often leading to an increased sense of coherence and self-agency. Farb et al. (2015) write,

> As the embodied self is more fully realized through awareness of ongoing interoceptive interactions, two complementary senses emerge: presence, one's connection to the moment, and agency, one's ability to effect change, which are both foundational in determining a person's sense of well-being.

Cultivating interoception is very important to transform the sense of bodily alienation, disconnection and somatic dysphoria which is so common with trauma. Participants discover that they can change how they feel by the act of paying attention, as well as by moving in response to what they discover. Participants often discover interoceptive experiences of, for example, empowerment or pleasure that physically contradict the more familiar interoceptive "signature" of overwhelm and hopelessness.

Autonomic Nervous System and emotional regulation

A healthy nervous system responds to threat by mobilising energy through the fight/flight response. That is, the activation of the sympathetic branch of the ANS, which involves a focus on external threat, high emotional arousal, and a range of physiological changes. Once the threat has past, a well-regulated nervous system can return to a baseline state of lower arousal. This involves the activation of the parasympathetic branch of the ANS, which is essentially energy-conserving. It allows the body to let go of the mobilisation, and to recuperate. If a threat continues in a way that leads to prolonged helplessness, the organism moves into a parasympathetic state of freeze, which shuts down interaction with the environment. Optimally, with the acquisition of self-regulatory skills in early childhood, the two branches of the ANS can work together in a coupled reciprocal mode, that is, they counterbalance each other. This involves the capacity to switch from one mode of functioning to the other, from arousal to relaxation to arousal, as required (Schore, 2003).

The ANS of traumatised people is often unable to flexibly respond to challenges and safety, and these people consistently live in a state of anticipatory vigilance about the possibility of future threatening events. Interpretations of external events, as well as internal "events" – thoughts, feelings and sensations – then become the triggers for new cycles of sympathetic arousal, or for some, activate both the sympathetic and parasympathetic states at the same time. This is toxic for the brain, and damaging to other systems of the body, and can lead to a range of secondary problems, such as substance misuse, in an effort to self-regulate.

Meditation and yoga practices can be thought of as generalised, non-specific exposure processes; when participants practise, unwanted experience may arise. For those who have suffered trauma, these experiences may involve substantial changes within the ANS. Participants are then, very gently, invited into many personal "experiments" through practise – the participant being both laboratory and scientist – to notice and explore their aversive experiences, and to consider multiple potential responses. Having an increased capacity to know and manage body experience, and its connection to thoughts and emotions, gives rise to increased self-efficacy and empowerment, including an increased sense of ownership and control over one's body (Dutton et al., 2013; Rhodes, 2015; West et al., 2016). In MBPs there is an emphasis on participants learning how to stay present with unwanted experience with some equanimity, allowing arousal to abate and a new relationship with the experience to arise. To assist this process of integration, people can be helped to make choices about where they place their attention in any moment. Because of TSY's commitment to non-coercion and choice, there is no encouragement to stay with unpleasant experience, but simply to notice or not notice and make whatever changes to the form and movement that feels right in the moment.

An example which captures this process is an MBSR participant – one who had experienced child sexual assault – who found the relative stillness of a "body scan" distressing. (A body scan involves shifting attention systematically through one's body with as much acceptance and curiosity as is possible in the moment.) She was however open to staying with the difficulty and making choices as she explored. Some of the adaptations she made included opening her eyes to orient to the present context, doing the practice sitting up, moving to gently release the impulse to flee and then coming back to stillness, and acknowledging that it was alright to feel both pleasant and unpleasant sensations in her body. In three weeks she found that by repeatedly being present to the body sensations of fear and agitation with maximum curiosity, and by recognising the reactive thoughts and impulses associated with it, that they slowly abated, and she eventually began to experience a sense of much needed rest and recuperation in that practice. She described it as a great relief to be able to drop into the parasympathetic state, and not be driven to constant activity to avoid her painful symptoms of trauma.

Change in perspectives on the self

Together with the "experiments" described above, practice can give rise to meta-awareness, or a sense of the self as a process rather than a fixed, permanent, static sense of self. In TSY this may be as simple as noticing that things change (the experience of sometimes feeling tense and sometimes feeling relaxed) or having a new palpable embodied experience of having some choice in the moment. In meditation practice in an experience-near and pragmatic way, moments may arise where participants can de-identify with the contents of experience and in so doing gain perspective and a sense of freedom from negative experiences, judgements and beliefs that they may previously have felt defined by. It is a very different experience to be able to say, "I am having a believed thought that I am worthless" to, "I am worthless". This capacity for reflection opens one up to the possibility of change. "Worthlessness", once experienced as a trait belonging to "me" in a rigid way, can be newly perceived as a state that is not a defining characteristic of "me"; it arises and passes under certain conditions and is associated with particular body sensations, thoughts and emotions.

Practising friendliness and compassion

In both approaches there is an implicit invitation to cultivate an attitude of friendliness and even compassion towards oneself and to others. This can enhance the capacity for emotional regulation and can also change one's relationship to oneself by undermining self-loathing and self-criticism (Germer and Neff, 2015). Explicit compassion practice is introduced in some MBPs; TSY prefers to leave this as an implicit discovery as the focus and emphasis is on providing a context for enhanced interoception within a shared authentic experience.

There is some debate in the field about the value of explicit compassion practice for trauma sufferers. Some studies have suggested that teaching compassion practice to people with developmental trauma can increase distress in unproductive ways as it evokes the attachment system leading to the potential "flooding" of negative affect, and that mindfulness skills need to be developed before undertaking generative compassion practice (Segal et al., 2012; Van den Brink and Koster, 2012). Other perspectives suggest that an explicit compassion focus can assist in developing the capacity to be present to painful material in a productive way (Gilbert, 2013; Germer and Neff, 2015). There may be many factors involved, including the individual's resources, timing and the immediate salience of the practice, the quality of the relationship between participant and teacher, and the context. The MBSR participant described above reported the impact of taking an active stance of kindness towards herself as initially alien, and unnatural, but gradually more and more soothing. She was eventually able to actively recognise her harsh inner critical voice when it arose in practice, see it as just a thought, and practise softening her body at the same time as offering an intention of tenderness and kindness to herself in these moments.

Group process

In MBPs and in TSY the classes are structured to be as non-hierarchical, non-pathologising and non-instrumental as possible (McCown, 2013; Emerson, 2015). In MBPs the group teaching method enables participants to see that their mind is operating in similar ways to that of most other people. This is often revelatory and can undermine shame and isolation with participants often declaring their relief in words like, "So I am not mad after all! Everybody has a mind like mine". Ideally, participants have an experience of their own "wholeness" or "good-enoughness" in a group that is deliberately benign and non-intrusive. This leads to the sometimes playful and creative nature of interpersonal exploration, and some surprising and enjoyable aspects of being in an "advice-free-zone" with one another. Participants often experience a spontaneous reduction of defensiveness which can sometimes be fruitfully expressed and acknowledged within the protected container of the class.

Even though there is a structured curriculum, the didactic elements ideally emerge from and are woven into participants' experiences of the practice, so there is a sense of contingency, aliveness and specificity in the process. As a result, rather than being a passive recipient, the participant has a sense of self-agency and can see their experience shaping the flow of the group. In both MBPs and TSY the teacher is not the holder of some "truth" or knowledge, but a co-explorer in facilitating and making space for the experiential truths of each participant.

In TSY, careful stewardship of the group facilitates a group experience which is predictable, and where participants can engage on their own terms, responding to their own needs. This can be a powerful experience of unspoken belonging and community for many people. There is an implicit embodiment of a shared authentic experience of all participants including the teacher, but there is no verbal sharing of personal experiences as the focus remains directly on the powerful experiences of interoception, choice, action-taking and rhythm-making. As an adjunctive treatment, it is recommended that most participants would have a therapy context in which to explore emotions and integrate their learning from TSY participation (Emerson, 2015).

Assessment and contra-indications

Assessment to ensure that potential participants have the necessary resources to attend and manage classes is central to the safety and efficacy of both approaches. A collaborative interview is important, and would include discussion of readiness and intentions, interest in practising, current physical and mental health, experience of trauma or addictions, and current supports, including the possible need for individual therapy while undertaking a program (Dobkin et al., 2011; Emerson, 2015). Individual differences in terms of timing, motivation and resources means an individual approach is recommended, rather than the application of rigid rules. The presence of dissociation and flashbacks need not generally preclude participation. People who are acutely unwell, psychotic, feel very unsafe, have unstable living conditions, or are not interested in a group program are however unsuitable, although they may benefit from one-on-one sessions using the methods.

Unpleasant and aversive experiences naturally arise in meditation and yoga practice for all humans, as participants come face-to-face with what is arising in the moment, for example, unpleasant sensations, boredom, frustration, anxiety, depression, pain, negative thoughts, or difficult memories, and this can be more pronounced for those who have experienced trauma. The teacher's capacity to embody openness, groundedness, compassion and equanimity is helpful for participants to feel safe to explore their experience.

Recent discussions of the dangers of mindfulness meditation most often refer to the intensive silent retreat experience where there may be an unclear hierarchy, many hours of silence and stillness, and no explicit permission or priority given to self-care and eliciting emotional support in the face of distress. Compson (2014) has suggested that contemporary secular approaches like MBPs may be better equipped to offer safe, titrated, responsive training, in comparison with Buddhist contexts in which teachers are not necessarily trained to work with those who have suffered significant trauma. This logic could well be extended to the TSY program in comparison with yoga classes that are not trauma-informed.

Adaptations for trauma

In both approaches, attention to the physical space of the room to ensure privacy, safety and a clear access to the exit is made available. Providing clear trauma-informed psycho-education for rationale of the practices early in either program is also important. A sense of safety can be encouraged by teaching specific self-regulation practices, and by teaching how to bring attention to an external focus when internal sensations become too difficult. Shorter sessions and longer courses may be helpful. It is also important to increase the emphasis on any positive experiences that arises in class, any sense of mastery, gratitude, acknowledging one's efforts, connection, or finding one's own wisdom, for example (Dutton et al., 2013; Magyari, 2015).

As discussed, TSY is already a trauma-sensitive skilful adaptation of basic Hatha yoga and includes care when inviting people into postures that may have connotations with abuse experiences. Participants are routinely offered alternatives to any posture being offered and are also encouraged to respond by moving out of a form that feels uncomfortable or distressing for them whenever they choose.

In MBPs, emphasis on flexibly responding to each person and making invitations to experiment is central for the growth of self-agency and curiosity. Teachers should be very explicit about participants taking actions to look after themselves and communicate these in ways that make it easy for participants to learn more about how to do this as the process unfolds. This might include not necessarily being in "sync" with the group, shifting focus at any time, and leaving the room to ground oneself and returning when able. An example of this flexibility is an MBSR participant who had had a traumatic experience with near-drowning and understandably found focusing on the breath activated fear and was quite unworkable. Through exploration he found that he could bring attention to his pulse instead, as an object of concentration. He then became more curious about seeing the movement of the breath as a kind of pulse, and slowly began to be able to explore this as an object of practice without as much reactivity.

Treleaven's book on trauma sensitive mindfulness (2018) offers a thorough review of many relevant issues including an understanding of the socio-political context, power dynamics, screening, theoretical frameworks for understanding experience and practical ways to bring this knowledge into the teaching and learning relationship.

Research

Given the infancy of this area of research, much of the literature available is exploratory in nature, and lacks rigour and generalisability. However, the results available show promise, suggesting that these approaches may provide safe and inexpensive benefits that can assist those who have experienced trauma to heal. These approaches may also assist in making psychotherapy more effective through both the development of greater emotional regulation and that participants have had some training in approaching negative thoughts, emotions and sensations with an exploratory attitude, rather than attempting to avoid them (Van der Kolk, 2014).

A wide range of positive psychological and physical outcomes from the practice of mindfulness meditation has been tabled in the literature (Grossman, 2004; Hofmann et al., 2010; Hölzel et al., 2011). Regarding MBPs specifically for those who have experienced trauma, these programs appear to have a significant effect in reducing Posttraumatic Stress Disorder (PTSD) symptoms across a range of trauma types and populations (Kimbrough et al., 2010; Niles et al., 2012; Bhatnagar et al., 2013; Dutton et al., 2013; Kim et al., 2013; King et al., 2013; Earley et al., 2014; Goldsmith et al., 2014; Gallegos et al., 2015; Polusny et al., 2015; Kelly and Garland, 2016; Wahbeh et al., 2016).

One longitudinal pilot study of 27 survivors of child sexual abuse in an eight-week MBSR class showed lasting decreases in all the major outcome variables of PTSD, anxiety and depression (Kimbrough et al., 2010). Participants were asked to practise mindfulness skills at home during the course, and three refresher classes were provided over the following 16 weeks. After eight weeks, a 65 per cent reduction was seen in depressive symptoms. In all three of the PTSD symptom criteria studied, symptoms levels decreased, with the greatest reductions in the avoidance cluster of symptoms. In this study, participant feedback was also consistent with respect to feeling more empowered and reconnected with their ability to grow and change. Many reported that they valued not having to "tell their trauma story", and that the curriculum focused on their current lives providing immediate strategies for living and going forward (Magyari, 2015).

To date, the TSY studies are limited in number but point to this approach being a feasible and effective adjunctive therapy for trauma. There have been three randomised controlled trials of TSY which found clinically significant decreases in PTSD symptomology following a yoga intervention of between eight and 12 weeks (Mitchel et al., 2014; Van der Kolk et al., 2014; Jindani et al., 2015). Follow-up studies suggest that continuing decrease in PTSD severity seems to be linked to ongoing practice after the study (Rhodes et al., 2016). Many participants also report TSY classes to be effective and beneficial to their recovery (Clark et al., 2014; Jindani and Khalsa, 2015; West et al., 2016) and that choice-orientation (Rhodes, 2015), the experience of the teacher and fellow participants, and the portable nature of the skills developed are the components seen as most helpful.

Training

Like many other therapies, it is important in both TSY and MBPs for the teacher to embody personal qualities such as genuineness, compassion, warmth, empathy and potency, so that participants can find safety and containment in the structure and delivery of the programs.

Though many therapists and counsellors are now integrating mindfulness practices into their work in an eclectic way with minimum immersion or training, international standards for mindfulness teaching of MBPs recommend specific professional training, supervision, in-depth personal practice, and experience of teacher-led silent mindfulness meditation retreats (Crane et al., 2017), and this is especially relevant in teaching trauma survivors (Magdari, 2015). Without this, teachers may prematurely decide that participants are unsuitable because of their own fear and unfamiliarity with the process, they may be unable to effectively titrate the practice in ways that do not lead to avoidance, and they may not have the expertise to respond with equanimity and confidence to the practice difficulties which invariably arise.

TSY also requires specific professional training and is made available to both yoga teachers, who are then trained in trauma theory and research, and to clinicians who have an in-depth experience of a yoga practice.

Conclusion

Trauma-specific programs which teach meditation, mindfulness and yoga can be both physically and psychologically useful and offer a way of creating a fresh relationship with painful experience and a platform to build a sense of self that is integrated within one's own body. Participants may also "open the door" to an ongoing exploration of what it means to be a human being in a community, and, perhaps optimally, the resource of a life-long practice that is less a "treatment" than a way of living.

References

Bhatnagar R, Phelps L, Rietz K, et al. (2013) The effects of mindfulness training on posttraumatic stress disorder symptoms and heart rate variability in combat veterans. *The Journal of Alternative and Complementary Medicine* 19(11): 860–861.

Cayoun BA (2011) *Mindfulness-integrated CBT: Principles and Practice*. New York, NY: John Wiley and Sons.

Clark CJ, Lewis-Dimello A, Anders D, et al. (2014) Trauma-sensitive yoga as an adjunct mental health treatment therapy for survivors of domestic violence: A feasibility study. *Complementary Therapies in Clinical Practice* 20: 154–158.

Compson J (2014) Meditation, trauma and suffering in silence: Raising questions about how meditation is taught and practiced in Western contexts in the light of a contemporary trauma resiliency model. *Contemporary Buddhism* 15(2): 274–297.

Cook A, Spinazzola J, Ford J, et al. (2005) Complex Trauma. *Psychiatric Annals* 35(5): 390–398.

Crane RS, Brewer J, Feldman C, et al. (2017) What defines mindfulness-based programs? The warp and the weft. *Psychological Medicine* 47(6): 990–999.

Damasio A (2000) *The Feeling of What Happens*. London, UK: Vintage.

Dobkin PL, Irving JA and Amar S (2011) For whom may participation in a mindfulness-based stress reduction program be contraindicated? *Mindfulness* 3(1): 44–50.

Dutton MA, Bermudez D, Matas A, et al. (2013) Mindfulness-based stress reduction for low-income predominantly African American women with PTSD and a history of intimate partner violence. *Cognitive and Behavioral Practice* 20(1): 23–32.

Earley MD, Chesney MA, Frye J, et al. (2014) Mindfulness intervention for child abuse survivors: A 2.5-year follow-up. *Journal of Clinical Psychology* 70(10): 933–941.

Emerson D (2015) *Trauma-sensitive Yoga in Therapy: Bringing the Body into Treatment*. New York, NY: WW Norton and Company.

Emerson D, Sharma R, Chaudry S, et al. (2009) Trauma-sensitive yoga: Principles, practice, and research. *International Journal of Yoga Therapy* 19: 123–128.

Emerson D and Hopper E (2011) *Overcoming Trauma Through Yoga: Reclaiming Your Body*. North Berkeley, CA: North Atlantic Books.

Farb N, Daubenmier J, Price CJ, et al. (2015) Interoception, contemplative practice, and health. *Frontiers in Psychology* 6:763. doi:10.3389/fpsyg.2015.00763.

Gallegos AM, Lytle MC, Moynihan JA, et al. (2015) Mindfulness-based stress reduction to enhance psychological functioning and improve inflammatory biomarkers in trauma-exposed women: A pilot study. *Psychological Trauma: Theory, Research, Practice, and Policy* 7(6): 525–532.

Germer CK and Neff KD (2015) Cultivating self-compassion in trauma survivors. In: Follette VM, Briere J, Rozelle D, et al. (eds) *Mindfulness-oriented Interventions for Trauma: Integrating Contemplative Practices*. New York, NY: The Guilford Press, pp.43–58.

Gilbert P (2013) *Mindful Compassion: Using the Power of Mindfulness and Compassion to Transform Our Lives*. London, UK: Hachette UK.

Goldsmith RE, Gerhart JI, Chesney SA, et al. (2014) Mindfulness-based stress reduction for posttraumatic stress symptoms: Building acceptance and decreasing shame. *Journal of Evidence-Based Complementary and Alternative Medicine* 19(4): 227–234.

Grossman P, Niemann L, Schmidt S, et al. (2004) Mindfulness-based stress reduction and health benefits: A meta-analysis. *Journal of Psychosomatic Research* 57(1): 35–43.

Hofmann SG, Sawyer AT, Witt AA, et al. (2010) The effect of mindfulness-based therapy on anxiety and depression: A meta-analytic review. *Journal of Consulting and Clinical Psychology* 78(2): 169–183.

Hölzel BK, Carmody J, Vangel M, et al. (2011) Mindfulness practice leads to increases in regional brain gray matter density. *Psychiatry Research: Neuroimaging* 191(1): 36–43.

Jindani F and Khalsa GFS (2015) A yoga intervention program for patients suffering from symptoms of posttraumatic stress disorder: A qualitative descriptive study. *The Journal of Alternative and Complementary Medicine* 21(7): 401–408.

Jindani F, Turner N and Khalsa SBS (2015) A yoga intervention for posttraumatic stress: A preliminary randomized control trial. *Evidence-Based Complementary and Alternative Medicine.* doi:10.1155/2015/351746.

Kabat-Zinn J (1996) Mindfulness meditation: What it is, what it isn't, and its role in health care and medicine. In: Haruki Y, Ishii Y and Suzuki M (eds) *Comparative and Psychological Study on Meditation.* Delft, Netherlands: Eburon, pp.161–170.

Kabat-Zinn J (2003) Mindfulness-based interventions in context: Past, present, and future. *Clinical Psychology: Science and Practice* 10(2): 144–156.

Kelly A and Garland EL (2016) Trauma-informed mindfulness-based stress reduction for female survivors of interpersonal violence: Results from a stage 1 RCT. *Journal of Clinical Psychology* 72(4): 311–328.

Kim SH, Schneider SM, Bevans M, et al. (2013) PTSD symptom reduction with mindfulness-based stretching and deep breathing exercise: Randomized controlled clinical trial of efficacy. *Journal of Clinical Endocrinology and Metabolism* 98(7): 2984–2992.

Kimbrough E, Magyari T, Langenberg P, et al. (2010) Mindfulness intervention for child abuse survivors. *Journal of Clinical Psychology* 66(1): 17–33.

King AP, Erickson TM, Giardino ND, et al. (2013) A pilot study of group mindfulness-based cognitive therapy (MBCT) for combat veterans with posttraumatic stress disorder (PTSD). *Depression and Anxiety* 30(7): 638–645.

McCown D (2013) *The Ethical Space of Mindfulness in Clinical Practice: An Exploratory Essay.* Philadelphia, PA: Jessica Kingsley Publishers.

Magyari T (2015) Teaching mindfulness-based stress reduction and mindfulness to women with Complex Trauma. In: Follette VM, Briere J, Rozelle D, et al. (eds) *Mindfulness-oriented Interventions for Trauma: Integrating Contemplative Practices.* New York, NY: The Guilford Press, pp.140–156.

Mitchell KS, Dick AM, DiMartino DM, et al. (2014) A pilot study of a randomized controlled trial of yoga as an intervention for PTSD symptoms in women. *Journal of Traumatic Stress* 27(2): 121–128.

Niles B, Klunk-Gillis J, Ryngala DJ, et al. (2012) Comparing mindfulness and psychoeducation treatments for combat-related PTSD using a telehealth approach. *Psychological Trauma: Theory, Research, Practice, and Policy* 4(5): 538–547.

Polusny MA, Erbes CR, Thuras P, et al. (2015) Mindfulness-based stress reduction for posttraumatic stress disorder among veterans: A randomized clinical trial. *Journal of the American Medical Association* 314(5): 456–465.

Rhodes AM (2015) Claiming peaceful embodiment through yoga in the aftermath of trauma. *Complementary Therapies in Clinical Practice* 21(4): 247–256.

Rhodes A, Spinazzola J and Van der Kolk BA (2016) Yoga for adult women with chronic PTSD: A long-term follow-up study. *Journal of Alternative and Complementary Medicine* 22(3): 189–196.

Schore AN (1994) *Affect Regulation and the Origin of the Self: The Neurobiology of Emotional Development.* Hillsdale, NJ: Lawrence Erlbaum Associates.

Schore AN (2003) *Affect Dysregulation and Disorders of the Self.* New York, NY: WW Norton and Co.

Segal ZV, Williams JMG and Teasdale JD (2012) *Mindfulness-based Cognitive Therapy for Depression, Second Edition.* New York, NY: The Guilford Press.

Siegel DJ (2001) Toward an interpersonal neurobiology of the developing mind: Attachment relationships, "mindsight," and neural integration. *Infant Mental Health Journal* 22(1–2): 67–94.

Treleaven D (2018) *Trauma-sensitive Mindfulness: Practices for Safe and Transformative Healing.* New York, NY: WW Norton and Co.

Van den Brink E and Koster F (2015) *Mindfulness-based Compassionate Living: A New Training Program to Deepen Mindfulness with Heartfulness.* East Sussex, UK: Routledge.

Van der Kolk BA (2014) *The Body Keeps the Score.* London, UK: Penguin Books.

Van der Kolk BA, Stone L, West J, et al. (2014) Yoga as adjunctive treatment for posttraumatic stress disorder: A randomized controlled trial. *Journal of Clinical Psychiatry* 75(6): e559–e565.

Wahbeh H, Goodrich E, Goy E, et al. (2016) Mechanistic pathways of mindfulness meditation in combat veterans with posttraumatic stress disorder. *Journal of Clinical Psychology* 72: 365–383.

West J, Liang B and Spinazzola J (2016) Trauma sensitive yoga as a complementary treatment for posttraumatic stress disorder: A qualitative descriptive analysis. *International Journal of Stress Management* 24(2): 173–195.

Williams JMG (2010) Commentary. Mindfulness and psychological process. *Emotion* 10 (1): 1–7.

21 Structured therapy versus psychodynamic therapy

Nick Bendit

Introduction

Patients with Borderline Personality Disorder (BPD) commonly present to mental health clinicians, accounting for approximately 15–25 per cent of inpatient and 10 per cent of outpatient presentations (Leichsenring et al., 2011). Although multiple factors contribute to the development of BPD, the most robust predictor is chronic attachment trauma in early childhood (Agrawal et al., 2004), frequently compounded by later traumatic experiences, for example, emotional neglect, violence or sexual abuse (Zanarini et al., 1997). Patients with BPD present with a marked intolerance of being alone, chaotic and overwhelming emotional instability, and desperate attempts to stave off unbearable negative feelings. Deliberate self-harm, impulsive acts, dissociation and suicide attempts may all be involved (American Psychiatric Association, 2013), and when these do not reduce overwhelmingly unbearable feelings, the patient may be left with chronic despair and hopelessness, overwhelming anger, and a feeling of deadness, often alternating with unbearable anxiety (Meares, 2004). Up until the 1990s, therapeutic nihilism with respect to the treatment of BPD was pervasive, as the usual mental health interventions were mostly unhelpful (National Institute for Health and Care Excellence, 2009).

In the early 1990s, controlled trials of two psychotherapy treatments showed surprisingly positive outcomes: a Cognitive-Behavioural treatment adapted substantially for patients with BPD, called Dialectical Behaviour Therapy (DBT) (Linehan et al., 1991), and an integrated psychodynamic treatment, called the Conversational Model of Psychotherapy (CM) (Stevenson and Meares, 1992). Since then, a diverse range of psychotherapies have been shown to be effective in a series of randomised clinical trials (RCTs). These include the more structured therapies such as DBT, Cognitive Therapy (Davidson et al., 2006; Weinburg et al., 2006) and Schema Focused Therapy, and relatively unstructured psychodynamic therapies, such as Transference Focused Therapy, Mentalisation Based Therapy and the CM (National Health and Medical Research Council, 2012).

Theoretical and practical differences between the structured therapies and the unstructured therapies are profound, and yet, when compared with each other in outcome studies in BPD, the results are not usually significantly different (Leichsenring et al., 2011). This has become a general truth in psychotherapy for all mental health disorders, according to Wampold, who, having reviewed thousands of psychotherapy trials for mental health disorders, states, "It appears, with some possible exceptions, that treatments intended to be therapeutic are generally equally effective, across disorders as well as for specific disorders. In general, no one theory is more effective than any other" (Wampold, 2010: p.83).

This chapter will describe a real-world, community mental health team approach to this conundrum, which has included developing an outpatient DBT program, then an outpatient CM program, and finally comparing the two in a RCT.

Introduction to DBT and the CM

DBT was developed by Marsha Linehan in the 1980s, as she worked to find an effective treatment for chronically suicidal female patients (Linehan, 1993). Initially she tried Behaviour Therapy, with some elements from Cognitive Therapy. This approach, focusing on changing behaviour patterns, seemed not only unacceptable to many of her patients, it was also of limited benefit. She then incorporated ideas of acceptance from Zen Buddhism, including focusing on awareness and description of the patient's feeling states, and the important communications that these feeling states provided, especially the painful ones. These fundamental, but opposite treatment mechanisms, change and acceptance, are then hypothesised to be held within a dialectical tension, such that there is maximal benefit in being able to skilfully balance these divergent treatment interventions. The strategies are taught in a weekly group program that supplements weekly individual therapy, over a 12-month period. Teaching concentrates on potential new behaviours in the areas of mindfulness, emotion regulation, distress tolerance, and interpersonal functioning. Individual therapy consists of understanding the emotional, cognitive and behavioural repertoires of the patient through a sustained here and now exploration – or "chain analysis" – and bringing solutions to the problems that unfold in these analyses, usually incorporating both the change and acceptance skills. Individual and group therapy are supplemented by 24-hour access via telephone to the therapist, although the actual amount of access is negotiated in each patient–therapist dyad. Finally, an essential part of DBT is the therapist's weekly consultation with other DBT therapists (Linehan, 1993).

The CM is an integrated psychodynamic model. First developed by Robert Hobson and Russell Meares in London in the 1960s, they attempted to treat the most intractable patients, now classified as having BPD (Meares, 2004). They incorporated ideas from Jungian and Winnicottian psychoanalysis, and linguistics, and privileged affect and feeling tones, so that this form of therapy more closely resembled an emotionally engaged conversation, whilst demonstrating an understanding that psychotherapy is an inherently complex and non-linear process. When Meares returned to Australia in the 1970s he continued to develop his theory around BPD, further incorporating ideas originally developed by Pierre Janet and William James. He conceptualised BPD as a disruption of the "self", where self is defined as a person's stream of internal awareness and consciousness (Meares et al., 2011). Such chronic disruption results in impairment of vital psychological functions, particularly those necessary to tolerate the feeling of aloneness. In practice, the CM requires the therapist to tune into micro shifts of affect and awareness and respond to them in a way that resonates with the patient, whilst attempting to establish what might seem a normal conversation. When breaks occur in this connection, the therapist's task is to explore the "disjunction" and attempt to repair it. Links may then be made between similar disruptions in both early relationships and the current relationship. Such implicit, and therefore largely unconscious, templates of how early caregivers responded to the patient will have been enacted throughout the patient's life, creating many of the problems of BPD. These early unconscious traumatic memories of interactions with others are described in the CM as the "expectational field", which is a subtle field of influence shaping the therapy relationship in powerful ways that are usually outside of awareness. The expectational field is analogous to but not completely the same as transference and countertransference, concepts which are central to all psychodynamic therapies. Furthermore, transference interpretations aimed at facilitating insight into these patterns, a central component of psychoanalysis, are never used, but the therapist uses knowledge of these complex patterns of interaction to inform his or her therapeutic responses, particularly to avoid unconsciously replicating earlier traumatic relationships.

Although both DBT and the CM share similarities such as close tracking and understanding of the emotional experience of the patient, there are significant differences in the "structure" of individual sessions. In DBT, a precise hierarchy of therapeutic goals is made for each session. Suicidal and self-harming actions during the week are given the highest priority for examination (Linehan, 1993). In the CM, the patient talks spontaneously while the therapist closely tracks and helps to expand the emotional and relational content of what is presented. Sessions in the CM are relatively "unstructured". However, in both therapies, the overall structure and conduct are laid out at the beginning; discussion of how the therapy will help the patient's problems is followed by an agreed contract of how the therapy will be conducted. This is called "the frame" in psychodynamic therapies such as the CM, and "agreements" in DBT (Linehan, 1993). These are explicitly discussed rules that enable therapy to be conducted safely and effectively.

Psychotherapy in practice

In Australia, Newcastle had one of the last "therapeutic community" inpatient wards, which was shut in 1998 after a 30-year history. The staff were retrained to provide DBT as an outpatient service for patients with BPD, as DBT was the only treatment at that point shown to be effective in an RCT (Linehan et al., 1991). A few years later, the CM was adopted as an alternative treatment after it had shown positive results in controlled trials (Meares, 2004), but not in an RCT. Although all practitioners in the team were trained in, and provided DBT, not all the practitioners wanted to be trained in a second model. After several more years of allocating patients to one model or other, it was decided to test the CM against DBT. By then, DBT was regarded as the "gold standard" treatment, as a result of a series of research RCTs showing efficacy in reducing deliberate self-harm and suicide attempts (National Institute for Health and Care Excellence, 2009). The therapeutic team wanted to investigate whether outcomes were as good in this general outpatient service with "real world" community mental health conditions as they are in research studies conducted by the developers of the models. Finally, there was an awareness of the inherent researcher bias in psychotherapy research studies, whereby studies where the lead researcher has a model preference tend to result in an outcome favouring that model (Luborsky et al., 1999). In this study, the two lead researchers had an interest in both models, but with contrasting preferences. Thus, there was a balance of research allegiance.

The study involved randomising 162 patients with BPD who had deliberately self-harmed or tried to commit suicide at least three times in the previous year. These patients were therefore severely unwell, and the study aimed to be as inclusive as possible, irrespective of multiple comorbidities the patients presented with (Posttraumatic Stress Disorder, Eating Disorders, Somatic Symptom Disorders, Substance Abuse Disorders, and so on). Patients were excluded if they had Schizophrenia or Bipolar Disorder as their primary diagnosis, or moderate to severe Intellectual Disability. The patients were treated twice weekly for 14 months, and the number of therapist hours per patient were roughly equivalent: the CM was twice weekly individual therapy, and DBT was one individual session per week, and one group session with six to eight patients for two and a half hours per week with two therapists. DBT and the CM required weekly supervision for all therapists. The one difference was that patients receiving DBT had access to an evening and weekend crisis phone line run by the service, whereas the CM patients did not.

Although the study was not designed to answer this question, it was hoped that the study would generate some secondary information that might help explain which treatment is likely to work best for each individual patient.

As an adult community mental health team offering psychotherapy, there was the advantage that this research could be generalised to other real-world community mental health teams, in comparison with research RCTs. However, there were several disadvantages and difficulties compared with a pure research team. These difficulties, and their solutions, included:

- Although approximately two-thirds of the team provided both therapies, there was a mix of allegiances within the therapists to one model or the other. This was impossible to control, so therapist allegiance was measured.
- Therapists were tempted to switch models during the treatment when the allocated model did not seem to work. Although this made clinical sense,

it was not possible from a research point of view, so there was sometimes tension between researchers and therapists.

- It was crucial to prove that the models were being delivered in an adherent and competent manner. To this end, all sessions were taped, and a percentage of tapes were randomly selected from each therapist in each model, and independently checked for adherence.
- Funding the study was difficult, as a large RCT requires a research assistant to do research interviews and code and enter the data. This was paid for by the delivery of training courses in DBT, as the team was unsuccessful in getting a grant to cover associated costs.

The results of the study were encouraging, but were roughly in line with the only other similar study, an RCT comparing DBT with psychodynamic therapy, where the research was done in a community mental health clinic and the study had two lead researchers with opposing allegiance. In that study in Toronto it was found that both treatments did well, but the outcomes for the two models were not significantly different over a range of parameters (McMain et al., 2009). Similarly, the Newcastle study found that deliberate self-harm and suicide attempts were profoundly reduced, but there was no significant difference between the models (Walton et al., submitted). This was important because there is a prevailing notion clinically in the Newcastle region that DBT is better for patients who are self-harming or attempting to suicide frequently. This was shown to be incorrect, both for suicide attempts and for non-suicidal deliberate self-harm. A second primary outcome was measuring depression scores. Because of previous studies (Stevenson and Meares, 1992; Verheul et al., 2003), there was the idea amongst clinicians that CM was effective at reducing depression, whereas DBT had a less robust and more variable effect on depression scores. This was also shown to be incorrect; although both models reduced depression convincingly, DBT was statistically significantly better at reducing depression at the endpoint. The secondary measures were also largely similar: symptom severity, dissociation, interpersonal functioning and sense of self all improved, but there was no significant difference between the models. For mindfulness and emotion regulation instruments, which measure constructs that are explicitly taught in DBT, there was also improvement with both models, but DBT did significantly better.

Data pooled from both treatment groups showed that almost all patients changed substantially over the period of treatment. In the first seven months of treatment, 74 per cent did not have a suicide attempt, and 83 per cent reduced their self-harm episodes. 77 per cent had a significant reduction in BPD symptom severity by the end of the treatment, and 38 per cent could no longer by diagnosed as having BPD. This latter outcome is particularly important: the notion that BPD is a diagnosis for life is prevalent amongst patients and health providers alike, and this study contradicts that belief.

As the patients can pursue any treatment options they wish after the 14 months of therapy, their naturalistic progress will be investigated by repeating the outcome measures at one, two and five-year post-therapy follow-up points.

As a result of this study, and the process of delivering two very different psychotherapy models in a community mental health team, the following conclusions can be drawn:

- Patients with BPD with high levels of deliberate self-harm and suicidal actions, including serious common comorbidities, can improve with well organised and time-limited psychotherapies.
- Regular community mental health team members who are willing to learn and deliver psychotherapy to patients with severe BPD can achieve excellent outcomes. Although individual therapists who delivered both models did have different allegiances for one model or the other, they were able to deliver effective treatment in both models. (At a later stage, the question of whether allegiance significantly affects outcome will be studied.)
- Service managers in Newcastle have conclusive proof of the benefit of psychotherapy for patients with BPD, and the effectiveness of the psychotherapy service. This has had a district-wide effect: after more than 15 years of treating patients with BPD, the team has been informed by the district inpatient units that many of the difficulties they used to have with intractable admissions for patients with BPD have become very unusual, whereas in the past such admissions were commonplace.
- Different models can be just as effective as each other, but one model may be better than another for an individual patient. The next phase of research needs to address which model is best for each individual patient. The study has also motivated the team to offer a third model, Schema Therapy, delivered almost entirely within a group setting. Two pilot groups have been completed. The team believes that choice and variety in models is likely to be better for patient outcomes in the real world of community mental health.

In summary, effective treatment can be delivered to patients with BPD who are commonly seen as either difficult or untreatable. However, these treatments require significant input by community mental health services. This level of therapeutic input is lacking in just about every mental health service in Australia. There is no compelling evidence that these treatments can be delivered in a few months, or that cost saving contractions, such as just delivering DBT by group, are effective (National Health and Medical Research Council, 2012). Therefore, a significant investment in long-term, yet still time-limited, psychotherapy is important. Both treatment models have treatment manuals that can be purchased and local training in Australia is available.

To effectively import either, or preferably both, models of therapy to a community mental health team requires three things. First, local champions, with relevant psychotherapy training and experience, are needed to drive the process. Second, managerial support is needed to acknowledge the need and to support the process, and to supply the funding for extra clinical staff and to protect adequate psychotherapeutic time. Finally, clinicians who wish to work with BPD patients and are willing to train in DBT or CM are needed. These clinicians need to be paid to have basic training, given relevant theory textbooks and psychotherapy manuals, and most importantly, be provided the intensive supervision necessary.

Why do different models result in similar outcomes?

As previously mentioned, there is increasing evidence that different models of psychotherapy result in equivalent outcomes. Why this occurs is not clear. One hypothesis, frequently cited (Barnicot et al., 2012), is that there are "common factors" in all psychotherapy treatments that have been specifically adapted to treat patients with attachment trauma. These common factors have been well summarised in a recent guide for generalist mental health professionals working with BPD (Bateman and Krawitz, 2016). They include:

- Welcoming, enthusiastic therapists. Such therapists actively choose to work with patients with BPD because they fundamentally believe that patients with BPD can recover, and they approach these patients with warmth and compassion. Such therapists engender hope and positive expectation that the therapist is safe to work with and that the treatment will work. Furthermore, the organisation supporting them is willing to treat patients with BPD with high intensity interventions.
- Therapeutic relationship. The therapist prioritises understanding the patient's emotional experience through active empathy and communicating with the patient in a way that the patient experiences that the therapist "gets it". When ruptures occur, and the patient experiences that the therapist "does not get it", there is a joint commitment to trying to work through this, usually initiated by the therapist recognising their part in this, and trying to acknowledge and repair the dysjunction. Finally, the therapist tries to be "an authentic person", rather than impersonal and remote.
- Features of the treatment model. The treatment is well structured, with a collaborative understanding of how the treatment will help the patient, and an active discussion at the start of treatment of therapeutic rules and boundaries. Sessions are regular, usually a minimum of once a week for 12 months, although with adolescents it is often necessary to be more flexible in regularity and shorter in length. During the treatment, the therapist is also active, rather than being passive or opaque.
- Supervision. Therapists are advised to be aware of their own feelings and reactions during the treatment. It is usually recommended to supplement this enhanced awareness with external observation by another therapist, through either peer or expert supervision. This is particularly important when working with patients who are actively suicidal, so that the therapist

does not become overly risk averse because of their own unmanageable anxiety.

- Patient self-reflection. Patients are encouraged to monitor their own experience both between and within sessions. In session, they are encouraged to identify and describe their own emotions and work through important events that have happened during the week. These may include self-harm or suicidal episodes, binge-drinking, relationship difficulties, and so on. An attitude of curiosity is highlighted, with both the therapist and the patient wondering "what happened" in a curious and non-judgmental way.

A vignette – "Jenny"

Jenny is a 28-year-old woman who has been cutting herself at least once a week since she was 14. She made many suicide attempts in her late teenage years in the context of a series of violent relationships with both men and women. In her 20s, the attempts stopped when she was in a relatively stable same-sex relationship, although her cutting continued. She found that the cutting temporarily reduced her unbearable feelings of shame, and the overarching feeling that she was nothing but evil. However, her female partner later had an affair, and Jenny became savage in her self-harm, and cutting became more about punishment, and, sometimes, she made active attempts to kill herself again.

Jenny had grown up in a very religious family, who, although committed to the "greater good", were unable to respond to Jenny's emotional needs. When she told the family the story of her increasingly confusing thoughts about whether to live or die when she was 14, her mother responded that "such thoughts are a sin", and exhorted Jenny's father to punish her with a strap, which he did. There was also a sexual assault by an older boy in her religious youth group when she was 15.

She reported having quite a few turbulent therapy experiences in her teenage years, which she felt were unhelpful. In the last three years, she had been seeing a private psychologist monthly for "support". However, with the increasing turmoil in the last year, and the extent and dangerousness of her self-harm, the psychologist told her, "You are too hard for me", and referred her to the Newcastle service. She was assessed and found to have BPD and more than three episodes of deliberate self-harm in the previous year. She was also episodically binge-drinking, and struggling with Bulimia and Social Anxiety Disorder.

About six weeks after she was referred a therapist became available, so a baseline research assessment was booked. Jenny didn't attend, and on follow-up via phone the next day she said that she had a panic attack in the car park. The research assistant made another appointment, and agreed to meet her in the car park, after Jenny told the research assistant the thought of sitting in the waiting room had led to overwhelming anxiety. After the research session, a clinician from the service rang her to help her with a temporary surge of shame, a result of answering some of the more difficult research questions, and also informed her that "Margaret", a psychotherapist social worker, would be ringing her in the next few days to organise the first session of CM therapy, which she had been randomly allocated to.

In the first session, Jenny described mixed feelings: she was disappointed that she didn't get DBT, because her psychologist had recommended that she, "Go to the mental health team and get DBT". On the other hand, she was also relieved that she did not get DBT, because she knew that she would struggle with social anxiety in group sessions. She also was a little annoyed, feeling like she had been "a rat in a maze" when doing the research questionnaires. But the hardest moment for the therapist was when Jenny sat down and said, with no preamble, "Are you religious?". It was clear from her stern demeanour that the answer would determine whether the patient could trust the therapist, and it seemed that the continuation of therapy hung in the balance. The therapist, with some apprehension, said "no", and Jenny breathed a sigh of relief, launching into details of her family life, and how her parent's religious attitudes had been so destructive for her.

At the mid-therapy point, around seven months, a further research assessment was done. Jenny arrived at the next session, telling the therapist that she had an unexpected and disorienting moment of pride, as well as sadness, when she told the research assistant that she had stopped self-harming. She struggled to explain, saying, "Cutting has been my only friend, the place I go when no-one in the world can help me". At the same time, although she was not sure that she was feeling better in terms of mood or emptiness, she could deeply feel that moment of pride, realising, "I'm on my way to something better".

Attending therapy continued to be difficult, particularly after she spent time on holiday with her family in the tenth month. She told her mother that she was not feeling suicidal anymore, nor was she self-harming, but her mother appeared disinterested, and then demanded to know, "What are you doing with your life?". Thereafter, Jenny became more depressed and confused about the benefit of returning to therapy. After her holidays, she cancelled the next two weeks of sessions, and the therapist became exceedingly anxious. Not just because Margaret was concerned that Jenny would become suicidal again, but also because Margaret wanted to talk about termination, as there were only three months remaining of the therapy contract. When Jenny returned, there was a difficult and painful discussion about finishing therapy, with Jenny finally admitting that she was frightened of finishing with Margaret, and had thought it was better to finish now.

At the end of the 14 months, the length of the therapy contract, they discussed the possibility of further treatment. Jenny recognised how much she had improved, particularly after the post-treatment research interview. But she also recognised how far she had to go. In the Newcastle service, therapy is capped at two years, although the therapist will help the patient try and find further therapy, if needed, in the private system. The issue of needing Margaret arose again, but with less intensity, so Jenny requested a further six months of once-weekly therapy, followed by three sessions at monthly intervals. This process did not go smoothly: just before they started the monthly sessions, Jenny had a serious fight with her partner, and cut herself. Once again, the therapist was very anxious at the next session, as she was worried that the whole therapy had been for nothing. However, Jenny worked hard in that session on understanding what had happened, and realised that cutting was not her "friend" any more, and it was time "to throw all of that in the bin forever".

Vignette discussion

Would DBT has been any better or any worse for Jenny? It is not possible to accurately answer this question, but from the Newcastle experience of assessing and randomising a large number of patients, the following suggestions are worth considering:

- Social anxiety. CM therapy was probably easier for Jenny because she didn't have to face her social anxiety by going to the DBT group. However, in the long run, the DBT group may have been beneficial, if Jenny could tolerate the initial overwhelming anxiety, and then realise that the others in the group would not hurt her. Some patients drop out of DBT group because their social anxiety is unmanageable, and others find that their social anxiety improves. It is difficult to predict outcome for any individual who is socially anxious prior to treatment.
- Structure within therapy. The other issue is one of more structure in DBT versus less structure in the CM. As Jenny had been significantly traumatised growing up in a fundamentalist community, which involved excessive structure, she may have struggled with DBT, as that implicit trauma system may have been activated by the extra structure. For patients who like structured learning within psychotherapy, however, DBT is likely to be a better "fit".
- Single versus multiple therapeutic attachment relationships. Another major difference between DBT and the CM is the sharing of the therapeutic attachment within DBT; one individual therapist and two skills trainers are involved in DBT, whereas in the CM the therapeutic attachment is with the individual therapist. The shared therapeutic attachment within DBT may have made the termination phase easier. There is also a type of attachment relationship to learning a set of life skills in DBT, such that when the therapeutic relationship finishes, the felt experience of the relationship can continue through the use of the DBT skill set. On the other hand, some patients with BPD who are particularly poor at forming the therapeutic bond may struggle with the more diffuse therapeutic relationships in DBT.

The strongest predictor of outcome in psychotherapy in mental health disorders, over thousands of studies, is the strength of the therapeutic relationship (Wampold, 2010). This "fit" between two people embarking on a process that generates profound intimacy, requiring ongoing moment-to-moment trust, is even more crucial in working with patients with BPD. Patients with BPD are more likely to have mistrust of emotionally significant others than most patients with other disorders (Fonagy and Allison, 2014), so building trust is the most important part of any therapy with patients with BPD. However, measuring that complex, dynamic and subtle process of trust-building is extraordinarily difficult to capture in research studies. Yet, it is the centrality of this process that may underpin why different treatments result in similar outcomes in patients with BPD.

Conclusion

Psychotherapy is the main treatment for patients with BPD, and there is now a range of empirically validated treatments, with no clear indication that one is better than the other, and no research data to determine which model is best for which patient. An Australian effectiveness RCT shows that completely different models, DBT and CM, can be effective for patients with histories of severe and chronic trauma. These complex models can be delivered in regular community mental health teams, and the benefits are likely to have a wider impact. Furthermore, it is found that the same therapist can deliver different models. The purpose of this chapter is to encourage mental health clinicians and managers within public community mental health teams to offer diverse effective treatments for patients with BPD, some of the most poorly serviced and stigmatised patients within mental health services.

References

Agrawal H, Gunderson J, Holmes B, et al. (2004) Attachment studies with borderline patients: A review. *Harvard Review of Psychiatry* 12: 94–104.

American Psychiatric Association (2013) *Diagnostic and Statistical Manual of Mental Disorders, Fifth Edition*. Arlington, VA: American Psychiatric Publishing.

Barnicot K, Katsakou C, Bhatti N, et al. (2012) Factors predicting the outcome of psychotherapy for borderline personality disorder: A systematic review. *Clinical Psychology Review* 32: 400–412.

Bateman A and Krawitz R (2016) *Borderline Personality Disorder: An Evidence-based Guide for Generalist Mental Health Professionals*. Oxford, UK: Oxford University Press.

Davidson K, Norrie J, Tyrer P, et al. (2006) The effectiveness of cognitive behaviour therapy for borderline personality disorder: results from the borderline personality disorder study of cognitive therapy trial. *Journal of Personality Disorders* 20: 450–65.

Fonagy P and Allison E (2014) The role of mentalizing and epistemic trust in the therapeutic relationship. *Psychotherapy* 51: 372–380.

Leichsenring F, Leibing E, Kruse J, et al. (2011) Borderline personality disorder. *Lancet* 377: 74–84.

Linehan MM (1993) *Cognitive Behavioral Treatment for Borderline Personality Disorder*. New York, NY: Guilford Press.

Linehan MM, Armstrong HE, Suarez A, et al. (1991) Cognitive-behavioral treatment of chronically parasuicidal borderline patients. *Archives of General Psychiatry* 48: 1060–1064.

Luborsky L, Diguer L, Seligman DA, et al. (1999) The researcher's own therapy allegiances: A "wild card" in comparisons of treatment efficacy. *Clinical Psychology: Science and Practice* 6: 95–106.

McMain S, Links P, Gnam W, et al. (2009) A randomised trial of Dialectical Behavior Therapy versus general psychiatric management for Borderline Personality Disorder. *American Journal of Psychiatry* 166: 1365–1374.

Meares R (2004) The Conversational Model: An outline. *American Journal of Psychotherapy* 58: 51–66.

Meares R, Gerull F, Stevenson J, et al. (2011) Is self disturbance the core of borderline personality disorder? An outcome study of borderline personality factors. *Australian and New Zealand Journal of Psychiatry* 45: 214–222.

National Health and Medical Research Council (2012) *Clinical Practice Guideline for the Management of Borderline Personality Disorder*. Canberra, Australia: National Medical Health and Research Council.

National Institute for Health and Care Excellence (2009) *Borderline Personality Disorder: Treatment and Management. National Clinical Practice Guideline*. Leicester, UK: The British Psychological Society and The Royal College of Psychiatrists.

Stevenson J and Meares R (1992) An outcome study of psychotherapy for patients with Borderline Personality Disorder. *American Journal of Psychiatry* 149: 358–362.

Verheul R, Van Den Bosch LM, Koeter MW, et al. (2003) Dialectical behaviour therapy for women with borderline personality disorder: 12-month, randomised clinical trial in The Netherlands. *British Journal of Psychiatry* 182: 135–140.

Walton CJ, Bendit NR, Lewin T, et al. (submitted) Dialectical Behaviour Therapy v. Conversational Model for Borderline Personality Disorder: Randomised clinical trial in a public sector mental health service. *British Journal of Psychiatry*.

Wampold BE (2010) *The Basics of Psychotherapy*. Washington, DC: American Psychological Association.

Weinberg I, Gunderson JG, Hennen J, et al., (2006) Manual assisted cognitive treatment for deliberate self-harm in borderline personality disorder patients. *Journal of Personality Disorders* 20: 482–92.

Zanarini MC, Williams AA, Lewis RE, et al. (1997) Reported pathological childhood experiences associated with the development of borderline personality disorder. *American Journal Psychiatry* 154: 1101–1106.

22 Working with trauma – implications for supervision and professional ethics

Elisabeth Shaw

Introduction

In recent years there has been considerable focus on trauma within the health and community sectors. Increased research and public awareness of the effects of war, migration, violence, and sexual abuse have emphasised that this is warranted. However, though it has been argued in Australia that the status of trauma-informed work can be described as "enthusiastic" in terms of the level of interest across sectors, it has also been described as "emergent" with respect to service delivery principles and practice, "opaque" in that materials and models are not widely available, and "piecemeal" in that leadership is without coordination and model development is idiosyncratic (Quadara and Hunter, 2016). Determining reliable signposts and anchor points for practitioners in this context is crucial to ensuring both competent and ethical practice with vulnerable clients.

The practice of clinical supervision has been afforded an important place across many sectors within health care, in an increasingly formal way, since the end of World War II (Milne, 2009). Contemporary clinical care models regard supervision as a key resource for practitioner support, development, quality assurance, and health and safety. Practitioners generally experience their supervisor as an expert, and as a reliable resource, with some evidence that, when practitioners need ethical guidance, they are more likely to turn to their supervisor than to their professional codes of conduct (Doyle et al., 2009).

When practitioners work with those who have suffered trauma, competent and ethical practice, self-care, and well-being must all be particularly safeguarded. Every practitioner needs to understand and be prepared for the potential effects of the work on them, and to be cognisant that "their own awareness, conduct and self-care have major implications for their interactions with clients" (Blue Knot Foundation, 2017: p.2). Indeed, it has been argued that the single most important factor in the success or failure of trauma work relates to the attention paid to the experience and needs of the helper (Saakvitne et al., 2000; Sommer, 2008), and, in this regard, the role of supervision and of the supervisor is critical.

This chapter explores supervision and ethical practice in relation to trauma. Specifically:

- What role does supervision play in quality, ethical practice?
- How do supervisors think about practice in relation to trauma? Would they apply their usual supervisory approach, or are any differences required?
- What are the individual professional responsibilities that are required of practitioners working with trauma?
- How do practitioners develop emotional and ethical maturity when working in a context of uncertainty?

A vignette – "Peter" and "Jane"

Jane has been Peter's external supervisor for six months. Peter has a varied professional background, having worked in a range of settings. He generally presents his work quite openly and is interested in ideas and feedback about clients. He is less open about his private life and his own personal connection to the work. However, Jane is aware that Peter is the youngest of three children, with both a brother and a sister, and that he grew up in a family where his father was very violent. Peter believes that his siblings were more affected by their upbringing than he was, because he was the "baby", and that he had come along at the "tail end" of the violence.

There is a strong focus on domestic violence and sexual assault in the service where Peter now works. Clients can attend the service for up to six months. Peter believes that his background has prepared him to have both understanding and compassion for his clients, and therefore the work suits him quite well.

Peter, however, told Jane in a supervision session that he had been reprimanded again by his manager for using the language of abuse and trauma too freely; he had told his manager that the removal of car parking for staff was, "unjust, abusive and disrespectful". He remarked similarly that the organisation's focus on data entry and key performance indicators was "outrageous" in the face of "this very difficult work we do". Peter also argued that the six-month service limit was potentially "re-traumatising" for clients, cutting them off when they were most attached and in need. He was clearly distressed and angry when talking about these issues. When Jane asked him how he was managing, he said things like, "No-one cares how hard this work really is". Jane was aware that Peter had not had a holiday for four years, but he had changed jobs several times over this period, stating that each new job had created the "refreshment" that he needed.

Supervision

Milne defines supervision as "relationship-based education and training, that is work-focused, and manages, supports, develops and evaluates the work of colleagues" (Milne, 2009: p.439). This definition asserts that supervision is about the work done, distinguishing it from personal therapy. It also emphasises that education and development within the context of an ongoing relationship are important. It additionally notes the role of evaluation, which is often insufficiently emphasised outside of a training context, but which should continue throughout a practitioner's professional life. Fulfilling the roles of educator, developer, supporter, and evaluator, supervisors can have significant influence with their supervisees, not only in relation to competence but also to well-being.

A supervisory relationship should always commence with a contract for the terms of the relationship, including a learning contract. Effective supervision will involve focusing on the supervisee, the client, the supervisee's experience of working with the client, their countertransference responses, and their well-being (Pack, 2014). Although it can be argued that these guidelines are similar for any supervision, in trauma work it is crucial that the supervisor pursues conversations about therapist competence and responsibility (including its limits), the toll taken by the work, self-care, and frequent, diligent ethical reflection, perhaps more than would be generally required.

A supervisor's input must also relate to the mix of service context, practitioner capability, and client need (Knapp et al., 2012). For Jane, this means reconciling the client presentations with Peter's professional capability and personal resilience, within a limited service contract. Keeping Peter, the client, and the service safe are paramount. It would be easy to "rail" with Peter against the service limits. However, helping him to be competent at his work in this context, to develop his skills and talents, and to reflect on the work he undertakes in the particular service in which he is employed is professionally and ethically responsible.

Working in the counselling and psychotherapy fields means working regularly with trauma. This requires practitioners to repeatedly listen to and empathically respond to painful and disturbing stories. Few of those who have trained are prepared for the degree of trauma they will be exposed to, and this places practitioners at risk of being traumatised themselves; this is often referred to as "vicarious trauma", or secondary trauma. However, engagement in traumatic client disclosures and the practitioners' responses to them is quite paradoxical: both may be the source of vicarious traumatisation as well as the means of developing vicarious resilience, which is described as the ability to "bounce back" after engagement in traumatic work (Pack, 2014). With trauma work, the role of supervision as a preventative measure in vicarious trauma has been well established (Saakvitne et al., 2000; Vetere, 2012; Pack, 2014; Gil and Weinberg, 2015).

Although supervision is considered private, so that the clinical, professional, systemic, and sometimes personal issues at play for practitioners can be explored, it is not realistic or useful to see the supervisory space as completely protected or confidential (Fisher, 2013). In fact, supervision is an arrangement that has public accountability, so that supervisors and supervisees may have to outline their work to management, and file notes, including those from supervision, may be the subject of lawsuits (Houser and Thoma, 2012). A wide range of other stakeholders may also be indirectly involved in the supervision: work colleagues, managers, industry bodies, insurers, employers, courts, and the government. In the vignette above, some of Peter's colleagues were worried about how he was managing, and one of them alerted Jane to how reactive he was in staff meetings. The service manager also asked Jane to encourage Peter to take some leave from work, worried that Peter's dedication to his clients might be an unhelpful over-investment in his work.

Readiness to supervise and be supervised – in relation to trauma

Despite the pivotal nature of supervision in a practitioner's development of competence and therefore client outcomes, it is often the case that supervisors have not received formal training in supervision, and that supervisory practice has developed independent of, and not at the same pace as, evidence-based treatments (Falender et al., 2013). Supervisors should not only undertake specific training in supervision, they should also undergo relevant training with respect to trauma and should be in individual and/or group supervision themselves, so that complex issues can be openly discussed.

For supervision to work effectively, it is also important to note that a supervisee's stance needs to be one of openness in relation to their own strengths and weaknesses, with a willingness to learn about oneself from others (Carroll and Shaw, 2012; Knapp and Gavazzi, 2012). It is the role of the supervisor, however, to create an atmosphere of both trust and curiosity in supervision, so that practitioners feel able to explore any matter that is relevant to their work, and therefore their practice can be improved. Supervision with more junior practitioners often needs to be more instructional, directive, and supportive, whereas supervision with more senior practitioners may be more reflective and collaborative. As trauma work can engender a great deal of anxiety, supervisors also need to provide a containment function, until supervisees have developed greater maturity. This is particularly important to note when junior practitioners start seeing clients with extensive trauma histories and difficulties across many domains.

The gender, status, cultural, historical, and professional backgrounds of the supervisor and of the supervisee may also affect how participants come together in their work, with the potential to re-enact unhelpful hierarchies of power, unless this is explicitly named and managed. Without conscious attention, training, and reflection, the ethnocentricity of Western perspectives can dominate, as can heterosexism, patriarchy, and other dominant social paradigms, leading to the viewing of clients (and supervisees) through a lens which may not be valid (Falendar et al., 2013, citing Marsella and Pederson, 2004). In the current mental health environment, this is particularly likely to lead to an inappropriate focus being given to "symptoms", "disease", and the delivery of "skills"; indeed, a lack of competence has been argued to have potentially devastating consequences for a diverse range of clients (Salter and Salter, 2012).

As a result, supervisors need to be aware of the very high prevalence of trauma in all clinical populations, with varied presentations across cultural and social contexts, and to assist supervisees to detect trauma and to respond empathically to it. Supervision also offers the potential to identify and reflect on bias, blind spots, and stereotypes. However, this will only be achieved if both the supervisor and the supervisee undertake personal and professional development in these areas, are surrounded by robust educational experiences and peer feedback, and contract for these to be openly discussed in the service of learning.

Practitioners experiencing occupational "burnout" are often less able to self-reflect and to access self-care. Discussion of these matters can be met with defensiveness and withdrawal in supervision. It is the role of the supervisor under these circumstances to both support and gently explore the pertinent concerns. To return to the example of Peter, he has shown signs of stress and frustration, and his outbursts have come to the attention of management, who have found his behaviour both worrying and disruptive. Jane has been repeatedly asked to address this, and to work with his distress and reactivity. However, when Jane raises Peter's outbursts, he argues that this is the fault of management, a problem which has nothing to do with him. Peter continues to show very little interest in exploring his own thoughts and feelings.

Jane had initially contracted in supervision with Peter to discuss emotional reactions, countertransference, and ethical issues required for reflective practice. She realised the need to persist with these issues with Peter, particularly his view that the service was unjust, to see if he could look at this from any other perspective; after all, Peter signed up to work in a service with known parameters. Effective supervision might be able to assist Peter to develop a new level of understanding about himself, and assist him to provide a clear, contained, and effective service within the organisation's usual parameters. The benefits of undertaking personal therapy, moving to another service, or away from this type of work, could all also be usefully discussed.

Ethical issues working with trauma

For robust ethical practice, practitioners need to be well trained, not because a model per se is "correct" or useful in every circumstance, nor teaches them about ethics, but the process of getting ready to practice helps them enter the profession from a more mature and considered position (Sprenkle et al., 2009). Practitioners must be well supported as well as appropriately challenged by supervisors and colleagues and have principles of practice well established and in the forefront of their minds. They must also continually strive to improve their emotional intelligence, and their self-awareness, which in many studies has been demonstrated to be linked to effective ethical decision-making (Smith et al., 1991; Betan and Stanton, 1999; Hauser, 2006; Krishnakumar and Rymph, 2012).

Peter's behaviour suggests a loss of reflective capacity as his distress escalates. His temptation to blame the system reinforces his sense of helplessness and blinds him to steps that he himself could take to feel more in control. Practitioners who feel like Peter may argue that they are unable to take leave as, "my clients need me". The position of management to limit sessions or encourage staff to take leave can confirm, in Peter's mindset, how little they understand. It can seem to be a "badge of honour" to put oneself aside in the face of the person in greater need. However, this perspective is unhelpful, and is implicated in poor and unethical practice, as the role of practitioner becomes more one of "rescuer".

To advance a safe framework of ethical practice, practitioners need personal skills and qualities, ethical awareness, a moral philosophy of practice, and skill in applied ethics (Carroll and Shaw, 2012; Shaw and Carroll, 2016). This includes consideration of their professional practice, and readiness to work in relation to the following key requirements.

Competence and context

In services providing specialist trauma intervention, the imperative to have attended highly focused and advanced training in trauma work is crucial (Knapp and Gavazzi, 2012). Proficiency in specific, evidenced-based trauma techniques and intervention strategies may be required, such as Schema Therapy, Dialectical Behaviour Therapy, or Eye Movement Desensitisation and Reprocessing. Increasingly, studies are showing evidence of the growing complexity of trauma, that no "one size fits all" treatment approach can be applied (Cloitre, 2015; Quadara and Hunter, 2016), so practitioners must be able to tailor treatment to individual clients, which involves the ability to skilfully utilise a range of clinical tools.

Practitioners must also have given thought to the physical and emotional resources they will need, the time they will require to provide effective therapy, as well as other important components, such as reading, training, and supervision (Knapp and Gavazzi, 2012). Therapists develop increasingly "broad shoulders" as they advance in their profession in terms of their skill set, experience, and emotional resilience. However, this also needs to be balanced with clear personal and professional limits in relation to work undertaken.

When determining the ethical issue of competency within a given context, there are four matters to consider. Firstly, the supervisor and the practitioner need to appreciate what the service is established to do. There should be clear guidelines and parameters regarding services on offer and working within those boundaries should provide a "bottom line" for discussions. For example, in Peter's case, there is a six-month limit of service, and all clinical planning needs to take that into account. Second, is the supervisor supporting the practitioner's decision to undertake the work? Indeed, is the allocated supervisor trained in trauma work? Without workplace support and endorsement, the practitioner's work can be rendered unsafe. Third, the practitioner must also consider what training and experience he or she has had that objectively qualifies them for the work. Finally, a practitioner needs to ask him or herself if he/she is "good enough" to carry out the work, from the perspective of client need. While learning on the job is part of every professional's journey to some degree, this should never occur at the expense of the client receiving effective service.

In the above vignette, Peter seems to have "lost his bearings". Several reasons for this can be considered. Is this an issue of skill? Perhaps Peter doesn't know how to contract and work effectively within a six-month contract, nor to case plan or conclude service effectively. Increased skills in case management and clinical planning could make him feel more settled in his role. Perhaps his personal and professional philosophy is at odds with what is required of him, and he might need to work in a different environment that is better suited to him. If the service is not providing enough containment, then this may need to be addressed, but in a more constructive way. Peter's reactivity is not helpful in the emotionally challenging area of trauma and could mean that he is not fit for the work at present, but this requires Peter's willingness to look at the emotional load he is carrying, and how it influences his reactions. These are all areas worthy of discussion in supervision.

Emotional competence and self-care

The ability to remain competent, that is, in the acquisition of skills, knowledge, tools and their appropriate application, is inextricably linked with the need to achieve emotional competence. Emotional competence refers to the practitioner's awareness of

> all the ways their emotional experience and functioning affects, both positively and negatively, their professional judgement and the performance of their job duties, as well as the capability to manage their emotional experience and functioning to maximise the benefit and minimise any harm for those for whom they work.
>
> (Tamura, 2012: p.175)

Research shows that vicarious trauma is a significant risk in the helping professions (Gil and Weinberg, 2015). This is closely related to emotional exhaustion, a warning sign of burn-out, signalled when practitioners start to, "feel less of everything: less valued, enthusiastic, competent, connected, idealistic, involved, energetic and creative" (Reynolds Welfel, 2013: p.101). It is of concern that research has demonstrated that 62 per cent of practitioners will continue to work when stressed, even though 85 per cent recognise that it is unethical to do so; research that has been replicated across a range of studies (Pope et al., 1987). Codes of ethics for most professions require practitioners to assess when they might be impaired and to restrict work duties accordingly. However, this is a significant bind: practitioners may need to work for the income, or because they have insufficient leave, and, in their distress, may not have the insight required to judge their level of impairment, yet may be at risk of harming both themselves and others. Moreover, studies have demonstrated that people tend to believe that colleagues are more in need of a break than they are themselves (Tamura, 2012). Peter when asked said he was coping quite well, but that it was management that needed help.

Key threats to emotional competence are a lack of self-reflection and self-assessment, personal factors and experiences (historical and current), professional factors and experiences (such as the burden of one-sided encounters, repeated exposure to traumatic material, the effect of the work on personal relationships, disappointment at clients remaining at risk despite best efforts to support them being safe), work-related factors (such as the claims made by Peter), an inflated sense of responsibility, and barriers to seeking help and care, such as feeling shame, fear of being vulnerable, difficulty being a client and difficulty accessing support in small communities (Tamura, 2012; Vetere, 2012). These are important considerations, but the degree to which they are discussed in supervision will depend on the quality of the supervisory alliance, the contract that has been established, and the openness of the supervisee to explore their own reactions and experience. Taking the necessary time initially to set up an effective and safe relationship in supervision increases the possibility of these important discussions taking place.

Emotional competence also demands a commitment to self-care that is proactive rather than reactive; indeed, this is an ethical imperative in itself (Norcoss and Guy, 2007; Tamura, 2012). Peter's accumulation of leave is one example of unhelpful behaviour in the face of the emotionally taxing work. However, multiple strategies for effective self-care are considered essential: a positive and hopeful approach to work, time to talk about things other than work, encouragement via supervision to leave work at the work-place, a range of personal health and mind strategies, and a good work–life balance, including a range of social and other activities outside of work. It is not inevitable that practitioners will experience burnout or vicarious trauma, but the evidence is that those who engage in career-sustaining activities and are committed to personal wellness will be better protected, better at self-monitoring, and will provide more competent services to clients (Reynolds Welfel, 2013).

In this context, Jane and Peter eventually made two breakthroughs. First, although Jane did not bring up Peter's childhood directly with him, she speculated about the link between Peter's violent father, Peter's choice of work, and Peter's anger at the system within which he worked. In supervision, she did ask Peter to think about his anger, in a curious way, and he did eventually come to think that it might be multifactorial and might not all be about "the system". Jane also helped Peter to see that he was deserving in his own right, and he finally agreed to take some long overdue annual leave. She also contracted with him to keep looking at his strengths and areas needing input, so that Peter could make the most informed decisions regarding suitable training and work for him into the future.

Maintaining appropriate boundaries

Relationships with clients who have experienced trauma offer an important opportunity for modelling safety and clarity about healthy relationships. Greeting the client, touch, distance, furniture placement, office décor, contracting around session length, gift-giving and sharing of food and drink, contact between sessions (social media contact, emails, phone calls), and management of fees and debts, are all potentially significant exchanges through which practitioners demonstrate their ethical position (Sommers-Flanagan, 2012). Clients who have significant trauma histories are often very sensitive about such matters, and so upfront clarity provides a new sense of safety and security, which constitutes an important part of the therapy.

With high-risk clients, multiple relationships should be particularly avoided, as they can confuse the terms of the relationship and result in either or both parties losing focus about the central contract. There is also the potential for practitioners to consciously or unconsciously re-traumatise clients via boundary crossings, for example, "becoming friends", which almost inevitably leads to later termination of either or both the "friendship" and the therapy with poor outcomes, or through boundary violations, particularly via sexual misconduct, which is universally damaging.

Self-disclosure is also particularly unwise, as its purpose or meaning could be more confusing for the trauma client, and open to misinterpretation (Knapp and Gavazzi, 2012).

Capacity to continually assess ability to consent

As informed consent is based on the moral principle of client autonomy and is in the service of empowering collaboration (Knapp and Gavazzi, 2012; Cloitre, 2015), it should be the basis of all therapeutic endeavours. It is an ethical duty to ensure that the client has the freedom to choose, or not to choose, the treatment that they are requested to participate in. This is especially crucial in cases of trauma, where the client may have had a history of being controlled or taken advantage of by others.

It is also important to note that informed consent is an ongoing process. Practitioners are trained to focus on consent at the establishment of the contract, as if all might be rendered clear from the outset. However, the needs of the client, such as complex presentations requiring lengthy input, can mean changes to treatment, case consultations, or referrals that require further discussion. New entrants into the therapy, such as a partner or parent, will also require renegotiation. An unexpected report for an employer or an outside body, being compelled to provide case notes or evidence in court, the need to complete a mandatory notification, or to intervene when a client becomes suicidal, are all events and circumstances that call for further dialogue in relation to consent. It is the practitioner's responsibility to adapt their approach and use relevant resources in relation to informed consent with their clients, taking into account their age, developmental, and contextual circumstances, rather than the client being a passive recipient of the practitioner's input (Corey et al., 2011; Reynolds Welfel, 2013).

For high-risk clients or those with more complex needs, informed consent is likely to mean that the practitioner needs to provide more details about the therapy in terms of methods, goals, and limitations (such as session numbers) especially in relation to roles, rules, and responsibilities of both parties in the therapy (Knapp and Gavazzi, 2012).

It is also important to know that the provision of informed consent does not release the practitioner from the duty to protect the client's information. In complex situations, practitioners can be required to be involved in report writing, advocacy, court support, and similar tasks, in ways that are not required of more mainstream presentations. Disclosure should always be limited to the extent that it is legally possible to do so, and to the extent needed to achieve the goal of disclosure (Bond and Mitchels, 2008; Corey et al., 2011).

The role of a supervisor is to support the practitioner to continually reflect on the client's capacity for informed consent and ensure that clients, particularly with a history of Complex Trauma, remain informed of all aspects of the therapeutic process.

Redefining the role of case records

Case records require special attention in relation to trauma work. Practitioners are more likely to have their work called upon for testimony in the public domain, whether that be in public hearings, criminal court, or for compensation claims. In Australia, case notes can be accessed under the Freedom of Information Act, the Health Records Act, and the Privacy Act. However, practitioners unaware of this can sometimes hold the belief that their records belong to them and can have difficulty with this requirement. Instead, records should be seen to be created in the service of clients, to document their experience, to plan for their treatment, to record contact and progress, to communicate with others about the client, and to ensure continuity of care (Cameron and Murray, 2012). Case records can offer crucial evidence for clients to have their experiences of abuse validated, such as the childhood, domestic, and/or other abuse or violence they may have suffered.

Given the greater potential in trauma work for case records to be made available to third parties, or requested to be viewed by the client, there is an increased responsibility for practitioners to reflect on what constitutes effective case records, an aspect of practice that is often insufficiently discussed in training and supervision.

Conclusion

Working with trauma presentations is challenging, taxing, and at the same time rewarding. Developing special skills in relation to trauma through focused learning, reading, training, and supervision can ensure professional standards of proficiency. Emotional competence is more difficult to achieve: it takes time, self-reflection, personal development, and ethical alertness, and is ultimately a journey, not a destination. Supervision is the key to keeping practitioners mindful of the quality of their work, their professional obligations, and the importance of self-care. Ultimately, practitioners are individually accountable for their work, and for themselves, and that requires active engagement in ethical and professional development throughout their clinical careers.

References

Betan EJ and Stanton AL (1999) Fostering ethical willingness: Integrating emotional and contextual awareness with rational analysis. *Professional Psychology: Research and Practice* 30(3): 295–301.

Blue Knot Foundation (2017) *Fact sheet for managers: Trauma-informed service delivery.* Available at: blueknot.org.au/Portals/2/Fact%20Sheets%20Info/Fact%20Sheet_Managers.pdf?ver=2016-2005-17-165542-350.

Bond T and Mitchels B (2008) *Confidentiality and Record Keeping in Counselling and Psychotherapy.* London, UK: SAGE.

Cameron J and Murray J (2012) *Take Note! A Practical Guide to Writing Case Notes.* Victoria, Australia: Turning Point Alcohol and Drug Centre.

Carroll M and Shaw E (2012) *Ethical Maturity in the Helping Professions: Making Difficult Life and Work Decisions.* Melbourne, Australia: PsychOz Publications.

Cloitre M (2015) The "one size fits all" approach to trauma treatment: Should we be satisfied? *European Journal of Traumatology* 6, doi:10.3402/ejpt.v6.27344.

Corey G, Corey MS and Callanan P (2011) *Issues and Ethics in the Helping Professions, Eighth Edition.* Belmont, CA: Brooks/Cole.

Doyle O, Miller SE and Mirza FY (2009) Ethical decision-making in social work: Exploring personal and professional values. *Journal of Social Work Values and Ethics* 6 (1): 14–48.

Falendar CA, Burnes TR and Ellis MV (2013) Multicultural clinical supervision and benchmarks: Empirical support informing practice and supervisor training. *The Counselling Psychologist* 41(1): 8–27.

Fisher MA (2013) *The Ethics of Conditional Confidentiality: A Practical Model for Mental Health Professionals.* New York, NY: Oxford University Press.

Gil S and Weinberg M (2015) Secondary trauma among social workers treating trauma clients: The role of coping strategies and internal resources. *International Social Work* 58(4): 551–561.

Hauser MD (2006) The liver and the moral organ. *Social Cognitive and Affective Neuroscience* 1(3): 214–220.

Houser RA and Thoma S (2012) *Ethics in Counselling and Therapy: Developing an Ethical Identity.* Thousand Oaks, CA: SAGE.

Knapp SJ and Gavazzi J (2012) Ethical issues with patients at a high risk for treatment failure. In: Knapp SJ (ed) *APA Handbook of Ethics in Psychology.* Washington, DC: American Psychological Association, pp.401–416.

Knapp SJ, Bennett BE and Vandecreek LD (2012) Risk management for psychologists. In: Knapp SJ (ed) *APA Handbook of Ethics in Psychology.* Washington, DC: American Psychological Association, pp.483–518.

Krishnakumar S and Rymph D (2012) Uncomfortable ethical decisions: The role of negative emotions and emotional intelligence in ethical decision-making. *Journal of Managerial Issues* 14(3): 321–344.

Milne D (2009) *Evidence-Based Clinical Supervision: Principles and Practice.* West Sussex, UK: BPS Blackwell.

Norcoss JC and Guy JD (2007) *Leaving it at the Office: A Guide to Psychotherapist Self-Care.* New York, NY: The Guilford Press.

Pack M (2014) Vicarious resilience: A multilayered model of stress and trauma. *Journal of Women and Social Work* 29(1): 18–29.

Pope KS, Tabachnick BG and Keith-Spiegel P (1987) Ethics of practice: The beliefs and behaviors of psychologists as therapists. *American Psychologist* 42(11): 993–1006.

Quadara A and Hunter C (2016) *Principles of Trauma-informed Approaches to Child Sexual Abuse: A Discussion Paper.* Sydney, Australia: Royal Commission into Institutional Responses to Child Sexual Abuse.

Reynolds Welfel E (2013) *Ethics in Counselling and Psychotherapy, Fifth Edition.* Belmont, CA: Brooks/Cole.

Saakvitne KW, Gamble S, Pearlman LA, et al. (2000) *Risking Connection: A Training Curriculum for Working with Survivors of Childhood Abuse.* Baltimore, MD: The Sidran Press.

Salter DS and Salter BR (2012) Competence with diverse populations. In: Knapp SJ (ed) *APA Handbook of Ethics in Psychology.* Washington, DC: American Psychological Association, pp.217–240.

Shaw E and Carroll M (2016) Ethics for Counselling Psychologists. In: Douglas B, Woolfe R, Strawbridge S, et al. (eds) *Handbook for Counselling Psychologists, Fourth Edition.* London, UK: SAGE, pp. 244–258.

Smith TS, McGuire JM and Abbott DW (1991) Clinical ethical decision making: An investigation of the rationales used to justify doing less than one believes one should. *Professional Psychology: Research and Practice* 22(3): 235–239.

Sommer CA (2008) Vicarious traumatisation, trauma sensitive supervision, and counsellor preparation. *Counselor Education and Supervision* 48: 61–71.

Sommers-Flanagan R (2012) Boundaries, multiple roles and professional relationships. In: Knapp SJ (ed) *APA Handbook of Ethics in Psychology.* Washington, DC: American Psychological Association, pp.241–278.

Sprenkle DH, Davis SD and Lebow JL (2009) *Common Factors in Couple and Family Therapy: The Overlooked Foundation for Effective Practice.* New York, NY: The Guilford Press.

Tamura LJ (2012) Emotional competence and well-being. In: Knapp SJ (ed) *APA Handbook of Ethics in Psychology.* Washington, DC: American Psychological Association, pp.175–215.

Vetere A (2012) Supervision and consultation practice with domestic violence. *Clinical Child Psychology and Psychiatry* 17(2): 181–185.

Part IV

Organisational approaches

23 The principles of trauma-informed care and the need for cultural and organisational change

Pam Stavropoulos

Introduction

Trauma-informed care is an emergent paradigm in mental health and human service delivery, the implications of which extend far beyond the mental health sector from which it derives. The paradigm stems from the recognition that trauma is highly prevalent, that most clients who access the public mental health system have trauma histories (Jennings, 2004), and that the current organisation of health and human services does not reflect this reality and is inadequate to cope with it. It also stems from an acknowledgment of the disturbing reality that far from providing safe environments for the many traumatised people who access mental health services, "trauma has often occurred in the service context itself" (Jennings, 2004: p.6).

Trauma-informed care and practice (TICP) can be defined as "an approach which recognises and acknowledges trauma and its prevalence, alongside awareness and sensitivity to its dynamics, in all aspects of service delivery" (Mental Health Coordinating Council, 2017). Grounded in a comprehensive understanding of the biological, neurological, psychological, and social effects of trauma and interpersonal violence, it involves "not only changing assumptions about how we organise and provide services, but creates organisational cultures that are personal, holistic, creative, open and therapeutic" (Mental Health Coordinating Council, 2017). Though regarding the traumatised person through the contextual and relational lens of harm – that is, the individual becomes traumatised via adverse overwhelming experiences – TICP is also a strengths-based framework, predicated on the philosophy of empowerment.

History and background

In contrast to the earlier recognition of the devastating impacts of trauma, the roots of TICP are more recent. It was not until the 1990s that health professionals drew attention to "the importance of the organisational context in the delivery of services" to people who have undergone traumatic life experiences (Wilson et al., 2013: p.5). The precursors to this development were concern about the high prevalence of physical and sexual abuse of women seen in the public mental health system and the re-victimisation experienced in inpatient and residential settings from practices such as seclusion and restraint (Wilson et al., 2013). However, the context in which services are provided has not traditionally been seen as important; the environment of service delivery has tended to be regarded, when it is considered at all, as the neutral backdrop to the service supplied. Crucial to reappraisal of this view was a conference convened in 1994 in the USA by the Substance Abuse and Mental Health Services Administration (SAMHSA) at which the need for organisational change in service delivery for survivors of trauma became apparent from survivor testimonies.

Dramatic illustration of health service re-enactment of prior client abuse if the service is not trauma-informed is provided in the table "Institutional Retraumatization" by American trauma educator and advocate Ann Jennings (Jennings, 1994). The first column of this table, "Early childhood trauma experience", lists a range of violations which typify the isolating, shaming, threatening, and betrayal of the child victim, and is based on the actual experience of Jennings' daughter, Anna, who suicided at age 32 in a long-stay ward of a US mental health facility. The second column, "Common mental health institutional practices", lists alongside how each of these violations was replicated, almost to the letter, by inpatient interventions which are frequently harmful and re-traumatising.

For example, during her sexual abuse as a child, Anna was tied up and held down with her hands and arms bound. The same subsequently occurred in mental health institutions via the practice of "take down" and restraint, during which her arms and legs were shackled to a bed. Her childhood abuser had taken her to places which were hidden from others; in mental health institutions she was forced, "often by male attendants", into a seclusion room. Stripped and penetrated by her childhood abuser, she was also stripped as a mental health patient, and forcibly injected (Jennings, 1994). The correlation of numerous standard institutional practices to which Anna was subjected as an adult with the abuse she experienced as a child is both striking and disturbing.

The need for systemic change was brought to the attention of wider audiences in October 1998, when the *Hartford Courant*, the largest daily newspaper in Connecticut, and regarded by many as the oldest continuously operated newspaper in the USA, published an investigative series on the brutalisation and death of involuntarily secluded and restrained patients. "The resulting public and professional furore prompted a spate of new [US] federal regulations and legislative initiatives, setting national standards for reporting and clinical oversight" (Busch and Shore, 2000).

In 2001, a major initiative between SAMHSA and the US Congress led to the emergence of the National Child Traumatic Stress Network. Initially, this body focused on improving access to services for children, families, and communities in the USA, as well as improvement in the standard of care (Wilson et al., 2013). By 2003, the role of systems in either supporting or eroding the treatment of those who had suffered trauma had become increasingly apparent, and, in response, in 2005, SAMHSA founded the National Center for Trauma-Informed Care which "suggested that every part of an organization seeking to be trauma-informed … be assessed and potentially modified to include a basic understanding of how trauma affects the life of an individual seeking services" (Wilson et al., 2013: p.6). SAMHSA has since become a major vehicle for the advocacy of TICP in the USA.

Since the genesis of TICP in the mid-1990s, recognition has grown that appropriate responses to trauma survivors require new knowledge and attitudes about the nature of care that should be provided, extensive workforce training in trauma, and cross-service collaboration between consumers, carers, and policy makers. To the extent that trauma is "an almost universal experience of public mental health and substance abuse consumers" (Havenga, 2010), the need for TICP is similarly universal.

Principles of trauma-informed care

Literature on TICP notes that it derives from a range of influences, that it combines several core principles, and that it is applicable to a wide range of contexts (Wilson et al., 2013). Recurrent descriptors are that it rests on a foundational understanding of the impacts of trauma, that it is strengths-based, fosters empowerment, and "emphasizes physical, psychological, and emotional safety for both providers and survivors" (Hopper et al., 2010: pp.81–82).

Importantly, the paradigm of TICP contrasts markedly with the biomedical model of psychiatry and mental health, which emphasises symptoms and deficits, and is therefore inherently pathologising (Moskowitz, 2011). By contrast, the strengths-based approach of trauma-informed care emphasises the adaptive function of behaviours which may otherwise be regarded as signs of pathology, primarily treated by medication. From this perspective, "symptoms" can also be viewed, as per the findings of the Adverse Childhood Experiences (ACE) study, as the outgrowth of coping strategies which have ceased to be adaptive because the underlying trauma has not been resolved (Felitti and Anda, 1998). The question of what has happened to a person – that is, the prior experience of overwhelming stress – rather than the biomedically driven question of what is "wrong" with a person, encapsulates the difference.

A trauma-informed approach does not comprise clinical treatment (in contrast to "trauma-specific" services) and is also applicable to services outside the health sector for this reason. It rests on a "do no harm" orientation that seeks to avoid compounding prior trauma. It is attuned to how institutions may re-enact trauma dynamics inadvertently and aims to minimise this risk by being "informed about, and sensitive to, trauma-related issues" (Jennings, 2004: p.15).

The extent to which policies and procedures of a service foster these core principles requires ongoing attentiveness to all aspects of the service through "a trauma-informed lens". The prevalence of trauma mandates the possibility of underlying trauma in all clients as a central organising premise (Jennings, 2004; Fallot and Harris, 2009). This is a multifaceted perspective which needs to be consciously prioritised and monitored. In stark contrast to a conventional understanding of service provision, trauma-informed care emphasises the "how" as well as the "what" of service delivery, that is, the way in which a service is delivered, not just what the service comprises.

The five core trauma-informed principles on which all interactions with people who experience the impact of trauma should be based are safety, trustworthiness, choice, collaboration, and empowerment (Fallot and Harris, 2009). These "bedrock" principles are of paramount importance for those who have survived trauma, many of whom have experienced violation of the most fundamental human values in contexts of abuse and breaches of duty of care.

The principle of safety is central and non-negotiable and underpins all trauma-informed values and priorities. All who have been traumatised may have safety concerns, including emotional, relational, and physical safety. Interpersonal interactions in a trauma-informed service should always be sensitive to safety concerns and be delivered to promote a sense of safety. This principle importantly requires that the geographical space of service settings should also be physically safe, welcoming, and functional (Fallot and Harris, 2009).

Many people who have undergone interpersonal trauma have had their trust betrayed in intimate relationships and the pervasive effects of trauma can include "the way people approach potentially helpful relationships" (Fallot and Harris, 2009: p.2). The principle of trustworthiness requires service sensitivity to client needs at all levels of contact, and attentiveness to ways in which the reliability of the service is consistently conveyed to clients, so that genuineness and predictability can be expected (Fallot and Harris, 2009).

The experience of choice is often unfamiliar to those who struggle with the impacts of trauma, as wishes and preferences have been overridden when control has been removed. The principle of choice means that services should provide options to clients at all the levels at which it is possible to do so. While taking care not to overwhelm clients with a confusing array of options, this requires the service to repeatedly consider ways in which choices can be offered, even and especially where the possibilities for the exercise of choice may seem minimal (Fallot and Harris, 2009).

People who experience trauma are often wrongly seen as unable to collaborate in decisions which affect them. Though there may be situations and times where it is not possible for traumatised people to have significant input into their treatment plan, the experience of trauma does not mean that people should be infantilised or regarded as passive and helpless. The principle of collaboration requires consistent imparting to clients of a sense of "doing with", rather than "to" or "for".

The principle of collaboration is closely related to the principle of client empowerment. For people who have been disempowered by the experience of trauma, the often predominantly biomedical and patriarchal nature of the health system can inadvertently reinforce this situation. The experience then of being able to exert some influence over one's immediate surroundings and to be part of the treatment planning process can be both welcome to those who have been traumatised and helpful to treatment providers, "People with Complex Trauma will respond better to treatment when they are empowered in ways that are unique to them, and the professionals and institutions should not underestimate the patient's ability to be very useful and active in their own treatment" (Stillwell, 2012: p.viii).

Although these principles apply to the approaches that should be taken to any person who may have experienced trauma and be in need of care in any setting, they are particularly applicable to those who require inpatient treatment and are especially relevant for those held against their will on mental health orders.

Operationalising trauma-informed care

An understanding of the five principles of trauma-informed care is necessary at all levels of service provision to enable transformational outcomes (Bateman et al., 2013). Substantial organisational change is required to achieve this. People who experience trauma have contact – both direct and indirect, formal and informal – with a range of personnel of diverse qualifications and skill bases. Recognition is needed that the achievement of "a truly trauma-informed" health system requires no less than "a process of reconstitution within our organisations top to bottom" (Bloom and Farragher, 2006: p.2) and involves all stakeholders in an organisation, from coalface staff to the upper echelons of management.

Introduction of TICP requires systemic, as well as interpersonal change;

> Changes to a trauma-informed organisational service system environment will be experienced by all involved as a profound cultural shift in which consumers and their conditions and behaviours are viewed differently, staff respond differently, and the day-to-day delivery of services is conducted differently.
>
> (Jennings, 2004: p.15)

The following question encompasses the many implications for the requisite changes to health service delivery on the ground:

> By looking at how the entire system is organised, and services are delivered through a 'trauma lens', what should be done differently? The answer can be used to guide practice, policy, procedures, and even how the physical caregiving environment is structured.
>
> (Wilson et al., 2013: pp.1–2)

Attention to the latter, the physical caregiving environment, is critical. At all times and in all its forms, client safety – the cardinal principle of trauma-informed care – should be upheld and safeguarded. This entails attentiveness to and introduction of measures to reduce the potential for clients to be triggered and overwhelmed. This includes the organisation of all relevant rooms and settings for care and treatment. Indeed, one study has found that enhancement of the physical environment in which a service is offered was more positively correlated with reduction of client stress associated with standard institutional practices than was staff education about the impacts of trauma (Borckardt et al., 2011). All areas of contact should also be as soothing and stabilising as possible. This increases the likelihood of uptake of more specific services by people who have trauma histories. If apprehension about interpersonal and institutional contact is not allayed by reassuring environments, and service culture and practices, traumatised people may not access or continue to access the wider service at all.

This also necessitates adherence to trauma-informed practice at the first client contact, irrespective of the medium, by first responders and by all reception staff. Without awareness of these principles, staff may unwittingly escalate client distress by mistaking anxiety for intentional non-cooperation or lack of courtesy, resulting in the client being labelled as "difficult".

The respect of the trauma-informed paradigm for the lived experience of clients, which, when traumatic and overwhelming, generates the need for coping strategies which serve adaptive purposes that the biomedical model risks subsuming within the lens of pathology, has several practical implications. For example, it means that trauma-informed services require not only the standard staff training around confidentiality, dual relationships, and respect for client diversity (culture, gender, age, ethnicity, sexual orientation, and so on), but that respect for and tolerance of diverse coping mechanisms is also required (Jennings, 2004; Fallot and Harris, 2009). More rigid, punitive responses on the other hand are much more likely to lead to the potential for client "triggering", re-traumatisation, and shame. Fallot and Harris also suggest that,

> There is need to determine if any policies or procedures are damaging and replicate past abusive practices. There is special need for alertness to 'traumatic re-enactments masquerading as benign practice', and policies and procedures that may inadvertently permit and rationalise abusive responses and relationships.
>
> (2009: p.9)

In a comprehensive but step-wise manner, trauma-informed principles can be introduced and disseminated throughout all domains of a health service setting. The following steps may be advised in this regard: (i) identify key formal and informal activities and settings; (ii) ask key questions about each of the activities and settings; (iii) prioritise goals for change, and, (iv) identify specific objectives and responsible persons (Fallot and Harris, 2009).

As systemic change is required, some of the necessary measures may be more challenging and take longer to implement than others, although, with staff training, some necessary steps can be operationalised quite rapidly. Identification of methods by which the core trauma-informed principles can be operationalised may be assisted by attentiveness to a number of key questions (Fallot and Harris, 2009). Are intake protocols and physical space welcoming, and more than just information gathering? Is the service setting sensitive to client needs at all levels of contact? Does the service provide choice to clients at all levels at which it is possible to do so? Does the service consistently communicate to clients a sense of "doing with" rather than "for" or "to"? How is client empowerment enabled by service systems, programs, and processes? The ways in which respect for client diversity – in all its forms – is conveyed and enacted should also be considered.

Helpful in translating from principle to practice is the establishment of a service-charter of trauma-informed care which emphasises a recovery orientation. Most important is a mechanism for the screening of underlying trauma that is implemented in a context which is fully trauma-informed. This helps ensure that all staff understand the impact of trauma. Staff also need to be given the time and training to proactively engage clients, to talk to them and to attempt to more fully understand them. They also need to learn how to assist clients to "de-escalate", to lower their arousal level, via a simple grounding exercise if necessary, to help them return to the "window of tolerance" (Siegel, 1999). Finally, communication and co-ordination between and among systems of care should be enhanced and promoted (Fallot and Harris, 2009; Kezelman and Stavropoulos, 2012).

Sources of resistance

Unless specifically subscribed to as a policy imperative, the introduction of TICP risks being subsumed by the pressures of daily service delivery. These include funding constraints, the demands of timetabling, and staff availability. Though the needs of clients comprise the basic rationale of service delivery, the nature of services is that they are often structured by the requirements of service provision itself. But the nature of the challenges posed by trauma-informed care to existing ways of operating are also separate and distinct from the day-to-day demands of the provision of care (Huckshorn and Lebel, 2013).

Another formidable impediment to the implementation of trauma-informed practice is the role of "mindsets", that is, the largely unconscious ideas and beliefs that dictate what humans think about and what they do not consider (Bloom and Farragher, 2011). Mindsets function largely to protect individuals and groups from anxiety, and they do so particularly in relation to trauma. As Herman elaborated a quarter of a century ago, "denial, repression, and dissociation operate on a social as well as an individual level" (Herman, 1997: p.2). In the context of trauma, potentially overwhelming even to contemplate, the social defence mechanisms elicited can be especially insidious (Bloom and Farragher, 2011). To the extent that the assumptive environment of the western intellectual tradition is predicated on "just world" theory and privileges agency, rationality, and consciousness (Brown, 2009), recognition of human vulnerability to trauma both individually and collectively can be especially challenging to concede.

It should be particularly noted the threat trauma poses to "the existing worldview and the mental models upon which human service delivery is built" (Bloom and Farragher, 2011: p.126) is a challenge that advocates of trauma-informed practice ignore at their peril. Stress radically impacts human reflective capacity, and the stress of trauma and fear is stress at its most extreme. The fact that humans are "highly susceptible to emotional contagion", and that "training, logic and intelligence are often no match for the power of groupthink" (Perry and Szalavitz, 2006: p.178), suggests that stressed systems, as well as the individuals which comprise them, are vulnerable, and may also struggle with reflective capacity and substantial change. This means that if the paradigm of trauma-informed care is to become standard practice, what is needed, as Herman predicted, are broad-ranging alliances strong enough to counteract the social pressures to deny (Herman, 1997). As Felitti and Anda have said of the findings of the Adverse Childhood Experiences study: "The potential is huge. So too is the likelihood of clinician and institutional resistance … . Actualising the benefits of this paradigm shift will depend on first identifying and resolving the various bases for resistance to it" (Felitti and Anda, 2010: p.86). This, they say, "will require far more planning than would be needed to introduce a purely intellectual or technical advance" (Felitti and Anda, 2010: p.86).

Key requirement – skilling a diverse workforce

All personnel, paid and unpaid, clinical and non-clinical, from senior management to clinicians, office juniors and volunteers, need to be trained in trauma-informed principles. Coherence of vision and integration of currently compartmentalised systems mandates a shared understanding and operationalisation of these principles, irrespective of occupation, skill base, and service type.

At the same time, the breadth of activities and services affected means that the changes required will affect different personnel and professions differently. To this extent, training may also be site and discipline-specific. For example, nurses who are directly responsible for the administration of medication have identified "a specific ethical dilemma" with respect to court-ordered or otherwise imposed medication regimes where this is against the client's wishes (Regan, 2010). Psychologists also face dilemmas. For example, the requirement to diagnose and conduct evaluations may limit opportunities to build trust with clients. This means that assessments arrived at, including via the use of assessment tools, may reflect "an incomplete understanding of the client's challenges if the analysis sidesteps etiology – how and why the behaviour developed in the first place" (Huckshorn and Lebel, 2013: p.79).

General and primary health care practitioners are often the first point of contact for people who experience a diverse range of health problems which may be trauma-related, and which remain undetected and sometimes inappropriately treated in the absence of practitioner awareness of the impacts of trauma. The current "symptom-based" orientation of the biomedical model –

according to which, medication is frequently the standard treatment response – is ill-equipped to address the prevalence of underlying trauma, and to understand that "symptoms" may be the outgrowth of coping strategies used to manage the after-effects of trauma that have ceased to be protective (Felitti et al., 1998; Felitti and Anda, 2010); psychiatrists may also view difficulties through the same biomedical lens.

The paradigm of trauma-informed care stands in clear contrast to the biomedical approach, and its introduction to the training curricula of relevant health care practitioners would have far-reaching positive effects. Clearly this is beyond the purview and purpose of health services themselves. As a marker of quality assurance, services should, however, promote education about trauma, provide relevant professional development opportunities, and foster both collaborative partnerships and relevant research.

Progress in Australia

In Australia, the comprehensiveness of the systemic change required for service delivery to become trauma-informed is specifically and explicitly stated by its major advocates (Bateman et al., 2013). Milestones in furthering this perspective were the final report of the Senate Standing Committee on Community Affairs, "Towards Recovery: Mental Health Services in Australia" (2008) and the landmark 2011 conference, "Trauma-informed Care and Practice: Meeting the Challenge", convened by the Mental Health Coordinating Council (MHCC), the Blue Knot Foundation (then Adults Surviving Child Abuse), the NSW Health Education Centre Against Violence, and the Private Mental Health Consumer Carer Network Australia.

Some important steps in the introduction of trauma-informed care in Australia are now in place. In 2011, the MHCC launched a microsite dedicated to TICP, in 2012 the Blue Knot Foundation released its acclaimed, "Practice Guidelines for Treatment of Complex Trauma and Trauma-informed Care and Service Delivery" (Kezelman and Stavropoulos, 2012), the Australian literature on trauma-informed care is growing (Muskett, 2014), and frequent requests from services, many generated by the Australian Royal Commission into Institutional Responses to Child Sexual Abuse, for staff training in the principles of trauma-informed practice are being received.

The National Trauma-informed Care and Practice Advisory Working Group continues to maintain and promote the need for trauma-informed care across service sectors. It also facilitates opportunities "for public, private and the community-managed mental health sectors to understand and embrace the principles of trauma-informed care and practice thereby adopting a shift in organisational culture and service delivery" (Bateman et al., 2013: p.7).

At one level, recent and current events, among which the Royal Commission, noted above, is very significant, are expanding awareness of the need for trauma-informed care as the necessary and indeed the only meaningful response to the prevalence of trauma. Yet, the diversity of service settings which need to become trauma-informed, for example, acute care, primary care, psychological and psychiatric private practices, indicates the enormity of the challenge.

In light of this necessary shift, "on the ground" implementation has been unsurprisingly uneven at best. As Bloom notes, "The emergence of radical new knowledge requires a capacity for innovative change and high-level integrative practices that are not available to significantly stressed systems" (2011: p.57). This is especially so when such systems are themselves founded on division, in a social and political context in which there exist powerful investments at multiple levels which serve as disincentives to change.

Conclusion

Despite the now extensive research which substantiates the frequently devastating effects of trauma, and the incontestable case at an intellectual and rational level of the need for implementation of trauma-informed services, resistance remains strong. As Middleton comments, "The issue is much more about society's willingness to know, and our at times extraordinary need to believe something, other than the unsettling truth" (Middleton, 2012: p.xiii). The paradigm of trauma-informed care however poses a formidable challenge to the biomedical model of psychiatry and mental health, and given the high individual and collective cost of trauma and its multiple impacts across a range of indicators – psychological, physical, financial, and social – the stakes for failing to comprehensively introduce the paradigm are high.

Urgently needed for implementation and embedding of trauma-informed practice across the full spectrum of health service delivery is:

- Prioritisation of trauma as a public health challenge,
- Expanded training programs for staff across all disciplines and sites, at both undergraduate and postgraduate levels,
- Trauma screening at multiple levels, including at the level of primary care,
- Significantly expanded treatment options for clients, both by choice and by geographical availability,
- Relevant cross-sectoral collaborative partnerships,
- Research, and
- Funding commensurate with the above.

The term "trauma-informed" is now increasingly invoked, and the paradigm is well supported, particularly in the USA, by readily available and accessible materials to assist in its implementation (Fallot and Harris, 2009; Guarino et al., 2009; Menschner and Maul, 2016). That services are now referencing this paradigm attests to a level of awareness that did not exist as recently as five years ago. It also prepares the ground for the comprehensive change which is necessary, but yet to come.

References

Bateman J, Henderson C and Kezelman C (2013) *Trauma-Informed Care and Practice: Towards a Cultural Shift in Policy Reform Across Mental Health and Human Services in Australia, A National Strategic Direction. Position Paper and Recommendations of the National Trauma-Informed Care and Practice Advisory Working Group*. Sydney, Australia: Mental Health Coordinating Council.

Bloom SL (2006) *Organizational Stress as a Barrier to Trauma-Sensitive Change and System Transformation*. Alexandria, VA: National Technical Assistance Centre.

Bloom SL and Farragher B (2011) *Destroying Sanctuary: The Crisis in Human Service Delivery Systems*. New York, NY: Oxford University Press.

Borckardt JJ, Madan A, Grubaugh AL, et al. (2011) Systematic investigation of initiatives to reduce seclusion and restraint in a state psychiatric hospital. *Psychiatric Services* 62(5): 477–483.

Brown LS (2009) *Cultural Competence in Trauma Therapy*. Washington, DC: American Psychological Association.

Busch AB and Shore MF (2000) Seclusion and restraint: A review of recent literature. *Harvard Review of Psychiatry* 8(5): 261–270.

Fallot R and Harris M (2009) *Creating Cultures of Trauma-Informed Care (CCTIC): A Self-Assessment and Planning Protocol*. Washington, DC: Community Connections.

Felitti VJ, Anda RF, Nordenberg D, et al. (1998) Relationship of childhood abuse and household dysfunction to many of the leading causes of death in adults: The Adverse Childhood Experiences (ACE) study. *American Journal of Preventive Medicine* 14(4): 245–258.

Felitti VJ and Anda RF (2010) The relationship of adverse childhood experiences to adult medical disease, psychiatric disorders and sexual behavior: Implications for healthcare. In: Lanius RA, Vermetten E and Pain C (eds) *The Impact of Early Life Trauma on Health and Disease: The Hidden Epidemic*. New York, NY: Cambridge University Press, pp.77–87.

Guarino K, Soares P, Konnath K, et al. (2009) *Trauma-Informed Organizational Toolkit*. Rockville, MD: Center for Mental Health Services, Substance Abuse and Mental Health Services Administration and the Daniels Fund, the National Child Traumatic Stress Network, and the WK Kellogg Foundation.

Havenga S (2010) Community psychiatric clinic. In: *Trauma Informed Care and Practice (TICP)*. Cited by the Mental Health Coordinating Council. Available at: mhcc.org.au/sector-development/recovery-and-practice-approaches/trauma-informed-care-and-practice.aspx.

Herman J (1997) *Trauma and Recovery*. New York, NY: Basic Books.

Hopper EK, Bassuk EL and Olivet J (2010) Shelter from the storm: Trauma-informed care in homelessness services settings. *The Open Health Policy and Services Journal* 3: 80–100.

Huckshorn K and Lebel JL (2013) Trauma-informed care. In: Yeager K, Culer D, Svendsen D, et al. (eds) *Modern Community Mental Health*. Oxford, UK: Oxford University Press.

Jennings A (1994) On being invisible in the mental health systems. *The Journal of Mental Health Administration* 21(4): 374–387.

Jennings A (2004) *Models for Developing Trauma-Informed Behavioral Health Systems and Trauma-Specific Services. Report*. USA: National Association of State Mental Health Program Directors and the National Technical Assistance Center for State Mental Health Planning.

Kezelman CA and Stavropoulos PA (2012) *The Last Frontier: Practice Guidelines for Treatment of Complex Trauma and Trauma-Informed Care and Service Delivery*. Sydney, Australia: Adults Surviving Child Abuse.

Menschner C and Maul A (2016) *Key Ingredients for Successful Trauma-Informed Care Implementation. Issue Brief.* Hamilton, NJ: Centre for Health Care Strategies.

Mental Health Coordinating Council (accessed 2017) *Trauma-Informed Care and Practice (TICP)*. Available at: mhcc.org.au/sector-development/recovery-and-practice-approaches/trauma-informed-care-and-practice.aspx.

Middleton W (2012) Foreword. In: Kezelman C and Stavropoulos P *The Last Frontier: Practice Guidelines for Treatment of Complex Trauma and Trauma-Informed Care and Service Delivery*. Sydney, Australia: Adults Surviving Child Abuse, pp.x–xiii.

Moskowitz A (2011) Schizophrenia, trauma, dissociation, and scientific revolutions. *Journal of Trauma and Dissociation* 12: 347–357.

Muskett C (2014) Trauma-informed care in inpatient mental health settings: A review of the literature. *International Journal of Mental Health Nursing* 23: 51–59.

Perry B and Szalavitz M (2006) *The Boy Who Was Raised as a Dog: What Traumatized Children Can Teach Us About Loss, Love, and Healing*. New York, NY: Basic Books.

Regan K (2010) Trauma-informed care on an inpatient pediatric psychiatric unit and the emergence of ethical dilemmas as nurses evolve their practice. *Issues in Mental Health Nursing* 3: 216–222.

Senate Standing Committee on Community Affairs (2008) *Towards Recovery: Mental Health Services in Australia*. Canberra, Australia: Australian Parliament.

Siegel DJ (2003) An interpersonal neurobiology of psychotherapy: The developing mind and the resolution of trauma. In: Solomon MT and Siegel DJ (eds) *Healing Trauma*. New York, NY: Norton, pp.1–56.

Stillwell T (2012) Foreword. In: Kezelman C and Stavropoulos P *The Last Frontier: Practice Guidelines for Treatment of Complex Trauma and Trauma Informed Care and Service Delivery*. Sydney, Australia: Adults Surviving Child Abuse, p.viii.

Wilson C, Pence M and Conradi L (2013) Trauma-informed care. In: *Encyclopedia of Social Work Online*. National Association of Social Workers and Oxford University Press. doi:10.1093/acrefore/9780199975839.013.1063.

24 Therapeutic services for traumatised children and young people – healing in the everyday experience of relationships

Joe Tucci and Janise Mitchell

Introduction

The past swirls and reverberates through children's experiences, shaping their present and influencing their future. Attuned, supportive, safe, and reliable early relationships create opportunities for children to learn, adapt, and connect as they grow. Young children develop to believe in themselves and those around them. However, when these relationships are experienced as abusive, violent, and disruptive, they are forced into developing self-protective states that shut them off from others, making them more resistant to change, and locking them into behavioural routines which repeat the very strategies they have used to survive the danger that has permeated their lives (Perry, 2002; Ogden et al., 2006; Baylin and Hughes, 2017).

In the face of chronic exposure to trauma, the brains and bodies of children become trapped in a highly vigilant state, constantly scanning their environment for threat. These children lose the capacity to respond creatively and flexibly. They crave consistency and routine. Their experience of relationships often amplifies their needs rather than reduces them. Any change in what they come to expect, good or bad, can quickly trigger cascading stress reactions that overwhelm them (Schore, 2001, 2002, 2003; Gunnar and Quevedo, 2007).

As children grow into young people, they face increasing demands. For those with early histories of destructive relationships and experiences of violence, adolescence often erupts into sequences of high-risk behaviour, intensifying relationship conflict, social isolation, and reduced levels of engagement with supportive adults. These adolescents often find school and structured opportunities for learning stressful and unrewarding. They frequently find it difficult to settle and experience comfort, even when it is offered to them. They may also be particularly reactive to small shifts in interpersonal dynamics involving family, peers, and others in their community (Van der Kolk, 2003a, 2003b; Schore and Schore, 2008).

These young people experience an adolescence that cycles through past patterns of distress and confusion that invades the present. They find themselves clinging to familiar responses, ill-equipped to navigate the challenges of this developmental phase with the adaptability required. In this context, the future trajectories for these young people often involve persistent, pervasive, and cumulative forms of disadvantage (McEwen, 2006). Their past continues to isolate them. Trauma disrupts their connections, and heightens the likelihood of other problems, such as homelessness, unemployment, substance abuse, mental health issues, problems associated with ongoing interpersonal violence, and an increased risk of engaging in crime or becoming victims of crime.

Trauma not only affects children and young people's functioning in everyday life, it also creates a vortex of reactions that often paradoxically reduces the degree of understanding and compassion provided by others; their networks and communities often blame them, and stand in judgement over them. They are held responsible for their behaviour and any damage they may cause, whilst the conduct of the adults who abused and hurt them is often ignored or minimised. Frustration and anger ripples through communities who may demand to understand why these challenging children and young people do not change, and why the support offered to them is not embraced. These children attract labels as defiant, oppositional, disinterested, unmotivated, hopeless, and criminal.

Children and young people are then doubly betrayed. They continue to suffer trauma deep in their hearts, minds, and bodies (Ogden et al., 2006; Porges, 2011). Their world is not safe. Relationships are untrustworthy. The meaning of what has happened to them is never acknowledged. When they turn to adults for help, they are not always believed, reinforcing their experience of shame (Tucci et al., 2010). Children and young people find their identity reconstructed, emphasising problem-saturated narratives that undermine not only their strengths, but also their own efforts to survive (Siegel, 1999, 2009; Perry, 2002; Baylin and Hughes, 2017).

Therapeutic interventions are at their most effective when they look beyond external behaviours and concurrently address the multiple layers of need that abused children and young people exposed to family violence present. The core dimension central to such work is the creation and strengthening of relational attachments that resonate backwards and forward through time, intentionally aiming to repair the past in the day-to-day experience of relationships in the present.

Trauma-integrative and trauma-transformative practice

There appears to be an in-built impatience in the child welfare sector to tolerate the time required to allow the power of attuned, sensitive, and secure relationships to heal the hurt that traumatised children carry with them (Tucci, 2016). In many ways, the field is at a crossroads. The original enthusiasm – offered by the exciting new knowledge in the neurobiology of trauma – is fading as the basis of service design for traumatised children and young people. Increasingly, forces are pushing to find that "next new thing", the innovation that will bring about change quickly. These forces are driven by a lack of an agreed definition of what the term "trauma-informed" means, by government reform agendas and funding restraints, and an urgency to be seen to be doing "something" about the often confronting and distressing behaviours of traumatised children and young people. As a result, there is a constant drive towards the provision of time-limited behavioural therapies, interventions that have not always served the best interest of these children and young people.

For these reasons, children's trauma services need to move beyond being trauma-informed. They need to be trauma-integrated and trauma-transformative (Tucci, 2016). According to the US Substance Abuse and Mental Health Services Administration (SAMHSA), a trauma-informed approach to service delivery is defined thus:

> A program, organization, or system that is trauma-informed realizes the widespread impact of trauma and understands potential paths for recovery; recognizes the signs and symptoms of trauma in clients, families, staff, and others involved with the system; and responds by fully integrating knowledge about trauma into policies, procedures, and practices, and seeks to actively resist re-traumatization.
>
> (SAMHSA, 2014, p.9)

In contrast, trauma-integrated services are not only familiar with the knowledge base about trauma, they have fused these principles with their own mission and vision. A trauma-integrated service combines its own value base with its commitment to achieving change. Knowledge of trauma is not separate to the operations of the service – it is at the centre. The evidence from the neuroscience of child development and interpersonal relationships offer resources to practitioners that build on other important principles which include being culturally strong, risk-responsive, rights-oriented, and strengths-based. Trauma-integrated services focus away from individual trauma symptoms, and toward the individual, as a whole person, and as part of a network of relationships that are strengthened as the basis for change (Tucci, 2016).

Trauma-transformative services embed two significant additional layers into their orientation. They have thought of, and committed themselves to, a theory of change that realistically supports how children, young people, and families affected by violence come to experience their lives differently. The service and its staff believe that the effects of trauma can be changed. They represent hope to service users and the community. They oppose broader community narratives that serve to trap those affected by the effects of trauma in identities that are shaming. Trauma-transformative services connect the community to the pain of violence and resource both understanding and compassion (Tucci, 2016).

Principles of therapeutic work with children and young people

The Australian Childhood Foundation (ACF) has a 30-year history of advocating for children's rights to protection, love, and care. The Foundation began providing child specific sexual assault therapeutic services in 1991, and now runs specialist therapeutic programs for children and young people who have experienced abuse and family violence nationally. Its aim is to be a child-serving and trauma-transformative organisation. Its practice framework has taken the knowledge base about trauma and attachment, and integrated it with beliefs about children's needs and how they can best be met by the communities of relationships which surround them. These principles are described below.

1 Respect for children's rights

Children and young people are entitled to have their needs for physical, emotional, and psychological care met by adults, and they have a right to be listened to and understood. They have a right to be safe from all forms of violation, including child abuse and family violence. The language used to describe children and young people should not disempower them, nor should it define their identity on the basis of the problems they cause or experience. Additionally, any language practices that label children and young people in ways that hold them responsible for their abuse should be actively resisted. Children and young people also have the right to access, know, practice, and value their cultural identity and heritage. They should also be entitled to opportunities to learn and develop positively, and meaningfully participate in decision-making processes which affect their lives. Intervention with children and young people should be sensitive to diversity of gender, sexuality, cognitive, and physical ability.

2 An understanding of the neurobiology of trauma and attachment is crucial

Trauma is a disintegrative experience for children, families, and communities (Siegel, 1999). Trauma reduces the capacity of children and young people to achieve complex adaptive self-regulatory states (Perry, 2002; Porges, 2011). In reaction to trauma, children and young people engage in initially adaptive responses to survive. If these responses continue, they can become maladaptive patterns of functioning. An understanding of the neurobiology of trauma and attachment disruption offers powerful and helpful explanations about the way that these experiences affect children and young people.

3 An appreciation of child development underpins all interventions

An appreciation of child development is critical to the recognition of the differential impact of trauma on children and young people. Children and young people who experience ongoing trauma frequently experience developmental delay across a range of areas, including cognitive, language, motor, and social skills. As a result, they may display complex clusters of behavioural, emotional, and relational difficulties, and they may often show a combination of appropriate developmental as well as developmentally inconsistent or inappropriate behaviours. Sensitivity to the developmental capacities and needs of children and young people is a respectful orientation to practices of assessment and intervention. Children and young people with disabilities require additional support to ensure that they are protected from abuse and supported to recover from traumatic experiences.

4 The experience of abuse sets the parameters for how the world is understood

Child abuse is the antithesis of attuned communication. Acts of abuse and violation negate children and young people's needs and rights. They communicate that the needs of the more powerful are a priority over the needs of children and young people. Violence establishes the parameters through which children and young people interpret other experiences. If children and young people's experiences of trauma have been through abusive interpersonal relationships, then they come to see people and the world in these abusive contexts. Conversely, respectful interpersonal relationships are the vehicle for transformation and change.

5 Healing for traumatised children and young people is embedded in their relational context

Children and young people rely on relationships to establish a sense of self, others, and their world. Families provide the platform for children and young people's development and their capacity to connect. Children and young people's understanding of their experiences is influenced by the beliefs and attitudes of their social network, including cultural and community discourses. The engagement of informal networks of support for a child or young person and his or her family greatly enhances the achievement of positive outcomes.

6 Children and young people's experience of their culture is a critical resource

Growing up "strong in culture" acts as a key protective factor for children and young people (Aboriginal Affairs Victoria, 2008; Aboriginal and Torres Strait Islander Healing Foundation, 2008, 2009, 2012). Cultural worldviews and ways of meaning-making in work with children, young people, and families should always be incorporated, and cultural knowledge about well-being and healing should be privileged and incorporated into Western understanding in meeting the needs of Aboriginal and Torres Strait Islander (ATSI) children, young people, and families. Attention should also be paid to the core ATSI values of interdependence, spiritual connectedness, links to land, group cohesion, and connection to community. This perspective can be achieved by adopting a position of informed curiosity about the cultural frames of references of others, and with the involvement of cultural knowledge brokers (ATSI Healing Foundation, 2008, 2009, 2012). Every effort should be made to ensure that caring references appropriate cultural norms, obligations, and responsibilities, and culturally strong parenting practices. Effective cross-cultural practice relies on reciprocal learning, facilitated by deep listening, and working in partnership with children, young people, and their families to design, develop, and test interventions that may be helpful (Morseu-Diop, 2013).

7 Supporting children and young people from Aboriginal and Torres Strait Islander backgrounds is vital

There should always be recognition and appreciation of the diversity of ATSI populations with respect to geography, language, culture, social, and economic circumstances (ATSI Healing Foundation, 2008, 2009, 2012). It is also important to recognise the history of colonisation of ATSI peoples, and the past and current practices of removal of children from their care. The consequences of these practices continue to resonate to the present time, and significantly affect the health and well-being of ATSI peoples across generations. Acknowledgment should also be given to the experiences of chronic sorrow and loss, cultural, community, and family disconnection, and dislocation, identity, and intergenerational trauma of many of the ATSI families in Australia. Self-determination and the empowerment of ATSI families and communities should always be overarching principles, as should working in partnership with families, community leaders, and community-controlled organisations to develop approaches to support, care, and build individual, family, and community values.

8 Collaboration within services and between services improves outcomes

There is a strong evidence base arguing for greater collaboration within services and between services to achieve best practice outcomes for vulnerable children, young people, and adults (Tucci and Mitchell, 2013, 2015a, 2015b). Collaboration is only the starting point for effective intervention for young people and families who have experienced trauma (Tucci and Mitchell, 2015c). The most effective responses occur when practitioners take responsibility to build sustainable coalitions of mutual respect with others, to ensure that the needs of children and young people are met consistently across the contexts in which they live, learn, and play.

Relational approaches are critical in the provision of services

The implementation of trauma-transformative services for children and young people requires a repositioning of how resources are focused. The ACF has come to use the phrase "therapeutic effort" to help describe the nature of how practitioners spend their time and energy to support healing outcomes for children and young people affected by trauma.

The starting point is to connect children and young people with the important adults in their network, so that relationships can be provided that care, educate, and support, relational safety being both a major goal of intervention and a major resource in the healing process (Tucci et al., in press). Relationships which heal are trustworthy and enduring; they stabilise and they help regulate. They also help interpret and re-interpret identity, and allow new meanings to emerge, based in the grounded visceral experience of comfort and love. Importantly, they brace and allow resistance to old neural activation and old habits to take hold, reinforcing children and young people gently, and allowing them to grow. They recruit phylogenetically new systems to connect and to stay connected (Porges, 2009), creating new memories of care and trust. They support the generation of narratives that make the world feel less dangerous, and help children feel more capable.

In the first instance, therapeutic effort is aimed at preparing the relevant adults in these relationships – parents, carers, extended family members, teachers, sport coaches, community members – to be open to tolerating the activated states of children and young people affected by trauma. This includes activities which support them to understand more about the impact of trauma on the neurodevelopment of children. It is, however, more importantly, the way in which these adults come to reflect on the meaning they hold about trauma and its consequences for children that takes the most effort, and has the potential to create the most change.

Therapeutic effort also involves integration of services provided, often by multiple professionals. This requires searching for and finding common ground, and a communal therapeutic purpose. This is frequently achieved when a shared understanding of children's behaviours and needs can be arrived at. Thereafter, the relational resources available to children and young people can be strengthened in the moment-to-moment interactions through which their traumatic experiences can be processed and integrated into their sense of self. The adults involved need to help validate children's past self-protective strategies, hold children's pain as they encounter the reverberations of their trauma, and offer responses that compassionately soothe and quieten children's activated neuro-physiological states of stress. Efforts need to be directed into facilitating comfort and safety that can be experienced through relationships in and around children in their daily lives. For this reason, the work needs to be undertaken in classrooms, in the homes of foster carers, in residential units with young people, and, sometimes, on the football oval or netball court.

The effort is worth making. As these relationships find their way closer and closer to the deeply embedded stories of hurt that children carry with them, they come to experience relief. Relationships stop being sources of terror, instead they become sources of care and hope. Children change. They begin to shed the habitual patterns of activation that have been defined by their trauma-based responses to the world, and their hearts open themselves to affection.

These connections are further deepened as they emerge. Adults and children are encouraged to find ways to match physiological states of safety. Opportunities for playful exchanges are facilitated which promote further collaboration between children and their important adults. This is followed by supported acts of turn-taking, and mutual acknowledgement of each other's responses. Each therapeutic moment ends with joint reflection that attempts to give reciprocal meaning to the relationship as it evolves.

Finally, efforts are made to work directly with children and young people therapeutically. Engagement is with symbols, and the form inherent in their play, and their connection to their therapists. Meaning is discovered and shared. Opportunities are explored to unearth the moments of opposition to trauma that children and young people may have experienced, who supported them, and the way they were helped. Pathways are discovered by which these almost inaudible whispers can be integrated into a strengthening communication between child and therapist, and child, network, and therapist.

Children's healing occurs in a milieu of relational transformation.

Service delivery description

The acceptance criteria for each of the programs delivered by the ACF vary according to the local context and needs of children and young people in a geographical area, and with the contractual obligations associated with service funders. An example of acceptance criteria for therapeutic services for children and young people affected by family violence include the child being 17 or younger, the presence of family violence, consent from a guardian for the child to receive counselling, active involvement of at least one responsible adult, and no involvement from other publicly funded counselling services.

The Foundation currently employs approximately 110 professionals with social work, psychology, and occupational therapy qualifications, often with substantial experience in their field. Services are delivered through small teams of five to six practitioners, working at a local level in community-based settings or on an outreach basis. Each team has a supervisor who provides regular fortnightly or monthly supervision. A number of programs are organised and managed under a senior program manager who oversees the quality of the work provided and supports the key relationships with partner agencies. The Foundation works in partnership with more than 40 other agencies nationally, many of whom are direct care providers. The services are currently delivered throughout metropolitan and regional Victoria, as well as in Western Australia, South Australia, Tasmania, the Australian Capital Territory, and the Northern Territory.

In general, the services are funded through a combination of state government contracts and the Foundation's own income-generating services. The most effective government contracts span five years. These allow for the appointment of therapists who are attracted to working flexibly and creatively. Job security is an important factor in recruitment of high calibre staff.

It is important to acknowledge that there are risks involved in working with some children and young people for whom the reality of abuse and violence is so significant that they require the involvement of statutory child protection services to keep them safe. This form of practice must put at its core the building and resourcing of a network of relationships around children as the vehicle through which healing occurs. It should involve both formal and informal decision-making processes between the people that relationally care for and protect children. The formation of care teams as a collective point of deliberation and planning supports a systemic focus with shared responsibilities.

It is also critical to appreciate in the establishment of these services that there is significant need to pay attention to embedding the service as partnerships in the networks of adults around children and young people. Services involved include schools, primary health, child protection, and various other government and non-government organisations. Partnerships with these organisations need to be made formal, using appropriate agreements and protocols. These documents and the process through which they come to be negotiated set the parameters for the way in which inevitable tensions in priority and approach can be negotiated on a continuing basis. Much like the care provided to children and their families, these relationships need qualities of compassion, understanding, joint purpose, and collaboration for them to be successful. The Foundation has learnt that the more time and energy is invested into making partnerships work, the more effective and sustainable the support that can be offered to children, young people and the important relationships around them.

Finally, these services require other processes that help move practitioners from seeing themselves as individuals working in a private practice to a more integrated collective that works from a similar practice framework with a shared set of values and principles. The internal support of staff for supervision, training, conference attendance, and other opportunities for reflective practice and growth, are all key ingredients in establishing and running complex therapeutic services for children.

Research and effectiveness data – ensuring the future

The Foundation has implemented an impact framework that captures critical data about the effectiveness of the services provided. It includes qualitative data that are used to describe the types and severity of trauma suffered, with the intensity of the intervention that is required. It also utilises basic psychometric data derived from a combination of the Behaviour Assessment System Checklist (BASC-3), Parent Relationship Questionnaire (BASC-3 PRQ), Trauma Symptom Checklist (TSCC), Trauma Symptom Checklist for Young Children (TSCYC), Strengths and Difficulties Questionnaire (SDQ), and others. It has been important to recognise that almost all these psychometric tools are limited in relation to the Aboriginal and Torres Strait Islander children and young people. As such, these tools are not used in practice with them.

In some of the programs, the preferred model of evaluating change is through the use of the Goal Attainment Scale (Mailloux et al., 2007). According to Arney and Brooke (2013), the use of the Goal Attainment Scale is a promising methodology for standardising an analysis of change in the functioning of children and their contexts (family and school) as a result of trauma-informed therapeutic intervention. It is of particular relevance to Aboriginal and Torres Strait Islander children and young people and their families. It operates on the basis of identifying changes in frequency and intensity of a specific behaviour over time, compared with the intensity and frequency of that behaviour prior to any intervention. The scale can be used for specific children and for specific behaviours. It can also include feedback from children and young people themselves, their families, and teachers. Because it is relevant to a specific child and their context, it does not compare children with a standardised norm which has inbuilt biases that are not appropriate for children and young people from Indigenous cultures. In addition, it averages ratings of change from different perspectives. As a result, it is able to provide a more comprehensive analysis of how change is translated across different relationship settings.

Evaluation and impact measures represent an opportunity for the Foundation to provide evidence about the ways in which traumatised children and young people can be supported in collaboration with their families and important network of adult relationships. This narrative of what children need to recover from the trauma they have experienced is significant in continuing to meet the broader objectives of the Foundation to create government and community agreement to continue to resource these types of services.

Conclusion

Healing starts when children are kept safe from further violation. It is sustained when the adults around children and young people are supported to be reflective and attuned to the needs of children and young people. These adults include parents or other caregivers, other friends and family, teachers, and therapists. These collective discussions are not psychoeducational in nature. Rather, they act to empower these adults to use their own lived experiences as physiological, metaphorical, and relational resources in their day-to-day interactions with their young. In so doing, these reflective moments help hold the systems around children and young people open and flexible, ensuring that the responses that they receive are transformative.

References

Aboriginal Affairs Victoria (2008) *Strong Culture, Strong Peoples, Strong Families: Towards a Safer Future for Indigenous Families and Communities*. Melbourne, Australia: Victorian Government.

Aboriginal and Torres Strait Islander Healing Foundation (2008) *Healing for Our Stolen Generations: Sharing Our Stories*. Canberra, Australia: Aboriginal and Torres Strait Islander Healing Foundation.

Aboriginal and Torres Strait Islander Healing Foundation (2009) *Voices from the Campfires: Establishing the Aboriginal and Torres Strait Islander Healing Foundation*. Canberra, Australia: Aboriginal and Torres Strait Islander Healing Foundation.

Aboriginal and Torres Strait Islander Healing Foundation (2012). *Our Healing, Our Stories*. Canberra, Australia: Aboriginal and Torres Strait Islander Healing Foundation.

Arney F and Brooke S (2013) *The Evaluation of the Holding Children Together Service in Alice Springs*. Darwin, Australia: Centre for Child Development and Education, Menzies School of Health Research.

Baylin J and Hughes DA (2017) *The Neurobiology of Attachment Focused Therapy*. New York, NY: Norton and Co.

Gunnar M and Quevedo K (2007) The neurobiology of stress and development. *Annual Review of Psychology* 58: 145–173.

Mailloux Z, May-Benson T, Summers C, et al. (2007). Goal attainment scaling as a measure of meaningful outcomes for children with sensory integration disorders. *American Journal of Occupational Therapy* 61: 254–259.

McEwen BS (2006) Protective and damaging effects of stress mediators: Central role of the brain. *Dialogues in Clinical Neuroscience* 8(4): 367–381.

Morseu-Diop N (2013) Indigenous yarning modalities: An insider's perspective on respectful engagement with Torres Strait Islander clients. In: Bennett B, Green S, Gilbert S, et al. (eds) *Our Voices: Aboriginal and Torres Strait Islander Social Work*. Melbourne, Australia: Palgrave MacMillan, pp.114–135.

Ogden P, Pain C, Minton K and Fisher J (2006) *Trauma and the Body: A Sensorimotor Approach to Psychotherapy*. New York, NY: Norton and Co.

Perry B (2002) *The Vortex of Violence: How Children Adapt and Survive in a Violent World*. Houston, TX: Child Trauma Academy.

Porges SW (2009) The polyvagal theory: New insights into adaptive reactions of the autonomic nervous system. *Cleveland Clinic Journal of Medicine* 76: 86–90.

Porges SW (2011) *The Polyvagal Theory: Neurophysiological Foundations of Emotions, Attachment, Communication, Self-regulation*. New York, NY: WW Norton and Co.

Schore AN (2001) The effects of early relational trauma on right brain development, affect regulation and infant mental health. *Infant Mental Health Journal* 22: 201–269.

Schore AN (2002) Dysregulation of the right brain: A fundamental mechanism of traumatic attachment and the psychopathogenesis of posttraumatic stress disorder. *Australian and New Zealand Journal of Psychiatry* 36: 9–30.

Schore AN (2003) Early relational trauma, disorganised attachment, and the development of a predisposition to violence. In: Solomon MF and Siegel DJ (eds) *Healing Trauma: Attachment, Mind, Body and Brain*. New York, NY: WW Norton and Co, pp.107–167.

Schore J and Schore AN (2008) Modern attachment theory: The central role of affect regulation in development and treatment. *Clinical Social Work Journal* 36: 9–20.

Siegel DJ (1999) *The Developing Mind*. New York, NY: Guilford Press.

Siegel DJ (2009) Emotion as integration: A possible answer to the question, "What is emotion?". In: Fosha D, Siegel DJ and Solomon M (eds) *The Healing Power of Emotions: Affective Neuroscience, Development and Clinical Practice*. New York, NY: WW Norton and Company, pp.145–172.

Substance Abuse and Mental Health Services Administration (2014) *SAMHSA's Concept of Trauma and Guidance for a Trauma-Informed Approach. HHS Publication No. (SMA) 14-4884*. Rockville, MD: Substance Abuse and Mental Health Services Administration.

Tucci J, Mitchell J and Goddard C (2010) *Doing Nothing Hurts Children: Community Attitudes About Child Abuse and Child Protection in Australia*. Melbourne, Australia: Australian Childhood Foundation and Child Abuse Prevention Research Australia.

Tucci J and Mitchell J (2013) *Collaboration is the key to practice in supporting traumatised children and their families*. Melbourne, Australia: Australian Childhood Foundation.

Tucci J and Mitchell J (2015a) The collective endeavour of interpreting neuroscience – A collection of Australian-based trauma-informed research and practice. *Children Australia* 40: 165–166.

Tucci J and Mitchell J (2015b) Consilience in Action: Lessons from an International Childhood Trauma Conference. *Children Australia* 40: 93–94.

Tucci J and Mitchell J (2015c) *Safe and Secure – A Trauma-informed Practice Guide for Understanding and Responding to Children and Young People Affected by Family Violence.* Melbourne, Australia: Australian Childhood Foundation.

Tucci J (2016) What comes after trauma-informed practice? *Prosody*. Available at: childhoodtrauma.org.au/2016/december/what-next.

Tucci J, Weller A and Mitchell J (in press) Realizing "deep" safety for children who have experienced abuse: Application of polyvagal theory in therapeutic work with traumatised children and young people. In: Porges S and Dana D (eds) *Clinical Applications of the Polyvagal Theory: The Emergence of Polyvagal-Informed Therapies*. New York, NY: WW Norton and Co.

Van der Kolk BA (2003a) The neurobiology of childhood trauma and abuse. *Child and Adolescent Psychiatric Clinics of North America* 12: 293–317.

Van der Kolk BA (2003b) Post-traumatic stress disorder and the nature of trauma. In: Solomon MF and Siegel DJ (eds) *Healing Trauma: Attachment, Mind, Body and Brain.* New York, NY: WW Norton and Co, pp.168–195.

25 Setting up a "whole of culture" trauma-informed care model in Australia

Matthew Spicer and Veronica Burton

Introduction

The Sanctuary Model, a "whole of culture" trauma-informed care model, originated in the Philadelphia area of the USA in the 1980s. It was developed by psychiatrist Sandra Bloom and her colleagues Joe Federaro and Ruth Ann Ryan. The origins of the model can be found in Dr Bloom's care of a young college student whom she referred to as "Dawn", who suffered with unexplained memory losses, chaotic relationships, sexual difficulties, anxiety, bouts of depression, and feelings of worthlessness. Dawn disclosed having grown up in a family where her father was physically and emotionally abusive towards both her mother and her brother, but she denied suffering any abuse herself. Dr Bloom treated Dawn with a form of "non-directive therapy" for several years, with Dawn taking the lead in sessions. Eventually, Dawn moved away to another city, where she found another therapist when her difficulties re-surfaced.

In 1985, Dr Bloom was contacted by Dawn's mother for help, as Dawn was using drugs and had become suicidal, and Dawn was admitted to Dr Bloom's psychiatric unit. Expecting to see an embarrassed version of the young woman she had seen so many times before, she was shocked to see a more childlike version of her, sitting cross-legged on the floor, with a tiny voice, and a mischievous grin. Over a period of a few weeks, Dr Bloom realised that Dawn was suffering from what is now known as Dissociative Identity Disorder. During conversations with Dawn's alter personality, "little Dawn", and with confirmation from Dawn's mother, Dr Bloom discovered that Dawn had indeed been a victim of sexual and emotional abuse at the hands of her father, although the adult Dawn had no conscious memory of this.

Dr Bloom reflected,

> I knew about child abuse from my work in the emergency room and pediatrics … but I never really thought about those same abused children grown up. Incest was certainly known to exist but was said to be exceedingly rare … . We rarely if ever asked people about their

> history of abuse assuming, perhaps, that any major traumatic experience would be volunteered willingly by the patient.
>
> (Bloom, 2013: pp.xiii–xiv)

Thinking about abused children as adults requires conscious recognition that abuse occurs, questioning individuals about a history of abuse whether they disclose it or not, understanding the impact of abuse experiences on the individual in the present, including an inability to recall events, and acting to assist victims to heal and recover. As Dr Bloom and her colleagues looked more deeply into trauma, they became convinced that abuse-related trauma was not the rare experience it was once thought to be, not simply an additional or a peripheral problem, rather it was the central problem for these patients, with profound impacts on a person's thoughts, feelings and behaviours.

Dr Bloom came to see that the neurotransmitter impairment model of psychiatry was inappropriately reductive, that the psychiatric facilities available to treat patients who had been traumatised were both unsuitable and ineffective and, in many cases, created further distress for patients as their expectations of help were met with rigid procedures and rules, and often disempowering, judgmental, and confusing systems. As a result, Dr Bloom and her colleagues considered alternative models that would provide treatment experiences in a place of safety that normalised behavioural responses to abnormal stress, that understood personal vulnerabilities, but that also held expectations and prosocial group norms that supported healing and recovery.

The Sanctuary Model

A recognition that adversity, trauma and chronic stress are widespread within the experience of people in communities forms the basis of the Sanctuary Model. The model acknowledges that the impact of such events is present, not only for those people who seek services, but also for the people and organisational systems that deliver those services. Furthermore, there is also a recognition of the inherent resilience of people, and an understanding that people can heal and recover from such experiences.

The Sanctuary Model provides a structured approach for creating a wholly trauma-informed culture, supporting both organisations and their staff to engage with each other and their clients in emotionally intelligent ways. The overall objective of the model is to provide an environment within which healing from traumatic experiences can be addressed (Esaki et al., 2013). One of the most important elements is a focus on the development of positive relationships with those who have been traumatised, with these relationships forming a foundation for the development of resilience. In partnership with Dr Bloom, the Sanctuary Institute in the USA has adapted the Sanctuary Model for use in several countries, including Australia, with more than 350 organisations delivering human service programs within foster care, residential treatment, schools, group homes, juvenile justice, and community-based settings.

Within Australia, the Sanctuary Model is provided via the Sanctuary Institute Australia at MacKillop Family Services. Formed in 1997, MacKillop traces its origins back 160 years to the Sisters of Mercy, the Christian Brothers, and the Sisters of St Joseph. Their work in Victoria established homes for orphaned, destitute or neglected children, and for mothers in need of care and support. With a workforce of more than 1200, MacKillop is now a leading provider of specialist and trauma-informed services for vulnerable children, young people, and families across Victoria, NSW, and Western Australia. MacKillop works to support vulnerable families to build skills for safe, strong, nurturing relationships with their children, to develop their full potential and to have a sense of belonging. In Australia, there are currently nine separate and independent organisations using the Sanctuary Model within foster care, therapeutic residential care, group homes, schools, and community-based settings. These organisations also constitute the Sanctuary Network within Australia and are part of the broader network internationally.

Key elements of the Sanctuary Model

Comprised of "four pillars", the Sanctuary Model provides a framework of trauma-informed practices. Importantly, the first pillar involves trauma theory. In helping to develop an understanding of trauma, the first pillar provides a platform for the provision of more empathic responses to a person's struggles, asking the fundamental question, "What has happened to this person", rather than trying to label, "What is wrong with them?". The second pillar involves the philosophy necessary for creating safe environments through community adherence to the "Seven Commitments" or values. The third pillar involves a trauma-informed problem-solving framework based on the categories Safety, Emotions, Loss, and Future, or "SELF", and the fourth pillar includes a set of practices within the Sanctuary "Tool Kit".

The "Seven Commitments" are the guiding values of the Sanctuary Model, and all members and clients of an organisation using the Sanctuary Model are supported to act in a manner that is congruent with the commitments. The first commitment, non-violence, encourages people to strive to behave in a manner that avoids or minimises words and actions that lead to violence and associated harm. Emotional intelligence involves learning how to recognise and manage the impact of emotions on one's self and on others. The social learning commitment requires an understanding that actions are always a model for one's self and for others. Open communication with others involves teaching healthy techniques by which both success and difficulty can be communicated, aiming to ensure that "unspeakable" issues do not develop, whilst also ensuring that difficult truths are shared openly with kindness. The ability for open communication within ourselves is also vitally important for improving internal understanding, because disconnection from feelings can significantly impair the ability to work with others via a healing relationship. The commitment of social responsibility aims to foster a sense of shared responsibility for values and practice and supports group connection. The commitment of democracy supports the requirement that all voices should be heard. Finally, a commitment to growth and change involves being open to ideas in support of life-long learning and holding hope that change can occur for recovery and healing.

The SELF framework provides a simple organising structure for treatment planning and support, and a problem-solving approach for organisational and individual issues. It also creates a shared language for all members of the therapeutic community to use, whether they are staff or clients with differing experience, areas of training, or practice. Safety is of paramount importance, and involves physical, emotional, moral, and social safety. Experiencing and managing emotions, working through loss and grief, and focusing on the future and healthy new behaviour make up the remainder of the SELF framework. The Sanctuary Institute in Australia implements the Sanctuary Model with an additional explicit focus on cultural safety. This recognises the importance of a practice that considers traditions, ceremony, and cultural connections to family and to country. It represents a deliberate response to diversity and the implications of historical and cultural trauma experienced by Aboriginal and Torres Strait Islander people in Australia since British colonisation.

The Sanctuary Model Tool Kit provides a set of strategies to support both individuals and organisations in becoming more effective in understanding the impact of trauma, adversity, and chronic stress, at managing strong emotions, in strengthening relationships, and in discussing and dealing with difficult situations. The Tool Kit includes community meetings, safety plans, self-care plans, SELF team meetings, SELF service planning, red flag meetings, Sanctuary core teams, and a range of other initiatives.

Community meetings are very important as they aim to immediately break down power hierarchies and engender openness and trust. They are utilised by staff, clients, or a combination of both. They involve a set of three questions as a means of connecting participants in an authentic and mindful way. The question, "How are you feeling today?" promotes the identification and expression of feelings in words, increasing emotional intelligence and alternatives to the violent expression of feelings. "What is your goal for today?" helps participants to focus on the future rather than the past and supports self-efficacy, thereby assisting growth and change. The final question, "Who can you ask for help?", promotes trust, a sense of connection with others, and use of the group as a resource, supporting social responsibility. Neural networks within the human brain change in a use-dependent manner in response to external stimuli, where repeated experience is required to underpin such change (Perry, 2006). Community meetings provide a powerful means of engaging in structured, frequently repeated, and adaptive behaviours that are aimed to counteract the impact of stressful and traumatic events upon individuals and the organisation. Clients are encouraged to engage in a community meeting twice daily. Clarke and Royes (2014) describe the association between the use of, and attachment to, the community meeting, and healing from trauma. For example, building trust with others can help people overcome the impact of poor attachment experiences. Similarly, identifying and naming feelings in a group setting can help to build the internal resources necessary to deal with past events and future adversity.

A vignette – use of community meetings in a residential program

In a residential program for young people, when community meetings were introduced, one young person participated willingly from the start, a second was curious and at first participated by observing and later joined in, and a third would not participate at all, but over a period of weeks began to observe, and finally participated in the process with staff. On one occasion, after assisting the young people to separate after a dispute, staff became concerned that the house had become unusually quiet. Upon investigation, they found the three young people, sitting together. One of them turned to the staff member and said, "Will you nick off, we're trying to have a community meeting to sort our stuff out!". Weeks of repeated modelling and practice resulted in the young people generalising the use of the tool and using it as a way of connecting. Social learning principles such as imitative learning can improve social behaviour, by observing others engaging in adaptive and prosocial behaviour (Liberman and LaVigna, 2016).

Safety plans are developed by the individual and provide strategies that assist them to avoid behaving in unsafe ways when they are overwhelmed by strong emotion. People are encouraged to carry their plans around with them and they can be shared with peers to harness their support. The process of developing the plan is empowering and enhances autonomy. The repeated use of safety plans assists people to develop a new repertoire of coping methods for stressful periods. Self-care plans address longer term well-being. SELF team meetings privilege democratic decision-making, use positive language to exercise the principle of non-violence, support participation of all staff regardless of their role, use the SELF framework to focus on the clients and the community, and discuss both problems and solutions.

"Red flag" meetings are a key feature of the Sanctuary Model, supporting organisational responses to important events or urgent community needs. The meetings provide an opportunity for clients and staff at all levels of the organisation to have equal power in that any individual can identify the need for, and request, a meeting. Red flag meetings recognise and harness both the wisdom and resources of the group. Upholding the commitment to open communication, they also serve to strengthen the community by relieving fears and reframing problems, from those of individuals to those of the team or group. Furthermore, they place the responsibility of working through the problem with the entire team.

A vignette – a "red flag" meeting

A young person living in foster care with their three siblings was growing concerned about the lack of planning and support for their mother who was soon to give birth again. Knowing that their mother could not care for the baby, and that the foster carer also had insufficient resources to do so, the young person grew increasingly concerned at the likely break-up of the family. The young person called a red flag meeting which led to the development of a case plan and the allocation of additional resources; the newborn was then placed with their siblings within the existing placement. The young person was empowered by a system that recognised and responded to their concerns and came to see themselves as both protector and unifier of the family.

The Sanctuary core team involves regular meetings of members who represent groups and programs within a Sanctuary organisation. The team focusses on implementation and monitoring of the model. The teams are particularly helpful in harnessing the wisdom inherent within a service. Direct service delivery staff are involved in all processes, and the incorporation of the suggestions of staff assists in lowering resistance to change.

Implementation of the Sanctuary Model

Implementation of the Sanctuary Model typically commences with an evaluation of service strengths and opportunities, followed by five days of training in the model for leaders and key staff within an organisation. This group then becomes responsible for the formation of a "core team" that will represent groups of employees and programs, with the aim of supporting implementation of the model. Within Australia, the core team receives ongoing telephone and face-to-face support from a Sanctuary Institute Australia consultant. In addition to the contracted support with the identified consultant, organisations can also access support from the Sanctuary Network as required.

Service providers have indicated that several factors are helpful in supporting implementation of the Sanctuary Model. These include a congruence between espoused organisational values and the seven commitments, the inclusion and support of senior operational and clinical leaders, including boards of management, an internal allocation of resources to specifically support and monitor implementation, regular review and evaluation of progress, implementation at all levels of service delivery areas, and, for some, across the entire organisation. Usefully, the model provides a framework and strategies that can be tailored to many settings and populations, with organisations and staff encouraged to be innovative in adapting them to their service context. Funding for implementation is typically sourced from an organisation's training budget, although some agencies make application to trusts or foundations for support.

A case study – implementation of the Sanctuary Model in an Australian school

In 2014, MacKillop transformed a small activity-based day program for young people disengaged from mainstream educational settings into a school. An initial needs assessment identified three notable challenges. First, staff were feeling under pressure, and demonstrated some resistance to the change of management, including a sense of loss as the new systems began to replace previous methods of operating. Second, there was a need for an adjustment to values held and attributions made about student behaviour. Discussions revealed two themes amongst staff, one where staff held a more positive regard to students and stated that, "Students do well if they can", and a second less helpful belief by some staff that, "Students 'chose' their behaviour, and that incidents of acting out were attempts at manipulation". Third, the concept of referring on a difficult student's issues to others would need to be replaced by an approach whereby staff who were part of any "problems" needed to be part of any solutions, with a focus on relationships as a key context for learning. These early adjustments saw some staff depart.

The Sanctuary Model's training in trauma theory was helpful for staff because it provided a new way to understand that young people impacted by trauma would relate and behave differently because of their experiences. For example, a common statement from young people was that they didn't feel heard or understood. Teachers wanting to be supportive often made what they thought were complimentary statements about the students such as, "You're smart, so you should be at school more". However, what young people reported hearing was, "You should be good at this, and you're not". They often worried they weren't good enough, and that they had let others or themselves down; their experiences had created a filter to how information was heard.

Further implementation of the Sanctuary Model required considering its implications for policy. One example included approaches to managing circumstances where students did not comply with school rules, and where there were issues related to discipline. A relevant change made was the development of a more flexible approach to managing difficulties based on understanding the meaning or function of a student's behaviour. For example, in dealing with young people who came late to school, staff might have previously sought to introduce sanctions, and advised the student to cut down their computer usage and to go to bed earlier. Understanding trauma theory assisted teachers to be curious about what was happening, and to recognise that sleep disturbance is common because of the impact of past experiences. Staying up late on computers, or computer gaming, may be a way to manage unpleasant feelings or symptoms related to what had happened to the students in the past. Understanding these facts helped lead to better problem-solving approaches being taken. Instead of focusing on breaches of rules and using sanctions, teachers sought to focus on improving relationships and connecting with students in the development of solutions. The importance of listening, understanding, and taking a collaborative approach to students on the part of teachers cannot be overstated. This particularly allows teachers to focus on the underlying issues and needs, and not on the presenting behaviour, and in this example led to much improved punctuality and compliance with rules on the part of the students as they learnt new coping skills and felt more connected to staff, school, and the program. Furthermore, the staff's ability to read student behaviour and needs increased, avoiding many escalations and potential incidents. Discussing these strategies with students was also helpful in raising their awareness of emotions, modelling coping abilities and, importantly, improving their ability to self-regulate.

Staff reported that several tools from the Sanctuary Tool Kit were particularly useful. Most notable were the trauma training delivered to all staff, the related psychoeducation curriculum, and the repeated use of community meetings. They reported initial resistance to the latter, describing concern at the idea of "airy-fairy sharing", a reference to the meetings being an impractical or a non-action-based task. It was perhaps also a reaction to the fear of discussing personal feelings in public. The logic for the use of these tools was presented to staff by asking the question, "How could the students self-regulate if they do not know where they were themselves?".

Persistence with the use of the Sanctuary Tools presented several benefits: improving personal skills involving emotions, creating safety using the SELF model to develop and practice a common language, with increasing trust amongst staff stemming from the repeated use of the strategies throughout each day, including the use of two community meetings. This increased the competency of both staff and students alike in their ability to discuss, identify, and manage strong feelings.

It is acknowledged that, when student outbursts are characterised by violence, it is difficult for other students and staff not to exhibit a typical "fight or flight" response. In the Sanctuary Model, the focus is not on avoiding emotions but acknowledging and managing them, and then selecting an effective way of supporting the student. The foundation for these abilities is the practised use of community meetings, the development and use of safety plans, reflective supervision, and self-care plans.

A vignette – a knife at the school

One young male student entered a classroom with a butter knife brought from home. The student was asked to leave the knife outside as other students may not have felt safe with a dangerous item brought into the room. The student struggled with the request and left the class, became angry, and banged against the classroom windows. The teacher thought that it would be unsafe for the student to re-enter the classroom at this point. Drawing on attachment and trauma theory, the teacher also thought that trying to enforce rules might re-enact difficult experiences from within the student's home, and that what the student needed was to connect with a safe person to regulate their emotions, not to face a repeat of the usual sense of rejection and worthlessness they had come to expect. Prepared with this knowledge, the teacher responded counter-intuitively – to the student's need, not to their presenting behaviour – by keeping the other students in class and leaving the room to attend to the student. To do so the teacher needed to enact their own safety plan to manage their emotions, remaining calm, not over-reacting, and risking further escalation and a potentially punitive response. By modelling how to be calm and attending to the student's need for security and connection, the teacher allowed the student to settle, and to return to class without shame or sanction. Such needs-based responding is shown to be effective in resolving behavioural crisis (Spicer and Crates, 2016) without reinforcing the behaviour of concern (Crates and Spicer, 2016).

Fluency in these skills and practices increased open communication and, over time, led to the development of an environment and culture that supported both students and staff. The information coupled with the routine, repeated, and predictable practice of the tools each day supported the development of a trauma-informed culture. Changes were often small and slow, but change accumulated over time. Throughout Sanctuary Model implementation, staff numbers increased from 10.5 full-time equivalent (FTE) positions in 2015, to 12.8 FTE positions in 2016 and 12.1 FTE positions in 2017, while student numbers increased from 46, to 58, to 57 over the same period. Related outcomes, such as total school behaviour incident data - for example, dangerous, disruptive, and violent behaviour - reduced from 51 in 2015, to 19 in 2016, and to only 10 in 2017. Perhaps more importantly, students also progressed with improved reading and mathematics scores on Australian Council for Educational Research (ACER) compass tests, and on measures of wellbeing. Furthermore, many graduating students also maintain an ongoing connection with the school.

Sanctuary Model effectiveness

Within Australia, organisations implementing the Sanctuary Model report anecdotally, or from internal reviews, improvements including greater staff satisfaction, improved staff retention, decreased numbers of client incidents, and improved client outcomes. These reports are consistent with the findings of several studies noting outcomes related to implementation of the Sanctuary Model. Elwyn et al. (2015) demonstrated an increase in safety for residents and staff within a secure juvenile facility for girls, and favourable comparisons of safety indicators with other services after implementation of the Sanctuary Model. However, given the many potential variables within an organisational change model, it can be difficult to determine exactly which factors brought about gains in safety, and to conclude a direct causal link with implementation. In earlier work, Rivard and others (2005) reported effectiveness of the implementation of a Sanctuary Model. Their application within a youth residential treatment service found that safety issues and scores indicating a therapeutic community environment were better when compared with non-implementation control units, and young people experiencing the model developed better coping skills. The model has also received a Scientific Rating of three, or "Promising Research Practice", by the California Evidence-Based Clearinghouse for Child Welfare (California Evidence-Based Clearinghouse for Child Welfare, 2011) and the model is currently recognised as the only organisational and clinical intervention to reach the standard of "Promising Practice" by the National Child Traumatic Stress Network (National Child Traumatic Stress Network, 2008). More research is necessary to determine how effective the model might be in various settings, and what are the most important variables.

Notwithstanding these limitations, and certainly of great value, is the acceptability of services under the Sanctuary Model. Stakeholder and service users of the MacKillop school report a range of benefits. The parents of one student reported, "The environment, the safety plans and the connections are predictable. Community meetings set up his day. We were struggling to keep him in school but now we see a future for him". One teacher said, "The Sanctuary Model supports building rapport which is fundamental to working with young people impacted by trauma", and another, "The environment is safe, supportive and nurturing; emotional development is as important as educational outcomes". The principal said, "The Model supports an environment where teaching is based on relationships that support a growing, living exploration with others". Finally, two students said, "It's better because I get supported, I don't get in trouble", and, "It's better because you're not getting distracted … I feel happy … I get my work done".

Conclusion

Given the importance of the work in supporting children, young people, and adults in recovering from experiences of trauma and adversity, the demands of such work, and the current socio-political climate within Australia, it is not surprising that interest in cultural change interventions such as the Sanctuary Model is increasing. As an organisational and cultural change intervention, the Sanctuary Model is intended to support the development and use of processes, staff and clients' actions and behaviours, and systemic operating procedures that lead to the development of a "whole of culture" community that aims to assist in the recovery from the effects of trauma and adversity. Many models address the treatment needs of individuals and groups impacted by trauma, adversity, and chronic stress. A unique strength of the Sanctuary Model is the extensive framework and guidance it provides for staff and managers in the delivery of services to their clients, and in creating safer, better-functioning workplaces and organisations. The literature base for the effectiveness of organisational and cultural interventions for the recovery from trauma is not yet complete. However, qualitative reports and implementation reviews indicate many likely benefits, including the views of clients experiencing services within the model.

The Sanctuary Model supports people by understanding the person and the impact of their past experiences of trauma, adversity, and chronic stress, delivering support consistent with a clear set of prosocial commitments conforming to a common framework, language, and set of tools. Staff commitment to, practice and implementation of the "four pillars" enables humane and compassionate behaviour that aids recovery and healing for individuals, whilst nurturing staff and supporting the organisations involved. The Sanctuary Model "comes to life" through the behaviour of those that implement it. Their development and the role modelling of emotionally intelligent behaviour are invariably taken forwards from the workplace into the homes and communities of those who benefit, improving resilience to the effects of trauma, adversity, and chronic stress, offering hope for increased community connection, and enriching society.

References

Bloom S (2013) *Creating Sanctuary: Toward the Evolution of Sane Societies, Revised Edition.* New York, NY: Routledge.

California Evidence-Based Clearinghouse for Child Welfare (2011) *Sanctuary Model.* Available at: cebc4cw.org/program/sanctuary-model/detailed.

Clarke A and Royes M (2014) The Sanctuary Model® and Community Meeting. *Therapeutic Communities: The International Journal of Therapeutic Communities* 35(4): 143–149.

Crates N and Spicer M (2016) Reactive strategies within a positive behavior support framework for reducing the episodic severity of aggression. *The International Journal of Positive Behavioral Support* 6(1): 24–34.

Elwyn L, Esaki N and Smith C (2015) Safety at a girls' secure juvenile justice facility. *Therapeutic Communities: The International Journal of Therapeutic Communities* 36(4): 209–218.

Esaki N, Benamati J, Yanosy S, et al. (2013) The Sanctuary Model®: Theoretical framework. *Families in Society: The Journal of Contemporary Social Work* 94(2): 87–95.

Liberman R and LaVigna G (2016) *New Directions in the Treatment of Aggressive Behavior for Persons with Mental and Developmental Disabilities, First Edition.* New York, NY: Nova Publishers.

National Child Traumatic Stress Network (2008) *Trauma-Informed Interventions. Sanctuary Model: General Information.* Available at: nctsnet.org/nctsn_assets/pdfs/promising_practices/Sanctuary_General.pdf.

Perry B (2006) Applying principles of neurodevelopment to clinical work with maltreated and traumatized children: The neurosequential model of therapeutics. In: Webb W (ed) *Working with Traumatized Youth in Child Welfare.* New York, NY: Guilford Press, pp.27–52.

Rivard J, Bloom S, McCorkle D, et al. (2005) Preliminary results of a study examining the implementation and effects of a trauma recovery framework for youths in residential treatment. *Therapeutic Community: The International Journal for Therapeutic and Supportive Organizations* 26(1): 83–96.

Spicer M and Crates N (2016) Non-aversive reactive strategies for reducing the episodic severity of aggression. *The International Journal of Positive Behavioral Support* 6(1): 35–51.

26 The trauma-informed inpatient facility

Ignatius Kim and Toni Ashmore

Introduction

Inpatient facilities are an important component of mental health care. They can be vital during a crisis, when an individual may become overwhelmed, and a place of safety, outside the home, with professional support, is needed. Such a refuge would be reasonably expected to focus on interpersonal safety, nurture meaningful collaboration between patients and clinicians, and deliver specialised therapies compassionately and professionally.

Currently, there are, however, very high levels of pressure on inpatient facilities, particularly those in public hospitals, generated by fundamental changes in psychiatric and mental health systems. The general shift away from inpatient care has resulted in concentrations of briefer, more acute admissions, with a reliance on biological and behaviourist interventions. Intrinsic to this is a paradox. On the one hand, inpatient facilities are environments of surveillance and control. Staff have the power to view people through the lens of both disease and risk, there is a clear hierarchy differentiating staff from patients, and forcible physical and pharmacological interventions occur frequently. On the other hand, people admitted to these facilities are at their most vulnerable, usually brought in urgently, many living with a legacy of trauma and its ongoing deleterious effects.

These people often report feeling unsafe when using inpatient facilities (Baker, 2000). Those with a history of interpersonal violence report feeling fearful, helpless, and distressed (Frueh et al., 2005). High rates of trauma are experienced during hospitalisation (Frueh et al., 2005), including sexual coercion and violence (Clarke, 2008). Past abuse heightens the risk of further abuse by leaving patients more vulnerable to boundary confusion and imbued with a sense of powerlessness (Reddy and Spaulding, 2010). Risk-focused practices involving people with trauma backgrounds may also heighten tension and increase the risk of harm in inpatient facilities.

A recognition of this paradox has led to the development of Trauma-informed Care (TIC) and Trauma-informed Care and Practice (TICP) in recent decades. This chapter privileges the latter term, to highlight the importance of actualising TIC consistently in daily practice throughout all levels of an organisation (Mental Health Coordinating Council, 2013). TICP adopts an empathic, curious stance that looks beyond immediate precipitants, presentations, and descriptive symptomatology. Trying to understand what has happened to a person, rather than what is "wrong" with a person, guides a search for the safest possible response to distress and crisis within an environment of physical and psychological safety. This involves an awareness that emotions of vulnerability such as fear, shame, and despair may be warded off by aggression and risky behaviour. On this basis, TICP works to avoid further harm.

TICP is relevant to all who experience trauma, but the approach is even more relevant with respect to those suffering with Complex Trauma, or Complex Post-Traumatic Stress Disorder (C-PTSD), because the symptoms of this condition may be severe yet still go unrecognised (Herman, 1992a). What defines Complex Trauma is its usual onset in childhood, within caregiving or other close relationships. The result is a syndrome of biopsychosocial ill-health, including psychiatric presentations and illness. The number of psychiatric symptoms and conditions associated with Complex Trauma is high, with even an association between childhood trauma and Psychosis (Varese et al., 2012), and between childhood sexual abuse and Psychotic Disorders (Cutajar et al., 2010). However, Complex Trauma remains neglected in health care (Adults Surviving Child Abuse, 2012). C-PTSD has only recently become an official diagnosis in the International Classification of Diseases 11th Revision, the ICD-11 (World Health Organization, 2018). It is still not recognised in the current, Fifth Edition of the Diagnostic and Statistical Manual of Mental Disorders, the DSM-5 (American Psychiatric Association, 2013), which is more widely used in Australia. As such, under the DSM-5, Complex Trauma alternately falls under a range of Personality, Dissociative, Psychotic, Mood, and Substance Abuse diagnoses, so that the link between trauma and presentation is often lost. This contrasts with the psychiatric sequelae of single-episode trauma which is formally recognised as Posttraumatic Stress Disorder by all government, non-government, and private agencies, entailing appropriate diagnosis and treatment.

Historical context

Understanding and treating the mind has always been prone to socio-political influences (Bromberg, 1975; Shorter, 2008), from the humanist era of William Tuke, Daniel Dafoe, and St Vincent de Paul, to the abuses of psychiatry in Nazi Germany and the Soviet Union. In late nineteenth-century Republican France, Pierre Janet however pioneered a trauma-informed approach to one psychiatric condition, then known as "Hysteria", at Paris's Salpêtrière Hospital. Sigmund Freud, a colleague of Janet's, extended this further by attributing the largely female disorder to childhood sexual abuse, before later recanting and retreating into his instinct-based psychoanalysis. This retreat was accompanied by the spreading influence of a "mechanistic behaviourism" in the age of Henry Ford and the assembly line (Meares, 2004); an influence that significantly impacted the field of psychiatry and mental health, leading to a diminished interest in the complexities of the mind and consciousness for many decades, particularly the relationship between trauma and mental and physical health.

Social upheaval in the 1960s saw a feminist rediscovery of Janet, the original Freud, the traumatised unconscious, and the emergence of a trauma-informed psychiatry (Herman, 1992b). This contributed to another wave of reform in inpatient psychiatric care – even while it was being phased out – leading to the introduction of therapeutic communities and multidisciplinary teams. Large residential institutions, hived off from wider society, had been the mainstay of treatment in Australia and internationally until reforms, bolstered by the pharmacological discoveries of the 1950s, gradually led to the "deinstitutionalisation" of long-stay patients and a new focus on community-based care (Fakhoury and Priebe, 2007). The Australian Government expanded community mental health centres in the 1970s as part of a larger investment in community health services (Henderson, 2008). A further impetus for deinstitutionalisation was the 1983 Richmond Report which exposed gross abuses in Australia's psychiatric institutions (Department of Health, NSW, 1983). This sweeping shift, however, proved inadequate for a population once accustomed to institutions that were like self-contained villages. Melbourne's Mayday Hills Hospital in the 1960s, for example, housed approximately 1000 residents. Today, the legacy of deinstitutionalisation has been the splintering of care across health, mental health, alcohol and other drug services, housing, disability, welfare, criminal justice, and correctional systems.

Focus on risk

The number of psychiatric beds in Australia continues to fall: in 1992–93, there were 45.5 beds per 100,000 people in public inpatient facilities in Australia; by 2014–15, this number had fallen to 29.2 (Australian Institute of Health and Welfare, 2016). In 1980, the average length of hospitalisation for a person with Schizophrenia in the Australian state of NSW was 134.5 days (Andrews et al., 1985). By 1998–99, this figure for acute public hospitals had fallen to 19.9 for those on involuntary orders and 16.6 for voluntary patients (Australian Institute of Health and Welfare, 2001). By 2014–15, the average length of an acute stay had fallen to 14 days (Australian Institute of Health and Welfare, 2016).

Faced with increased acuity, shorter admissions, and higher turnover, and in the context of under-resourced community services, mental health services have shifted the goal of treatment from symptom resolution to immediate risk management and stabilisation (Harris and Fallot, 2001). This new focus relies largely on biological and behaviourist interventions. In a study of 1035 articles dealing with the aetiology of mental illness in the *Australian and New Zealand Journal of Psychiatry*, Henderson (2008) found that the proportion based on a biological model went from 26 per cent in 1971–80 to 53 per cent in 1996–2000. This corresponds to an increasing use of pharmacological treatments worldwide (Ilyas and Moncrieff, 2012).

This bio-behaviourist model takes at face value the manifest behaviours of an individual; there is little regard for the "mind", the unconscious, or any underlying psychodynamic explanations. As such, the model is unable to explain the crises generated by trauma and Complex Trauma, leaving the vacuum to be filled by reactive, often coercive practices. The ensuing pattern is well-known in acute inpatient environments: crises amplify, leaving clinicians feeling less equipped to deal with situations, and often frightened, irritable, and distressed. Attempts to rapidly understand such events often spiral into a frustrated search for immediate answers, which can result in pejorative and often-times hostile conclusions being made about the patient and those clinicians seen to be more allied with them. Conflicts often erupt and escalate, while the patient's symptoms worsen, as iatrogenic elements compound the existing trauma. Such experiences impact on current and future acceptance of treatment (Reddy and Spaulding, 2010; Bloom, 2013). In this culture, a distressed person with a trauma history is often misdiagnosed, as behaviours conditioned by trauma arise in reaction to environmental stressors and present in ways that can be pathologised as psychiatric symptoms (Herman, 1992a; Harrison and Fowler, 2004; Lysaker and LaRocco, 2008).

A relational alternative

TICP aims to not just critique inpatient treatment, but to introduce a whole new perspective to mental health care. Since the 1980s, US psychiatrists such as Judith Herman and Bessel Van der Kolk have advocated for the inclusion of Complex Trauma in the Diagnostic and Statistical Manual. Reformers have also succeeded in reducing coercive interventions and reforming mental health laws across the world to better protect patient rights. For TICP to be truly effective in inpatient settings, however, it must be embedded throughout the organisation's daily culture, from that of its executive and senior management, through to its clinical and operational staff. Issues such as understanding the relational underpinnings of the background theory, the role of relationships in treatment and healing, issues surrounding enactments, workplace issues, power imbalances, the needs of individual clinicians and the therapeutic milieu, all need to be considered.

Working from a developmental perspective, TICP recognises that what makes people human is the drive to attach, to internalise those to whom a person attaches, and to transform those experiences into each unique individual's mind, self, and mode of relatedness (Stern, 1985). As such, relationship is seen to be the key in TICP, both the vehicle for treatment and the treatment itself. Any therapeutic intervention values the process of building "safe enough" relationships, as much as the content of the therapy. This includes an awareness that relationships can be influenced by the lived experience of trauma among both patients and clinicians. In this, the personhood and vulnerabilities of the clinician are also acknowledged.

Inpatient staff face particular challenges in managing relationships with those in their care. The inpatient setting has the natural 24-hour rhythm of residential living, much like a home. This lends itself to the unconscious enactments of family dynamics (the repetition of an unhealthy behaviour, derived from previous family experiences), among and between staff and patients (Bloom, 2013). Such enactments occur against a backdrop of past harmful practices and reverberations of trauma, leaving inpatient staff susceptible to emotional over-involvement. This may take the form of rigid, punitive attitudes, as well as the overstepping of professional boundaries. These actions constitute traumatic repetitions, not only for the patient, but also for the clinician. Such repetitions can stem from the chronic organisational stress prevalent in public mental health systems, often involving autocratic styles of leadership, conformism in team dynamics, and interpersonal stress between staff members. In short, this is a parallel process of acculturated organisational trauma, mirroring the experiences of the patients (Bloom and Farragher, 2013).

Trauma-informed systems of practice, supervision, training, and management offer safeguards against these challenges. TICP normalises the strong emotional reactions that staff may experience and recognises that vicarious or secondary trauma is a real possibility for staff, more so for those who have their own trauma history. TICP promotes the use of debriefing and reflective practice to continually address care for self and other. The ingraining of TICP further assists staff to better tolerate clinical uncertainty and complexity. TICP also promotes a non-judgemental inclusiveness towards different perspectives. This is important when a patient's fractured internal world manifests in "splits" of emotion, mood, and behaviour. Such patients often evoke contrasting responses in staff, from sympathy to indifference to hostility. A team that openly discusses these fractured responses can form a more integrated understanding of what is occurring clinically. The very process of engaging in this approach can offset the tensions, frustrations, and apathy that contribute to escalation of risk (Gabbard and Wilkinson, 1994).

This sort of cultural change also needs trauma-informed clinical and managerial leaders who recognise the interrelationship between the safety of clinician–patient relationships and the safety of the facility's management, resourcing, and organisational structure. As such, workplace conditions and issues of professional fatigue, conflict, under-resourcing, communication breakdown, inadequate training, and unclear roles are equally a focus for TICP (Bloom and Farragher, 2013).

Trauma-informed leaders address power imbalances between the various health professions, as well as between clinicians and patients. At present, many well-intentioned individuals feel impotent to challenge the potentially unsafe power relations in inpatient systems. In the face of serious incidents that erupt amid the cycle of crisis behaviours and custodial practices, these clinicians are caught in a difficult dilemma: how to safely give patients more control and decision-making. This is impossible at the individual level without systemic change and collective managerial commitment (Bloom and Farragher, 2010).

Trauma-informed leaders also approach deficits in individual practice in a supportive way. Nonetheless, they also protect, not only patients, but the team from the corrosive effects of any member persistently practising unsafely. This culture is strengthened by the practice of recruiting staff with the necessary professional and interpersonal values. Statements of duty should incorporate the need to be trained in TICP principles, and the need to adhere to these principles. Selection criteria and interviews should also test for trauma-informed traits and attitudes. This culture is reinforced by making TICP an important feature of continuing professional development and mandatory training.

Need for a therapeutic milieu

The scale and depth of organisational change needed for TICP also requires a renewal of the therapeutic community or therapeutic milieu. This was a concept and practice that reached its peak in the 1960s and 1970s, but which faded as inpatient treatment became more medicalised in the context of shorter, more acute admissions. However, some have advocated for the adaptation of the therapeutic milieu for shorter admissions as well (LeCuyer, 1992). Essentially, the therapeutic milieu considers all facets of an organisation to be of direct therapeutic relevance, including the attitudes of staff, the interactions between all individuals, the facility's programs and routines, and the physical environment. The therapeutic milieu, encompassing both patients and staff, has a whole-of-organisation and whole-of-admission perspective on inpatient recovery, rather than seeing treatment as particular, discrete events during an admission (such as medication administration, therapy session, or psychiatrist review). As such, not only does it encourage the active participation of patients in their treatment, the therapeutic milieu also facilitates a level of collective democracy, utilising methods such as community meetings and formal roles for patients. By the same token, staff members see themselves as facilitators of recovery, not only during specific "treatment interventions", but also by the manner in which they generally conduct themselves within the milieu.

The physical setting of the inpatient facility

The physical environment of any inpatient facility is critical. TICP cannot be properly and consistently implemented in small, poorly-designed wards, with insufficient beds and space, and where turnover is high. A refuge for acute crisis requires spacious buildings at ground level, with large common areas, high ceilings, abundant natural light, individual bedrooms, separate quiet areas, soft furnishings, greenery, and parklike grounds. The use of sound-absorbent materials, soothing colours, and artwork can also alleviate distress (Curtis et al., 2007). It is also important to note that risk-focused barriers, such as sealed-off nursing stations and staff-centred sightlines in floorplans, can paradoxically erode emotional and relational safety (Golembiewski, 2015).

An important safety feature is the segregation of women-only bedrooms and bathrooms, with policies and procedures on males entering these spaces. In some services, the use of a changeable ward design, whereby women-only sections can expand or contract depending on need, has reduced sexual assaults on vulnerable women (Ashmore, 2013). This model can also be applied to other vulnerable patient groups.

"Universal precautions" and safety planning

The principle of "universal precautions" in TICP is the presumption that every patient has been traumatised in some way, until proven otherwise. Similarly, there should be a working assumption that the facility will not necessarily feel safe for everyone. Each person should be routinely and sensitively screened for trauma. All disclosures – of historical abuse and of any that occur during hospitalisation – are voluntary and should be believed unless proven otherwise (Ashmore et al., 2015), and safely handled, with suitable staffing and training to continue therapeutic support during the admission (Substance Abuse and Mental Health Services Administration, 2005).

Trauma screening is recommended as soon as possible upon admission, as part of a general history-taking process (Read et al., 2007). The person's trauma history should then be incorporated into an individualised safety plan that is collaboratively completed. This plan details triggers for re-traumatisation, early signs of distress, safe coping methods, and supportive contact persons. Collaboratively completing a plan helps further break down power hierarchies and enhances trust, and the plan itself offers an opportunity to explore new coping methods available in the facility, such as resources for sensory modulation (Harris and Fallot, 2001).

Safety planning also includes meaningful activity scheduling, with the availability of an array of diversional and recreational activities. Boredom in restrictive settings can intensify the feeling of emptiness that afflicts people with a history of Complex Trauma. Distraction is a practical way of addressing the effects of trauma during an admission. Structured opportunities for socialising with others, such as ward meetings and group programs, can also be helpful. There should also be opportunities to participate in individual and/or group therapy to better understand the effects of trauma, to have experiences recognised and validated, to work through trauma-based interpersonal and emotional difficulties, and to learn new ways of coping.

Ideally, safety planning begins well before an admission. Recent reforms in mental health legislation in Victoria, the Australian Capital Territory, and Queensland have mandated the use of advance care statements. When people are well and have decision-making capacity, they can specify the nature of their care in the event of crisis and incapacity, including identifying what they find helpful and unhelpful. A trauma-informed advance care statement takes this an important step further by incorporating a person's trauma history and triggers, much like a safety plan. Mental health services can use this information to avoid re-traumatisation, as well as to identify and implement strategies to manage crises appropriately.

What is important with respect to advance statements, trauma screenings, and safety plans is not just the procedure or the document, but the safety of the relationships within which they are completed and implemented (Substance Abuse and Mental Health Services Administration, 2005). Patients need to feel safe enough to share their trauma histories with the treating team. It is essential that clinicians of all disciplines set aside protected time to actively listen to patients who, when in inpatient facilities, repeatedly complain that they are not listened to or heard. The art of deep listening and attunement, so fundamental to good patient care, has been lost in the shift to risk-focused, bio-behaviourist practices (Stickley and Freshwater, 2006). An increase in nurse–patient ratios, as well as a reform of the roles of nurses and nurse training, would help address this. Currently, the great majority of nursing time is devoted to non-care demands and routines (McAndrew et al., 2014), which is antithetical to safe, trauma-informed or indeed therapeutic care.

Sexual and cultural safety

Gender-sensitive practices are integral to TICP, not only with respect to women, but also those who identify as lesbian, gay, bisexual, transgender, intersex, and queer. The allocation of clinicians to a person's care should take into account any gender sensitivity stemming from their trauma history. Similarly, gender-specific therapy groups should be considered for all, especially those who have suffered sexual and other forms of gendered abuse.

Recovery is also culturally mediated. Inpatient services need to be trauma-informed in a wider, sociocultural sense, in relation to marginalised groups such as Indigenous people, refugees, other racial and ethnic minorities, and those with different ages, religions, and abilities, as well as those of diverse sexual orientation. It is particularly important to recognise the history of culturally traumatic practices by health agencies toward Aboriginal and Torres Strait Islander peoples and, as a result, their lack of confidence in mainstream services. This may impact on treatment adherence and inpatient stays. Wherever possible, TICP facilities should include designated Indigenous mental health workers and staff from differing cultural backgrounds, as well as easy access to the outdoors and cultural representations. Training in transcultural mental health should be provided to all staff, including an awareness of the sociocultural contexts for complex and intergenerational trauma.

Safe response to crisis

TICP guides clinicians to view crises as learning opportunities for themselves, rather than as threats or examples of personal failure. TICP aims to handle crises calmly and sensitively, by prioritising a listening and attuned presence. Importance is placed on avoiding power struggles, maintaining boundaries, defusing escalations, and exploring issues collaboratively. Nominated support persons should also be actively involved. The goal is to help people feel physically and emotionally safe, so that they may regain personal control. Staff should regularly workshop safe, trauma-informed communication strategies

(Isobel and Edwards, 2017), strengthened by ongoing attentiveness to reflective practice.

The use of de-escalation or sensory modulation suites is also gaining momentum in inpatient settings. These spaces help people maintain or regain control by reducing stressful stimuli and increasing those that are pleasurable, such as calming imagery, soothing music, weighted blankets, soft toys, and objects with pleasant scents or textures. Such spaces are useful for those who may be highly sensitive to noise, motion, or activity within the ward. Staff can support their use and reduce any fear of being alone by accompanying or remaining near the affected person. For people who are unable to verbalise their emotions or distress, the use of creative modalities such as art, music, and drama can also be therapeutic.

It is finally important to note that a common source of conflict and crisis in inpatient facilities are the "ward rules". These are frequently confusing, as they have usually evolved ad hoc on the basis of the needs of the staff and of the facility (Isobel, 2015), are not always well-known by patients, and do not make intuitive sense. In TICP, staff collaborate with patients to develop and periodically review rules that are clear and reasonable. They also allow room for appropriate negotiation rather than rote compliance, with a focus on the "spirit" rather than the "letter". Rules are explicitly communicated to the patient at the outset, both verbally and in writing, with an invitation to raise questions and concerns.

Ending seclusion and restraint

Although it is understood that, on occasion, physical restraint, involuntary medication, and seclusion may be necessary, TICP recognises that these practices are seriously harmful and traumatic. They should be used as an absolute last resort only, to prevent greater harm. Ultimately, TICP works to eliminate them altogether (Watson et al., 2014). Early interventions, such as meeting the patient's basic needs, trauma screening, safety plans, and advance statements, can meaningfully reduce the circumstances that engender a routine use of these harmful measures (Kontio et al., 2012). Considerable reductions have already been achieved. In 2008–09 Australia's rate of seclusions per 1000 bed days in public acute facilities was 15.6; by 2015–16 this was nearly halved to 8.1 (Australian Institute of Health and Welfare, 2016).

If absolutely necessary, injectable medications are administered in the ventrogluteal area of the hip, and vastus lateralis, or outer thigh, sites. Some can be administered in the deltoid, or upper arm, site. If the dorso-gluteal, or buttock, site is required, the person is held in the recovery position and with minimal bodily exposure. The prone position is always avoided because of the risk of asphyxiation and death. Methods of restraint do not use holds based on "pain compliance", which involve the intentional imminence of pain to control the person. A designated clinician continues to talk to the person with care and professionalism, including informing them of each step being taken. Whenever possible, males do not restrain females. If they do, they hold the less gender-sensitive parts of the body, such as the arms and lower legs, and in full view of the woman. Secluding a person should similarly be a measure of last resort, only to avoid greater imminent harm, and for the shortest duration necessary. Any person in seclusion should also continue to be offered the opportunity to therapeutically engage with staff (Kontio et al., 2012).

All forced interventions should be formally recorded and accounted to an external body, ideally chaired by a consumer representative (Watson et al., 2014). Staff and patients should also be given adequate time to debrief. Following an incident, the safety plan should be collaboratively revised with the patient. The enduring aim is to prevent the recurrence of such interventions.

A vignette – "Leah"

"Leah" was a 19-year-old woman with a diagnosis of Borderline Personality Disorder, in her second, prolonged admission. Both admissions occurred after serious suicide attempts. She was under indefinite, arm's-length observation, even during bathroom visits, despite which she continued to self-harm. Some of these incidents resulted in Leah being physically restrained, forcibly medicated, and locked in a seclusion room.

Following each incident, the supervising nurses variously experienced guilt, self-blame, and anger, along with recrimination from colleagues. Each nurse dreaded the prospect of a critical incident on their watch. The psychiatrists and managers were also reluctant to relax the arm's length supervision. At times, this highly charged situation spilled over into frustrated and accusatory discussions among staff about Leah's motives. Leah was a high achiever at school and university, but she said she often felt unable to meet her parents' high expectations. The treating team also felt unduly scrutinised by Leah's parents.

Eventually, the seemingly unending gridlock in treatment compelled the team to change direction and move towards a gradual reduction of supervision. A careful, stepwise plan of collectively taking and managing risk was developed in consultation with Leah and her parents. Intensive therapeutic sessions were conducted by a senior nurse, focused on deeply listening to and attuning to Leah's tumultuous internal world. Staff attended regular support sessions in small groups, to process the complex emotions and psychodynamics they had been involved in, as well as understand how the restriction of Leah's personal agency and privacy had exacerbated the situation. Leah was discharged within a few weeks to community care.

Conclusion

TICP can help maintain hope for recovery, even under very trying circumstances. In the face of difficult and challenging presentations, staff trained and supervised in TICP can use trauma-informed relational and emotional skills, as well as team support and systemic resources, to maintain their professionalism and compassion. In so doing, they can focus on a person's strengths while working collaboratively to resolve traumatic disturbances. The ever-present aim is to facilitate resilience and independence.

TICP requires a durable commitment at all levels of inpatient services. The extent and complexity of change in organisational culture, power relations, clinical philosophy, and professional practice necessitates fundamental reforms in how services are designed, managed, and staffed. Without such a comprehensive, strategic commitment, there is a risk that TICP will never be fully incorporated into inpatient care, and people like Leah will continue to be misunderstood and treated inappropriately.

References

Adults Surviving Child Abuse (2012) *Practice Guidelines for Treatment of Complex Trauma and Trauma Informed Care and Service Delivery*. Sydney, Australia: Adults Surviving Child Abuse.

American Psychiatric Association (2013) *Diagnostic and Statistical Manual of Mental Disorders, Fifth Edition*. Arlington, VA: American Psychiatric Publishing.

Andrews G, Hall W, Goldstein G, et al. (1985) The economic costs of schizophrenia: Implications for public policy. *Archives of General Psychiatry* 42(6): 537–543.

Ashmore TR (2013) *The Implementation of Trauma-informed Care in Acute Mental Health Inpatient Units: A Comparative Study. Unpublished Masters' Thesis*. Wellington, New Zealand: Massey University.

Ashmore T, Spangaro J and McNamara L (2015) "I was raped by Santa Claus": Responding to disclosures of sexual assault in mental health inpatient facilities. *International Journal of Mental Health Nursing* 24(2): 139–148.

Australian Institute of Health and Welfare (2001) *Mental Health Services in Australia 1998–99: National Minimum Data Sets – Mental Health Care*. Canberra, Australia: AIHW.

Australian Institute of Health and Welfare (2016) *Mental Health Services in Australia: Specialised Mental Health Care Facilities*. Available at: mhsa.aihw.gov.au/resources/facilities/.

Baker S (2000) *Environmentally Friendly? Patients' Views of Conditions on Psychiatric Wards*. London, UK: Mind.

Bloom SL (2013) *Creating Sanctuary: Toward the Evolution of Sane Societies*. New York, NY: Routledge.

Bloom SL and Farragher B (2010) *Destroying Sanctuary: The Crisis in Human Service Delivery Systems*. New York, NY: Oxford University Press.

Bloom SL and Farragher B (2013) *Restoring Sanctuary: A New Operating System for Trauma-informed Systems of Care*. New York, NY: Oxford University Press.

Bromberg W (1975) *From Shaman to Psychotherapist: A History of the Treatment of Mental Illness*. Chicago, IL: Henry Regnery Company.

Clarke H (2008) *Nowhere to be Safe: Women's Experiences of Mixed-sex Psychiatric Wards*. Melbourne, Australia: Victorian Women and Mental Health Network.

Curtis S, Gesler W, Fabian K, et al. (2007) Therapeutic landscapes in hospital design: A qualitative assessment by staff and service users of the design of a new mental health inpatient unit. *Environment and Planning C: Politics and Space* 25(4): 591–610.

Cutajar CM, Mullen PE, Ogloff JRP, et al. (2010) Schizophrenia and other psychotic disorders in a cohort of sexually abused children. *Archives of General Psychiatry* 67(11): 1114–1119.

Department of Health, New South Wales (1983) *Inquiry into Health Services for the Psychiatrically Ill and Developmentally Disabled*. Available at: nswmentalhealthcommission.com.au/sites/default/files/Inquriy%20into%20Health%20Services%20for%20the%20Psychiatrically%20Ill%20and%20Developmentally%20Disabled%20-%20Richmond%20Report%20-%201983.pdf.

Fakhoury W and Priebe S (2007) Deinstitutionalization and reinstitutionalization: Major changes in the provision of mental healthcare. *Psychiatry* 6(8): 313–316.

Frueh BC, Knapp RG, Cusack KJ, et al. (2005) Special section on seclusion and restraint: Patients' reports of traumatic or harmful experiences within the psychiatric setting. *Psychiatric Services* 56(9): 1123–1133.

Gabbard GO and Wilkinson SM (1994) *Management of Countertransference with Borderline Patients*. Washington, DC: American Psychiatric Publishing.

Golembiewski JA (2015) Mental health facility design: The case for person-centred care. *Australian and New Zealand Journal of Psychiatry* 49(3): 203–206.

Harris M and Fallot RD (2001) Trauma-informed inpatient services. In: Harris M and Fallot RD (eds) *Using Trauma Theory to Design Service Systems*. San Francisco, CA: Jossey-Bass, pp.33–45.

Harrison CL and Fowler D (2004) Negative symptoms, trauma, and autobiographical memory: An investigation of individuals recovering from psychosis. *The Journal of Nervous and Mental Disease* 192(11): 745–753.

Henderson J (2008) Biological psychiatry and changing ideas about "mental health prevention" in Australian psychiatry: Risk and individualism. *Health Sociology Review* 17 (1): 4–17.

Herman JL (1992a) Complex PTSD: A syndrome in survivors of prolonged and repeated trauma. *Journal of Traumatic Stress* 5(3): 377–391.

Herman JL (1992b) *Trauma and Recovery*. New York, NY: Basic Books.

Ilyas S and Moncrieff J (2012) Trends in prescriptions and costs of drugs for mental disorders in England, 1998–2010. *British Journal of Psychiatry* 200(5): 393–398.

Isobel S (2015) "Because that's the way it's always been done": Reviewing the nurse-initiated rules in a mental health unit as a step toward trauma-informed care. *Issues in Mental Health Nursing* 36(4): 272–278.

Isobel S and Edwards C (2017) Using trauma-informed care as a nursing model of care in an acute inpatient mental health unit: A practice development process. *International Journal of Mental Health Nursing* 26(1): 88–94.

Kontio R, Joffe G, Putkonen H, et al. (2012) Seclusion and restraint in psychiatry: Patients' experiences and practical suggestions on how to improve practices and use alternatives. *Perspectives in Psychiatric Care* 48(1): 16–24.

LeCuyer EA (1992) Milieu therapy for short stay units: A transformed practice theory. *Archives of Psychiatric Nursing* VI(2): 108–116.

Lysaker PH and LaRocco VA (2008) The prevalence and correlates of trauma-related symptoms in schizophrenia spectrum disorder. *Comprehensive Psychiatry* 49 (4): 330–334.

McAndrew S, Chambers M, Nolan F, et al. (2014) Measuring the evidence: Reviewing the literature of the measurement of therapeutic engagement in acute mental health inpatient wards. *International Journal of Mental Health Nursing* 23(3): 212–220.

Meares R (2004) From neurosis to trauma: Charting the currents in psychotherapeutic thinking from the nineteenth century on. *Meanjin* 63(4): 16–25.

Mental Health Coordinating Council (2013) *Trauma-Informed Care and Practice: Towards a Cultural Shift in Policy Reform Across Mental Health and Human Services in Australia, A*

National Strategic Direction, Position Paper and Recommendations of the National Trauma-Informed Care and Practice Advisory Working Group. Sydney, Australia: Mental Health Coordinating Council.

Read J, Hammersley P and Rudegeair T (2007) Why, when and how to ask about childhood abuse. *Advances in Psychiatric Treatment* 13(2): 101–110.

Reddy LF and Spaulding WD (2010) Understanding adverse experiences in the psychiatric institution: The importance of child abuse histories in iatrogenic trauma. *Psychological Services* 7(4): 242.

Shorter E (2008) History of psychiatry. *Current Opinion in Psychiatry* 21(6): 593–597.

Stern DN (1985) *The Interpersonal World of the Infant: A View from Psychoanalysis and Developmental Psychology*. New York, NY: Basic Books.

Stickley T and Freshwater D (2006) The art of listening in the therapeutic relationship: The role of the modern mental health nurse is becoming more technical when, argue Theodore Stickley and Dawn Freshwater, what would really benefit patients is the often misunderstood art of listening. *Mental Health Practice* 9(5): 12–18.

Substance Abuse and Mental Health Services Administration (2005) *Roadmap to Seclusion and Restraint Free Mental Health Services*. Available at: store.samhsa.gov/shin/content/SMA06–4055/SMA06–4055-A.pdf.

Varese F, Smeets F, Drukker M, et al. (2012) Childhood adversities increase the risk of psychosis: A meta-analysis of patient-control, prospective- and cross-sectional cohort studies. *Schizophrenia Bulletin* 38(4): 661–671.

Watson S, Thorburn K, Everett M, et al. (2014) Care without coercion – mental health rights, personal recovery and trauma-informed care. *Australian Journal of Social Issues* 49(4): 529–549.

World Health Organization (2018) *International Classification of Diseases, 11th Revision*. Available at: www.who.int/classifications/icd/en/.

27 Trauma-informed mental health care for Australian Defence Force personnel and veterans

John Cooper and Nicole Sadler

> This issue is bigger than us. It is a community issue … Australia must accept that when we ask ordinary people to do extraordinary things on our behalf we owe them a duty of care. But more than that, we owe them a debt of gratitude and compassion.
>
> Air Chief Marshal Mark Binskin, Chief of the Defence Force
> Order of Australia Oration, July 2015

Introduction

Military and veteran psychiatry have contributed significantly to the field of mental health over the past century. These contributions include descriptions of syndromes, additions to the prevailing systems of classification of psychiatric disorders, development of treatments, and more highly informed management of personnel. There is now a clearer and more consistent understanding of psychological trauma, its impact on mental health, and an expanding range of trauma-focused evidence-based treatments. More broadly, the treatment and service systems that interact with military personnel and veterans who have been psychologically traumatised have become trauma-informed and, as a result, more effective and better able to engage their stakeholders.

Background history

World War I produced many casualties presenting with physical symptoms, confusion, or amnesia without obvious physical injuries. There was much debate and uncertainty about the understanding of these symptoms. Some argued for a physical basis caused by explosions, whereas others interpreted these presentations as forms of cowardice or malingering. Myers used the term "shell shock" and concluded that these presentations were due to psychological trauma. He advocated for psychological treatments that included attempts to reintegrate traumatic memories (Howorth, 2000; Jones et al., 2007).

Combat stress reactions, battle fatigue, and combat or war neurosis were the ascendant constructs used to understand psychiatric casualties during World

War II. In addition to the direct impact of warfare, a greater understanding emerged of related factors, including duration of frontline deployment, unit cohesion, the meaning of the conflict, and news from home arriving by mail. Though this reflected a clear shift towards a stress-related and psychological understanding of the presenting mental health problems, the medical records of the time refer to psychiatric presentations attributed to defective personalities or characters. These derogatory formulations are perhaps more understandable when seen in light of Winston Churchill's views about the "charlatanry" of mental health practitioners, whose work he thought should be restricted as much as possible because of the immense harm they were capable of inflicting (Ellard, 2000).

Following the Vietnam War, American veterans presented for treatment with symptom clusters labelled "post-Vietnam syndrome" (Friedman, 1981) that had distinct similarities to civilians diagnosed with gross stress reactions and other trauma-related syndromes such as "Rape Trauma Syndrome" (Burgess and Holmstrom, 1974). This resulted in the major contribution from veteran psychiatry to the development and inclusion of Posttraumatic Stress Disorder, or PTSD, into the Third Edition of the Diagnostic and Statistical Manual of Mental Disorders, the DSM-III (American Psychiatric Association, 1980). The DSM-III reflected a paradigm shift in the way psychiatric disorders were diagnosed and classified by using operationalised criteria for improved rigour and reliability. Although the diagnostic criteria for PTSD have changed with each of the subsequent editions, the core features remain.

Modern warfare and psychological risk factors

Since the era of the Vietnam War, and particularly since the September 11, 2001, terrorist attacks in the USA, the nature of modern warfare has increased in complexity, impacted by various political, economic, climatic, technological, and cultural factors. Because of highly interconnected global relations and the increasing scarcity of natural resources, countries remain engaged in global and regional matters to maintain their own national security and prosperity. Over recent years there have been significant advances in the range and lethality of weaponry, and new technologies such as cyber warfare and unmanned aerial weaponry have emerged, providing methods for instigating attacks from remote locations. In addition, modern conflicts are often not between conventional militaries but rather between intra-state forces and non-state actors, such as insurgents, terrorists, and criminal networks. Involvement in this type of asymmetrical warfare results in the additional stress of trying to distinguish between combatants and civilians, and exposure to non-conventional tactics such as suicide attacks and improvised explosive devices. Conflict zones have also become increasingly urbanised, resulting in widespread devastation to vital infrastructure, and military personnel are often required to deal with humanitarian crises and large populations of displaced civilians. The decisions that are made and the actions that are taken by military commanders and personnel in these often dynamic, ambiguous, and ethically complex settings are then subject to intense public scrutiny through the 24-hour media cycle and social media. Threats to security are also increasingly occurring domestically. Terrorists have demonstrated their willingness to launch attacks anywhere in the world, with individuals or very small groups able to inflict mass casualties and devastation in non-combat zones (Australian Government Department of Defence, 2016a).

These factors have contributed to the emergence of new psychological risk factors for military personnel and challenges for the health care systems which support them. Similar to other Western countries, Australia's military has been in a period of "high operational tempo" since the late 1990s. The majority of Australian Defence Force (ADF) personnel have been deployed on at least one operation and around 40 per cent will have been deployed multiple times (McFarlane et al., 2011). By virtue of the nature of their training and work, personnel may be exposed to potentially traumatic events through war and war-like operations, peace-keeping and peace-monitoring missions, border protection, counter-terrorism and surveillance activities, disaster and humanitarian relief or support to national security tasks, as well as training accidents and other lifetime traumatic events experienced in either their personal or work lives.

Contemporary mental health issues for Australian Defence Force personnel

In this complex setting, understanding of the mental health problems faced by ADF personnel and veterans has improved. The 2010 ADF Mental Health Prevalence and Wellbeing Study (McFarlane et al., 2011) estimated that 22 per cent of the ADF will experience a mental disorder in a 12-month period, and just over half will experience a mental disorder in their lifetime. This lifetime rate of disorder, 54.1 per cent, is significantly higher than a matched Australian community sample at 49.3 per cent. The most common disorders in the ADF are Anxiety Disorders. Consistent with the community, PTSD is the most prevalent of these, and ADF males report significantly higher rates of PTSD at 8.3 per cent than a matched community sample at 5.2 per cent. This study also revealed that the incidence of Alcohol Disorders is significantly lower across both sexes in the ADF compared with the Australian community (McFarlane et al., 2011).

Though PTSD remains a core concept in understanding typical clinical presentations, there is a greater appreciation of the breadth of posttraumatic problems. For example, there is greater recognition of the cumulative effect of exposure to lifetime traumatic experiences, rather than a more restrictive focus on single incident or single deployment impacts. For some individuals there will be a progressive increase of symptoms with repeated trauma exposures, while those with sub-syndromal posttraumatic stress are at risk of delayed onset PTSD (McFarlane et al., 2011). Further, "moral injury" is an emerging construct in the posttraumatic mental health literature, whereby witnessing or experiencing an act that conflicts with or violates core moral values or deeply held beliefs leads to internal moral conflict (Drescher et al., 2011). It has been argued that this problem may be more prevalent in war zones where there may be greater exposure to experiences that cause crises of conscience. However, further work is required to clearly define the construct and how it may be related to PTSD, and to identify evidence-based treatment protocols. An international collaboration is currently underway to develop a moral injury outcome scale that will aim to operationalise the phenomenology of moral injury in ADF personnel and veterans. Similarly, the complex association between PTSD and mild Traumatic Brain Injury continues to be debated (Bryant, 2011).

The period of transition from full-time military service, and the impact of this on the health and wellbeing of military personnel and their families, is another growing field of international research (Sheilds et al., 2016; Van Hooff et al., 2017). A recent study of the health needs of ADF personnel during the first five years of transition from full-time military service highlighted the increasing rates of psychological morbidity as individuals leave. It was estimated that almost one in two transitioned personnel met the diagnostic criteria for a 12-month mental disorder, and more than half of these had at least one other mental disorder co-morbidly. Approximately one quarter were estimated to have met diagnostic criteria for PTSD in their lifetime, and just under one in five in the last 12 months (Van Hooff et al., 2017).

Another study comparing the number of deaths by suicide in full-time, reserve, and ex-serving ADF personnel between 2002 and 2014 revealed suicide rates were 53 per cent lower among full-time ADF and 46 per cent lower among reservists compared with the matched Australian population sample. However, the suicide rate in ex-serving ADF men was 13 per cent higher than men in the Australian community, with the greatest difference reflected in rates of suicide in young veterans aged 18 to 24 that were double the rate of the age-matched community group (Australian Institute of Health and Welfare, 2017). Increases in suicide rates in serving and ex-serving military populations is a significant issue for many countries, with devastating and enduring consequences for families, colleagues, and friends (National Mental Health Commission, 2017).

These studies of military personnel and veterans highlight that despite treatment advances there remains a significant minority with posttraumatic mental health problems that defy the best efforts to facilitate recovery. Research is increasingly targeting this group. Of equal importance, there is a growing recognition of the need to consider broad trauma-informed approaches to care, alongside specific trauma treatment.

Health care services for Australian Defence Force personnel

There are almost 60,000 current serving ADF members and around 5,000 are discharged from the ADF every year (Australian Government Department of Defence, 2016b). Both groups, ADF personnel and veterans, have access to mental health support and treatment that endeavours to be well informed about the nature of traumatic experiences, the common sequelae, and the best practice responses that are required.

Throughout their military career, full-time ADF members have access to a dedicated health care system, inclusive of health and mental health treatment, and occupational rehabilitation. Much like the situation in the Australian community, primary health care services are provided via a General Practitioner (GP) model of care, supported by a mixture of uniformed, civilian, and contracted mental health professionals. Mental health support is provided through a stepped care model, and individuals continue to be employed during their treatment and rehabilitation and given the opportunity to recover and return to their previous or new work within the ADF. If employment is not possible, the provision of health care and rehabilitation is transferred to the Department of Veterans' Affairs (DVA) or specialist providers.

Because of the relatively high levels of exposure to traumatic events, ADF personnel are also embedded in a broader work and support system that openly plans for and acknowledges this fact and facilitates early identification and pathways into care. This system also actively involves the protective factors associated with military service, including identity and sense of purpose, camaraderie, a clear command structure, and opportunities for mental health surveillance and targeted mental health awareness training (Australian Government Department of Defence, 2017).

The Department of Veterans' Affairs system of trauma-informed mental health care – from provider to purchaser

The Australian Government through the DVA is responsible for the health needs of veterans. The DVA service system has moved away from a provider model to a purchaser model, and there are both strengths and vulnerabilities associated with this model.

From World War II to the 1990s, the Australian Government maintained Repatriation Hospitals that provided comprehensive health services to veterans, similar to the current US Veterans Affairs system. Veterans with posttraumatic mental health problems could access a variety of hospital-based services including emergency departments, acute inpatient units, outpatient programs, drug and alcohol treatment, psycho-social rehabilitation, aged care services, and allied health treatments. From the early 1980s, this service system was complemented by a DVA-provided community-based counselling facility (the Vietnam Veterans Counselling Service, or VVCS). The name of this program was changed in 2007 to the Veterans and Veterans Families Counselling Service (also the VVCS).

Since the 1990s, there has been a progressive move away from DVA providing health services to DVA funding those services. Many of the functions of the Repatriation Hospitals are now provided by either private or state-based hospitals. Some of the functions are provided in the community by private psychiatrists, psychologists, and other allied health professionals. The VVCS is the only treatment service still directly provided by the DVA.

Despite the change to the new model, and relative to mental health services available to the general Australian community with posttraumatic mental health problems, the mental health service system for veterans has many strengths. From administrative policies and practices through to specialist clinical programs, the system has been developed through a "trauma-informed lens". The term "trauma-informed care" has been defined as

> A strengths-based framework that is grounded in an understanding of and responsiveness to the impact of trauma, that emphasises physical, psychological and emotional safety for both providers and survivors, and that creates opportunities for survivors to rebuild a sense of control and empowerment.
>
> (Hopper et al., 2010: p.82)

Although there is still some work to do, there has been a sustained effort to improve the mental health service system for veterans in Australia from the perspective of trauma-informed care, including the training of staff at multiple levels in this paradigm.

The strengths of the purchaser model are several: those needing assistance are "mainstreamed" to usual care, they also have access to a much more diverse group of providers than the ADF or DVA could directly provide, clinical services are provided by experts in the area, government is able to focus on its administrative strengths, and efficiencies are brought to bear. Importantly, there remains a comprehensive service system that can provide treatment responses to those in need. This change has also brought with it several challenges. These include the loss of veteran-specific clinical expertise, greater potential for disconnections and fragmentation of the service system, and the potential influence of commercial pressures on clinical practice.

Having outlined the potential advantages and disadvantages of the purchaser model, there has been little actual empirical research or evaluation that examines the effectiveness of the DVA mental health service system. It is therefore difficult to make informed comparisons with the non-veteran community-based mental health service system. Many relevant insights into the strengths and weaknesses of both the ADF and DVA health systems were obtained by the National Mental Health Commission (NMHC) that undertook a Review into the Suicide and Self-Harm Prevention Services available to current and former serving ADF members and their families (NHMC, 2017). The review noted the absence of "robust evaluative data". A range of negative veteran experiences were reported that reflected feelings of distrust and loss. However, the experiences and perspectives elicited were mixed, and the review noted the similarity with "many health services in the general community". Recommendations from the review included the need for better collaboration between the ADF and the DVA, ongoing work to improve the experience of transition from military to civilian life, more effective engagement with families, and the need to make the administration of compensation claims simpler and more efficient.

Opportunities for stepped trauma-informed care for veterans

The DVA explicitly endeavours to provide veterans with evidence-based treatment that is accessible, coordinated, and arising from thorough individualised assessments. Flowing from these principles is a service system that has the potential to be comprehensive, targeted, and delivered through a model of stepped care.

The intent of a stepped care service model is to provide interventions that are graded so that through assessment an individual's needs can be carefully matched to the most suitable treatment option (Bower and Gilbody, 2005). This enables resources to be targeted to where they are most needed. Within the Australian veterans' mental health service system, there are typically five levels of intervention available. These include: self-help, primary care, generalist mental health care, specialist mental health care, and case management of complex cases. It is apparent that most of these elements exist within the health systems in both the ADF and DVA. Anecdotal reports and more systematic examinations such as the above review conducted by the NMHC illuminate the areas within the existing model that can be improved. These areas include improving the visibility of services available to veterans, better care co-ordination, and systematic methods of evaluating the effectiveness of services.

Self-help strategies can be sufficient and stand-alone as well as underpin all other levels of care. Increasingly, web-based and mobile applications can be used that provide psychoeducational material, self-monitoring, and specific symptom management tools. When professional help is required, GPs are the entry point, and they are often the most readily accessible resource. Triage, assessment, referral, initiation of treatment, and integration of physical and mental health issues are some of the usual and relevant interventions for veterans.

Consequently, GPs will facilitate and coordinate referrals of veterans into the generalist and specialist mental health treatment domains. Private psychiatrists, allied health professionals, and the VVCS can provide evidence-based psychological and pharmacological treatments. This will usually be through episodes of care when specialist treatment is needed. Continuity of care is provided by the veteran's GP. The DVA also funds specialist mental health treatment programs for veterans. Since 1995, this has mainly been in the form of accredited PTSD treatment programs and trauma recovery programs. More recently, the DVA has approved a range of other mental health day programs to better meet the needs of veterans accessing private hospitals.

The following vignette demonstrates how the current service system can operate, acknowledging most of the levels of stepped care.

A vignette – "Jack"

Jack joined the Army aged 18, trained as an Infantry Rifleman, and later underwent Commando training. He had two deployments to Afghanistan in that role and served there for a total of 10 months. Following the first deployment he noticed increased difficulty with sleep, and his girlfriend commented that he was more "sensitive and jumpy". He wanted to re-deploy with his unit, so he said nothing of these issues to his commander or the medical officer during a routine medical check.

During both deployments Jack and his unit engaged with enemy combatants and came under enemy fire. He witnessed the aftermath of a suicide attack, and, during the second deployment, sustained a concussion after the vehicle he was in triggered an improvised explosive device.

After returning from leave following his second deployment, Jack found that he had lost interest in his work and training. He increased his alcohol consumption and he was criticised by his Commanding Officer on occasions for lateness and more frequent use of sick leave. Jack's sleep had deteriorated further, and he was experiencing nightmares most nights, usually reliving his exposure to the carnage after the suicide attack. His girlfriend left him saying she no longer felt safe around him, and that he was a changed person. At the age of 26, Jack decided to leave the Army, believing he was young enough to commence a second career as a fitness trainer.

Jack returned to his parents' home but made little progress with his vocational goals. He began to experiment with illicit drugs, specifically ecstasy and methamphetamine, he slept poorly, and often was unable to get up before lunchtime. He became socially isolated as his childhood friends were busy with study and work. At the insistence of his mother, Jack went to see the family doctor who had known him since childhood.

The doctor raised concerns that Jack had features of PTSD and Substance Abuse. He referred Jack to a private psychiatrist familiar with veterans, and also to the VVCS. Jack raised his concern about costs, as he had not applied for help from DVA, and he was still unemployed. The doctor reassured Jack that he had confirmed the diagnoses in his referral letter and that the DVA would cover the costs of all his treatment.

Jack telephoned the DVA and as he had served at least one day of full-time military service he was identified as eligible for a mental health treatment card which would provide him with access to services. The claims officer informed Jack of the processes within the DVA, both online and face-to-face, that he could access to clarify his ongoing entitlements. He was also given details of ex-service organisations who could provide support through welfare officers and advocates.

Jack accessed the VVCS where he received a thorough assessment and was offered individual counselling. He was also referred to an alcohol treatment group that was starting the following month. Jack's counsellor had trained in

Cognitive Processing Therapy (a trauma-focused psychological treatment) and offered him a block of 12 weekly sessions.

The psychiatrist Jack saw confirmed the GP's diagnoses, endorsed the treatment at the VVCS, and started Jack on antidepressant medication to help his PTSD symptoms. They also discussed the prospect of a future referral to a private hospital that ran DVA-funded trauma recovery programs for veterans.

Jack found the early stages of psychological treatment difficult, particularly writing out in detail and focusing on his traumatic memories. Though he began to feel less anxious and hypervigilant with the antidepressant, he developed sexual side-effects and the medication had to be changed. Six months later, Jack was seeing his counsellor every month to reinforce the treatment principles and to help keep him focused on his day-to-day functioning. Jack was tolerating the second antidepressant and the psychiatrist had discharged him back to the care of his GP. By this time Jack had also enrolled with a DVA-subsidised employment agency and had begun volunteering at the local gym as a fitness instructor. Most of his PTSD symptoms had remitted apart from physical anxiety reactions that were triggered by reminders of his traumatic experiences in Afghanistan, and he still refused to watch news reports on the television.

Challenges to trauma-informed health care for ADF and veteran populations

As the current model of mental health care operates, there are barriers to service utilisation and potential gaps that reduce the likelihood that military personnel and veterans will receive needed mental health care. Foremost, despite the comprehensive health system available to ADF personnel and veterans, and consistent with international research (Kulesza et al., 2015), there is a nexus between the identification of mental health conditions and help-seeking (McFarlane et al., 2011; Forbes et al., 2017). Various stigmas and barriers to care contribute to this under-utilisation of services within military populations, including cultural values of self-sufficiency, masculine identity, concerns they will be treated differently, and the requirement for good occupational health for operational deployments (Greene-Shortridge et al., 2007; Gibbs et al., 2011; McFarlane et al., 2011). The organisational balance between providing treatment and support and protecting career prospects is difficult to achieve. Even if military personnel do engage in treatment, an additional consideration is whether they experience evidence-based treatment and the degree to which they remain in care long enough to receive an effective intervention (Rosen et al., 2011; Forbes et al., 2017).

When veterans transition from military to civilian life, there are likely to be discontinuities between the respective service systems. There are different medical records, service providers, and often there will be geographical considerations as veterans return to their original homes and families. With the current model where DVA purchases treatment for veterans, discontinuities can also arise as treatment will be accessed "organically" and idiosyncratically according to referral practices, location, and veteran preference. Though it is always ideal and consistent with good practice, there is no obligatory communication or coordination between GPs and mental health clinicians, hospitals, or VVCS.

Moving from a provider model to a purchaser model for veterans may also mean that service delivery in either the public or the private health care systems is not prioritised or guaranteed, and that access to assessment and treatment may be delayed, or, in some circumstances, declined. The latter situation may occur when a private clinician chooses not to accept, or to limit, the number of DVA clients they will treat. This situation may be even more difficult in regional and remote areas where fewer clinicians are available.

It is finally important to note that the DVA determines the entitlements of each veteran who applies for both financial and health care support. This has the potential to create an adversarial context that can exacerbate the distress of veterans who may interpret the process as a negative reflection of their integrity and the value of their service to their country. The trauma training provided to all staff has assisted in this area. Other practices undertaken by the DVA to assist include supporting and sponsoring ex-service organisations to provide advocacy and welfare support to veterans and expediting a veteran's access to treatment by paying for treatment of a range of mental health conditions without requiring the veteran to prove the relationship of the condition to military service. Despite these efforts, it should be acknowledged that the potential for an adversarial process remains and is often experienced acutely by some veterans.

Conclusion

Military and veteran psychiatry have made many contributions to the field of posttraumatic mental health over the past century. There are multiple aspects to the experiences of military personnel and veterans that contribute to the complexity and severity of their mental health problems. These include the developments in modern warfare, the tensions between help-seeking and career progression, moral conflicts, major adjustments required when transitioning out of the military, and elements of the compensation and welfare provision for veterans.

The current system for providing mental health care to ADF personnel and to veterans has increasingly become a stepped care, trauma-informed approach, and in doing so provides an example for other mental health sectors. A stepped care approach to the provision of mental health care is generally seen as the preferred approach, as it provides for a fair matching of resources to need. The material presented in this chapter has demonstrated the strengths and weaknesses of the military and the veteran mental health systems and has highlighted that improvements can continue to be made in areas involving access to treatment, coordination, and evaluation.

References

American Psychiatric Association (1980) *Diagnostic and Statistical Manual of Mental Disorders, Third Edition.* Washington, DC: American Psychiatric Publishing.

Australian Government Department of Defence (2016a) *2016 Defence White Paper.* Canberra, Australia: Department of Defence.

Australian Government Department of Defence (2016b) *Defence Annual Report 2015–2016.* Canberra, Australia: Department of Defence.

Australian Government Department of Defence (2017) *Defence Mental Health and Well-being Strategy 2018–2023.* Canberrra, Australia: Department of Defence.

Australian Institute of Health and Welfare (2017) *Incidence of Suicide Among Serving and Ex-serving Australian Defence Force Personnel. Detailed Analysis 2001–2015.* Canberra, Australia: Australian Institute of Health and Welfare.

Bower P and Gilbody S (2005) Stepped care in psychological therapies: Access, effectiveness and efficiency. *British Journal of Psychiatry* 186: 11–17.

Bryant R (2011) Post-traumatic stress disorder vs traumatic brain injury. *Dialogues in Clinical Neuroscience* 13(3): 251–262.

Burgess AW and Holmstrom LL (1974) Rape trauma syndrome. *American Journal of Psychiatry* 131(9): 981–986.

Drescher KD, Foy DW, Kelly C, et al. (2011) An exploration of the viability and usefulness of the construct of moral injury in war veterans. *Traumatology* 17(1): 8–13.

Ellard J (2000) Principles of military psychiatry. *Australian Defence Force Health* 1: 81–84.

Forbes D, Van Hooff M, Lawrence-Wood E, et al. (2017) *Pathways to Care, Mental Health and Wellbeing Study.* Canberra, Australia: Department of Veterans' Affairs.

Friedman MJ (1981) Post-Vietnam syndrome: Recognition and management. *Psychosomatics* 22(11): 931–942.

Gibbs DA, Olmsted KLR, Brown JM, et al. (2011) Dynamics of stigma for alcohol and mental health treatment among army soldiers. *Military Psychology* 23(1): 36–51.

Greene-Shortridge TM, Britt TW and Castro CA (2007) The stigma of mental health problems in the military. *Military Medicine* 172(2): 157–161.

Hopper E, Bassuk E and Olivet J (2010) Shelter from the storm: Trauma-informed care in homelessness services settings. *The Open Health Services and Policy Journal* 3: 80–100.

Howorth PW (2000) The treatment of shell shock: Cognitive therapy before its time. *British Journal of Psychiatry Bulletin* 24(6): 225–227.

Jones E, Fear NT and Wessely S (2007) Shell shock and mild traumatic brain injury: A historical review. *American Journal of Psychiatry* 164: 1641–1645.

Kulesza M, Pedersen ER, Corrigan PW, et al. (2015) Help-seeking stigma and mental health treatment seeking among young adult veterans. *Military Behavioral Health* 3(4): 230–239.

McFarlane AC, Hodson SE, Van Hooff M, et al. (2011) *Mental Health in the Australian Defence Force: 2010 ADF Mental Health Prevalence and Wellbeing Study.* Full Report. Canberra, Australia: Department of Defence.

National Mental Health Commission (2017) *Review into the Suicide and Self-Harm Prevention Services Available to Current and Former Serving ADF Members and their Families. Final Report: Findings and Recommendations.* Sydney, Australia: National Mental Health Commission.

Rosen CS, Greenbaum MA, Fitt JE, et al. (2011) Stigma, help-seeking attitudes, and use of psychotherapy in veterans with diagnoses of post-traumatic stress disorder. *Journal of Mental and Nervous Disease* 199(11): 879–885.

Sheilds DM, Kuhl D, Lutz K, et al. (2016) *Mental Health and Well-being of Military Veterans During Military to Civilian Transition: Review and Analysis of the Recent Literature*. Canada: Canadian Institute for Military and Veteran Health Research and Scientific Authority, Veterans Affairs Canada.

Van Hooff M, Lawrence-Wood E, Hodson S, et al. (2017) *Mental Health Prevalence, Mental Health and Wellbeing Study*. Canberra, Australia: Department of Veterans' Affairs.

28 Developing a state-wide service for the treatment of patients with Borderline Personality Disorder

Sathya Rao and Josephine Beatson

Healing is a matter of time, but it is sometimes also a matter of opportunity.
Hippocrates, c.460 – c.370 BC

Introduction to Borderline Personality Disorder

Borderline Personality Disorder (BPD) is a serious and complex psychiatric illness. It is the most commonly diagnosed Personality Disorder, with a community prevalence rate of at least 1 per cent (Grant et al., 2008). BPD is particularly common in mental health settings. Its prevalence in psychiatric inpatient facilities is approximately 20 per cent (Zimmerman et al., 2005) and in community mental health settings approximately 11 per cent (Kass et al., 1985). It also commonly presents in primary care settings, with a prevalence rate that is fourfold greater than in the general community (Gross et al., 2002).

People with BPD have high rates of mortality and morbidity. When their illness is active, their lives tend to be both miserable and painful. They experience a pattern of mood instability that results in hyper-reactive and hyper-responsive emotionality. They may also show marked lack of impulse control, instability of identity, and have chaotic interpersonal relationships. Many people with BPD also fear abandonment in interpersonal relationships due to insecure patterns of attachment. This fear becomes particularly intense in the context of romantic relationships. Some experience a chronic sense of emptiness, "identity-less-ness" (Zanarini, 1998), severe self-loathing, and chronic hopelessness. Self-harm is the behavioural signature of BPD. About 85 per cent of people with BPD self-injure, 70 per cent attempt suicide in their life time, and up to 10 per cent complete suicide (Paris et al., 1987; Kullgren, 1988; Paris and Zweig-Frank, 2001).

BPD usually emerges during adolescence (Chanen et al., 2009). The National Health and Medical Research Council (NHMRC) Guideline (NHMRC, 2012) for management of BPD suggests that BPD can be diagnosed from as early as age 12. A recent report highlighted evidence that BPD symptoms also persist in people over 65 years of age (Beatson et al., 2016). BPD impacts both men and women with similar prevalence, although women are more often diagnosed with BPD in clinical settings (Grant et al., 2008).

Up to 85 per cent of people diagnosed with BPD report a history of trauma – physical, emotional, or sexual – or neglect during childhood, which suggests that trauma is one of several life experience factors that can play a role in the development of the illness. However, trauma does not appear to be a prerequisite for the development of BPD. Current expert opinion suggests that a complex interplay of psychological and biological factors (genetics, temperament, life experience, and the attachment patterns that develop from these) are involved in the aetiology of BPD. The relative importance of these factors, including childhood trauma when it has occurred, varies from person to person.

BPD is however strongly associated with insecure attachment to significant others (Agrawal et al., 2004). Insecure attachment underlies the fear of abandonment and contributes to the difficulties in interpersonal relationships for people with BPD. When parental figures repeatedly respond with rejection, hostility, indifference, or fear to the child's emotional needs and distress, the child develops an insecure pattern, or internal working model, of attachment (Ainsworth et al., 1978). This pattern is stored in the child's mind as typical of interactions with significant others, which then influences expectations of other interpersonal relationships in adult life.

Inevitably, this insecure attachment pattern will also affect treating clinicians. This often results in BPD patients encountering negative reactions and emotions in their interactions with the helping professions. Because of this, the importance of the nature and quality of the therapeutic relationship cannot be underestimated in the treatment of BPD. It is critical that clinicians are aware that these negative reactions and emotions in the treating clinician, usually referred to as the countertransference, are regarded as important sources of information about the patient's internal world, and therefore help to provide a deeper understanding. Clinicians may, for example, experience painful feelings that reflect what the patient has felt in early life. Clinicians may also experience, and display, negative, abusive, denigrating, and dismissive feelings that parental figures originally experienced in relation to the patient, and which have been internalised. Supervision for clinicians treating people with BPD is important to help them reflect on, and manage, what can be overwhelming emotional states, their own, and those of their patients.

In spite of the growth of research and knowledge about BPD that has occurred since it was included in the DSM-III in 1980, BPD remains a misunderstood disorder. It is also one of the most stigmatised disorders in psychiatry and mental health. As Gunderson famously stated, "BPD is to psychiatry what psychiatry is to medicine" (Gunderson, 2009: p.535). Research has found that many clinicians, including mental health clinicians, actively dislike treating people with BPD (Sansone and Sansone, 2013). This usually relates to the patient's use of maladaptive behaviours in an endeavour to soothe dysregulated emotions, and/or to negative countertransference responses on the part of clinicians. It is worth noting that negative attitudes among clinicians to people with BPD lessen with education that leads to increased understanding of both the disorder and ways of dealing with it (Knaak et al., 2015).

Evidence base for treatment of Borderline Personality Disorder

Therapeutic nihilism with respect to the treatment of BPD prevailed until the early 1990s. Change began with the publication of two papers, the first by Linehan et al. in 1991, the second by Stevenson and Meares in 1992. Linehan in the USA went on to develop Dialectical Behaviour Therapy (DBT), arguably the most well-known empirically supported treatment for BPD, whereas Stevenson and Meares recorded the positive outcome of treatment with the Conversational Model of Psychotherapy, a treatment originally from the UK that has been extensively developed and practised both there and in Australia.

Other empirically supported effective treatments that can result in remission and recovery from BPD followed, including Mentalization-Based Treatment (MBT), Transference-Focused Psychotherapy (TFP), and Gunderson's General Psychiatric Management.

DBT regards BPD as a result of dysfunction of the emotional regulating system, which has developed from a combination of biological factors (primarily inborn temperament) and an invalidating childhood environment (Linehan, 1993). The treatment focusses on the development of emotional regulation skills via a combination of individual and group psychotherapy. It is extensively supported by randomised controlled trials (RCTs), and may be particularly useful for patients with chronic self-harm and/or suicidality.

MBT was developed by Bateman and Fonagy (2004), following recognition that people with BPD lack the ability to reflect on their own mind and on the mind of others (that is, to mentalise) when the attachment system is aroused in stressful situations. They suggest that the phenomenology of BPD can be explained by this deficit. MBT aims at improving the capacity of patients to mentalise when stressed and has been found to be effective for BPD in RCTs when compared with treatments as usual.

TFP was developed by Kernberg's group in the USA (Yeomans et al., 2002). Psychodynamically-based, the therapy was developed to address the difficulties encountered by people with severe Personality Disorders, including BPD. TFP focusses on the internal relational world of the patient as it unfolds in the therapeutic relationship, and particularly addresses the disparate, or split, views of self and others.

It is beyond the scope of this chapter to discuss all other empirically supported treatments for BPD. Suffice to say that no specific treatment for BPD has been shown to be significantly superior to any other, nor were they found to be significantly superior to treatment employing those factors common to specific approaches, providing that treatment was both individualised and well structured. This important finding led to the development of an evidence-based guide to treatment for BPD that includes factors common to the specific treatments, which is applicable in general, rather than specialised, mental health settings (Bateman and Krawitz, 2013).

It is however now clear that many patients with BPD can achieve symptomatic remission when appropriate treatment is provided. Research has shown that rates of remission (defined as no longer meeting the DSM criteria for BPD) are significantly higher than those achieved with "treatment as usual" in patients receiving evidence-based treatments such as DBT or MBT after 12–18 months of treatment (McMain et al., 2009; Bateman and Fonagy, 2013). Treatments for BPD have also demonstrated effectiveness in terms of outcomes and cost. A recent systematic review by Meuldijk et al. (2017) demonstrated an average cost saving of $USD2987.82 per patient per year for BPD when evidence-based interventions were provided. However, as Bateman and Fonagy state,

> The view often expounded by protagonists of particular models of therapy that patients with severe personality disorder improve adequately after 12–18 months of treatment to the extent that they require no further support is fanciful, and remains a part of research mythology rather than realistic clinical practice.
>
> (2016: p.149)

In reality, a significant proportion of patients need to be in therapy for many years, and, even then, may continue to struggle in multiple areas of their lives, particularly when early trauma has been severe and prolonged, and perpetrated by caretakers.

Access to services for Borderline Personality Disorder

Despite its high prevalence, people experiencing BPD have limited access to evidence-based treatments. A generation of clinicians, including mental health clinicians, have not had access to adequate training in the treatment of BPD. The combination of competing demands for resources and inadequate workforce training contributes to the stigma, denial of treatment, and overall poor quality of care for BPD in most mental health settings. Limited resourcing means that the management of the most acutely mentally unwell patients (for example, those with acute psychosis) is prioritised, with the caveat that their illness can be managed using biological interventions. Since BPD treatments are psychotherapeutic in nature, it is even less likely that their care is prioritised. Furthermore, patients who present with repeated self-harming behaviour and erratic moods are at risk of being rejected by public and private service providers. Indeed, BPD pathology, which includes anger dyscontrol, self-loathing, and impaired interpersonal skills, further reduces the capacity of patients suffering with this illness to successfully access and negotiate appropriate care for themselves.

In Australia, it is also unfortunate that the government rebate for psychological services in the private sector is generally only provided for 10 sessions in any calendar year. Budgetary considerations have prevailed over consideration of the best interests of people with significant and disabling psychological conditions, including BPD, in this area. A sense of abandonment when the 10 session treatment ends can also be overwhelming for patients with BPD, and can lead to increased self-harm or suicidal behaviours. It is possible that this problem could be better managed by providing a particular focus for the 10 sessions, developing mindfulness skills, for example. This approach could serve to reduce anxieties around abandonment because the focus and structure of the treatment is established from the beginning. Some patients "dose" the sessions with the psychologist by attending on a monthly basis. These sessions can then serve as a relational "thread" when the patient is unsure of the ongoing commitment of other services to their treatment. Other patients establish an enduring relational thread with their General Practitioner (GP). Providing education about the factors common to effective treatments for BPD applicable in general practice settings and providing access to expert advice at times of crisis are areas where more could be done to assist GP's treating patients with BPD. It is however important to note that patients seen infrequently, less than weekly, with a condition of this severity, should not generally be expected to be able to meaningfully change or grow.

Australia, like most countries, also does not have a population-based approach for managing BPD. Unfortunately, the stigma, discrimination, and further traumatisation and dehumanisation of BPD patients is likely to persist in mental health settings unless urgent changes are made. The Tolkien II Report (Andrews and the Tolkien II Team, 2007) stated that only 15 per cent of BPD patients receive treatment, and this in a chaotic manner. The report suggested that ideal treatment would provide 30 per cent coverage, using a stepped care approach, from primary care to specialist care. This recommendation is lower than those espoused by the NHMRC guidelines for BPD published in 2012.

National Health and Medical Research Council Clinical Practice Guideline for the management of Borderline Personality Disorder

The NHMRC published clinical practice guidelines for the management of BPD in 2012. They provide a comprehensive, state of the art approach to the diagnosis and treatment of BPD. The NHMRC Guideline describes an ambitious vision, strongly advocating for organisation and provision of appropriate health care for people with BPD across health sectors and settings. However, no concerted and empirically validated efforts have been made to date to implement these recommendations in Australia.

This guideline recommends that most of an individual's treatment for BPD should be provided by community-based mental health services, across both public and private sectors. The guideline also recommends that, "Health professionals should consider referring people with severe and/or enduring BPD to a suitable specialised BPD service (where available) for assessment and ongoing care, if appropriate" (NHMRC, 2012: p.99). However, the expert committee determined that there was insufficient evidence to formulate evidence-based recommendations for the role of specialised BPD services.

In making consensus-based recommendations, the committee did agree to the following:

- For most people with BPD, effective treatment with a structured psychological therapy can be provided within mainstream public or private community-based mental health services, via individual appointments (with or without group sessions), by therapists with access to peer consultation and clinical review.
- Referral to a specialised BPD service is not routinely indicated for all people with BPD. People with complex care needs may however benefit from treatment within a specialised BPD service.

The NHMRC guidelines have also suggested the following roles for specialised BPD services:

- Treatment of people with complex care needs or those at high risk for suicide or significant self-harm.
- Providing consultation to primary care services and mental health services.
- Education, training, supervision and support for health professionals, including support for rural and remote services; education for local general mental health services; and consultation and advice for GPs managing BPD.
- Health promotion and advocacy, for example, raising awareness of BPD and reducing stigma related to BPD.
- Providing education and support for families and carers.
- Undertaking research to develop better treatment models.

Although state-based initiatives exist in Victoria and NSW, a unified national approach to understanding and addressing Personality Disorder is required. At present, two state-based initiatives, the recently introduced Project Air Strategy in NSW and the Spectrum Personality Disorders Service in Victoria, are available. The South Australian government has additionally announced its commitment to develop a BPD specialist service to deliver treatment to patients with severe and complex BPD.

Given the high prevalence of the disorder, it is appropriate that treatment for most BPD patients is provided by local mental health services. The role of state-wide specialist services such as Spectrum is to manage the most complex patients with BPD, as well as to teach, train, and support other mental health services in their provision of on-site BPD-appropriate treatment.

"Spectrum", a state-wide Personality Disorder service for Victoria

In the mid-1990s, the then Victorian Department of Human Services recognised the need for expert support to assist area mental health services in their responses to patients presenting with severe BPD.

This initiative led to the creation of Spectrum in 1999, a service set up to both directly provide services for those people suffering with severe Personality Disorders and to assist Victorian public mental health services to better understand and provide treatment for individuals with severe BPD. Spectrum receives a recurrent annual block funding of approximately $AUD3.5 million dollars from the state government for a catchment population of just over 6.3 million people. At the time that Spectrum was first established, there was considerable stigma around BPD, significantly more than exists currently. Patients were often either refused services (partly because BPD was not regarded as a mental illness but was, "just a personality disorder"), or they were admitted to psychiatric facilities for prolonged periods because of the fear of suicide.

Spectrum has since emerged as a clinical centre of excellence for BPD. Staff strive to apply best available evidence to improve treatment and recovery for people with the disorder. The primary focus of Spectrum's direct interventions involves those patients most at risk of serious self-harm or suicide, and those who have particularly complex clinical needs.

In response to rapidly expanding knowledge regarding BPD, Spectrum has undergone numerous changes in its model of care. The initial inpatient treatment unit was replaced by a community day program model. Currently, Spectrum provides treatment for individuals, consultation to other clinicians, and training. The psychotherapeutic treatment and support is provided in both individual and group settings, for those patients at greatest risk of suicide and/or the most complex presentations and comorbidities. Of necessity, these patients are a central focus of the service's work. Spectrum also has other important roles, including secondary consultation, and the provision of training and support to a wide range of clinicians, in public mental health settings, as well as to primary and private sector staff. Prior to Spectrum's establishment, clinicians were inadequately trained in the treatment of Personality Disorders and there was significant therapeutic nihilism. Spectrum now has an important role in the provision of training to approximately 1000 clinicians each year, and has done so for 15 years. Clinicians come from all sectors, public, private and primary care. This training is gradually changing the landscape for Personality Disorder diagnosis and treatment in Victoria.

The Spectrum team also consults with other public service sectors including Victorian Mental Health Services, Corrections, Justice System, and Community Mental Health support services. Work with consumer and carer groups across Victoria and the Australian BPD Foundation are other important aspects of the service, providing outreach to the wider community.

The current Spectrum model of care has the following components:

1 The BPD Clinic:

   a Dialectical Behaviour Therapy Clinic,
   b Mentalization-Based Treatment Clinic,

   c Wise Choices Program, an Acceptance and Commitment Therapy for BPD,
   d Psychoanalytic Clinic,

2 Complex Care Service,
3 Psychiatry Assessment Unit for primary and private sectors,
4 Secondary Consultation Program,
5 Consumer and Carer psycho-education and support groups,
6 Research and Evaluation unit.

The Complex Care Service (CCS) was developed to assist public mental health services with patients whose personality pathology raises serious and complex problems in treatment and management. Many of these patients have multiple mental health problems, high chronic suicide risk, and/or engage in life-threatening self-harm behaviours that have not responded to usual treatment interventions, with accelerating risk of death. Increased anxiety within treatment teams in the face of escalating risk with this patient group can also lead to conflicts between clinicians and management about the treatment approach.

The role of the CCS is three-fold: assessment of the problems faced by the public mental health service, recommendations to address them, and regular and ongoing meetings with the treatment team to assist with ongoing management, including the provision of sufficient space for reflection on the intense emotions that often arise in these situations. In many cases, a second clinician from the CCS provides individual psychotherapeutic treatment for the patient for about two years or until the difficulties are contained. The combination of individual psychotherapy and regular consultations with public mental health clinicians can be crucial both to the containment of difficult situations and the prevention of potentially adverse consequences.

Spectrum treatment principles – humanising the care of patients with Personality Disorders

The NHMRC guidelines state that,

> many people with BPD have experienced significant trauma, either in the past or in their daily lives … people living with and suffering from the experience of past trauma need health care that is sensitive to their complex needs and makes them feel safe while they resolve their trauma.
>
> (NHMRC, 2012: p.34)

Spectrum recognises that most of its patient population have experienced and may have ongoing trauma in their lives, and need to be cared for in a clinical setting that is safe, kind, compassionate, and validating. It is not uncommon for patients to have experienced re-traumatisation during their engagement with other health services due to stigma and discrimination. These patients need long-term care using a collaborative approach, with less reliance on the medical model of care and more attention to the therapeutic relationship. Spectrum has compiled a list of important treatment principles. These are as follows:

1 Right to treatment,
2 Active and ongoing collaboration with patients,
3 Therapeutic relationship is central to change,
4 Self-responsibility,
5 Developmental perspective,
6 Learning from experience,
7 Valuing different perspectives,
8 Empathy, validation and empowerment,
9 Long-term perspective,
10 Service co-ordination and collaboration,
11 Staff support and supervision.

The importance of the therapeutic relationship to the outcome for patients suffering with BPD cannot be overstated. A good therapeutic relationship starts with a clear frame and/or contract. The principle of collaboration is particularly important, with the need for both parties to work together; giving advice to patients with BPD can be fraught with difficulty, as it can repeat early abuse dynamics. Critically, the patient must experience the therapist as empathic, someone who deeply wants to understand their difficulties, focused on their mind and on their emotional states, rather than their behaviours. The patient must also experience the therapist as someone who validates their history and their difficulties in a non-judgemental manner. When misunderstandings or disjunctions occur, the therapist must always endeavour to repair the relationship. Limit-setting may also be required, but it is always important to bear in mind again the possibility of inadvertently repeating adverse earlier experiences when doing so.

Support and supervision for clinical staff

Spectrum employs approximately 30 clinical staff representing a range of mental health disciplines. Spectrum clinicians develop a high degree of self-awareness and are familiar with the transference and countertransference phenomena common in BPD. They are also aware of their own psychological reactions towards patients and of how the work can potentially impact on them. The work is demanding and requires a high level of emotional literacy and emotional intelligence.

Clinicians are encouraged to be aware of the psychological impact their work has on their functioning. Peers are alert for signs of emotional burn-out and "empathy fatigue" amongst their colleagues, and it is common for clinicians to point this out to one another. Clinicians are provided with time to reflect and process the impact of the work on their emotional health. They are also encouraged to practise self-compassion. The structures in place to prevent and manage vicarious trauma are wide-ranging, with most clinicians spending about four hours each week in activities including:

- Weekly clinical review meetings where clinicians discuss challenging patients,
- Treatment modality-specific supervision (DBT, MBT, and so on) for every clinician,
- Discipline-specific supervision for every clinician,
- Peer consultation groups,
- Informal peer to peer supervision,
- A "reflective space" to discuss complex clinical situations,
- Widespread practice of mindfulness – maintaining a here and now approach,
- A culture of taking a non-judgemental approach to patients and other clinicians.

Clinicians can also access extra training in specific therapies and approaches.

Importantly, Spectrum has a "no blame" culture that does not judge clinicians based on clinical outcomes. It holds the belief that every clinician is doing the best work they can with their patients. This helps clinicians to work with chronically suicidal individuals and tolerate risk without being excessively apprehensive about adverse clinical outcomes.

A vignette – "Natalie"

Natalie, a 23-year-old single woman, who had a diagnosis of BPD, was referred to Spectrum for secondary consultation. She was case managed by a local rural mental health service in Victoria. A secondary consultation by telephone was requested as there was concern about her escalating suicide risk. Natalie had been treated by the service since the age of 16. In the last two years, Natalie had become increasingly isolated. She had conflicts with family and friends, and stopped communicating with them. She lived alone and binged on alcohol. She inflicted deep lacerations to regulate her emotions. She had made three suicide attempts by overdosing on medications in the past two months, resulting in brief psychiatric admissions. She told her case manager Judy that she was "beyond hope". She had known Judy for five years, but more recently had not been attending appointments with her. She called Judy by phone and was angry at her; it was at that point that she asked to be discharged from case management.

Secondary consultation was provided by a Spectrum psychiatrist. The rural health service training psychiatry registrar, case manager, psychiatrist, and the inpatient unit nurse attended the teleconference. The consultation revealed that the case manager felt hopeless about Natalie's prognosis and was very fearful of her suicide risk. The possibility of hopelessness as a countertransference phenomenon – perhaps predominantly reflecting Natalie's innermost fears – was discussed. Natalie's request for discharge and her increased suicide risk were also discussed, and understood as a way that she might be managing her fear of rejection, part of her abandonment dynamic, the reasons for which emerged later.

In response, and because of the increased risk of suicide, it was suggested that Judy offer Natalie more frequent appointments in the short term, and Judy seek regular supervision and support from Spectrum to overcome her own feelings of hopelessness. Natalie's crisis management plan was also modified to accommodate more frequent and slightly longer admissions. In sessions with Judy, it eventually became evident that Natalie had become more suicidal in the last few months because her uncle who had sexually abused her as a child was back in town, and her family was hosting his visit. Natalie told Judy that her family did not believe that her uncle had sexually abused her, and she felt betrayed and invalidated. She also had a strong sense of rejection, and as a result had felt hopeless and suicidal. Judy's unconditional acceptance of Natalie's emotions and thoughts regarding her uncle's visit helped her to feel validated and to contain her suicidal thoughts.

Research and evaluation

The effectiveness of Spectrum's treatment program was reported by Hulbert and Thomas (2007). The 12-month outcome data demonstrated a reduction in self-harm acts, suicide attempts, and overall medical risk. There was also reduction in anxiety, hopelessness, and dissociation; improved quality of life; and increased subjective wellbeing. Though these gains were maintained for one year at follow-up, the quality of life of these patients remained below that of other Australian psychiatric samples (Hulbert and Thomas, 2007). It is likely that the Spectrum patient cohort tends to be more severely disturbed, as the expectations of the service brief is to treat the most complex patients. Another study demonstrated reduced need for psychoactive medications when BPD-appropriate treatment was provided (Broadbear et al., 2016).

Spectrum also continues to develop and adapt novel treatments that expand the range of alternatives it can offer to patients and to improve the "fit" between patient and treatment to optimise recovery. Spectrum is currently addressing one of the most pressing issues regarding the provision of treatment for BPD: the prohibitive cost of most psychotherapeutic BPD treatments due to their long-term nature and specialised clinician training. As a result, Spectrum is trialling a time-limited intensive group treatment program that, if early indications are borne out, may provide an efficacious and cost-effective intervention that can be readily adapted to other mental health services. Spectrum has also piloted a BPD-specific risk assessment training program for mental health practitioners (Rao et al., 2017), and this risk assessment method has been incorporated into the NHMRC clinical practice guidelines for management of BPD.

In keeping with its status as a centre of clinical excellence, Spectrum also engages in collaborative research with universities, other health care agencies, and experts in the Personality Disorder field, to explore a wide range of questions relevant to the understanding, treatment and recovery of BPD. Spectrum publishes books (Beatson et al., 2010), primary research, reviews (Beatson et al., 2016; Elsner et al., 2018), and opinion papers, thereby expanding the reach of the expertise that has been developed at Spectrum. Spectrum staff are also encouraged to present research findings at national and international scientific conferences.

Conclusion

Spectrum's experience has demonstrated that specialist BPD services help increase awareness of BPD amongst clinicians, upskill the workforce, and dispel the notion that BPD is untreatable. It has also served to improve the clinical outcomes for people with complex and or severe BPD. Spectrum advocates for the establishment of Specialist BPD services across the country. One dollar per citizen per year would be a start in the right direction toward establishing specialist BPD services in every state and territory of Australia.

References

Ainsworth M, Blehar M, Waters E, et al. (1978) *Patterns of Attachment.* Hillsdale, NJ: Erlbaum.

Agrawal H, Gunderson J, Holmes B, et al. (2004) Attachment studies with Borderline Patients: A review. *Harvard Review of Psychiatry* 12: 94–104.

Andrews G and the Tolkien II Team (2007) *A Needs-based, Costed Stepped-care Model for Mental Health Services.* Sydney, Australia: World Health Organisation Collaborating Centre for Classification in Mental Health.

Bateman A and Fonagy P (2004) *Mentalization-based Treatment for Personality Disorders: A Practical Guide.* Oxford, UK: Oxford University Press.

Bateman A and Fonagy P (2013). Impact of clinical severity on outcomes of Mentalisation-Based Treatment for Borderline Personality Disorder. *British Journal of Psychiatry* 203: 221–227.

Bateman A and Fonagy P (2016) *Mentalization-based Treatment for Personality Disorders: A Practical Guide, Second Edition.* Oxford, UK: Oxford University Press.

Bateman A and Krawitz R (2013) *Borderline Personality Disorder: An Evidence-based Guide for Generalist Mental Health Clinicians.* Oxford, UK: Oxford University Press.

Beatson J, Broadbear JH, Sivakumaran H, et al. (2016) Missed diagnosis: The emerging crisis with Borderline Personality Disorder in older people. *Australian and New Zealand Journal of Psychiatry* 50(12): 1139–1145.

Beatson J, Rao S and Watson C (2010) *Borderline Personality Disorder – Towards Effective Treatment.* Melbourne, Australia: Australian Postgraduate Medicine.

Broadbear JH, Nesci J, Thomas R, et al. (2016) Evaluation of changes in prescription medication use after a residential treatment program for Borderline Personality Disorder. *Australasian Psychiatry* 24(6): 583–588.

Chanen A, McCutcheon LK, Germano D, et al. (2009) The HYPE Clinic: An early intervention service for Borderline Personality Disorder. *Journal of Psychiatric Practice* 15 (3): 163–172.

Elsner D, Broadbear JH and Rao S (2018) What is the clinical significance of chronic emptiness in borderline personality disorder? *Australasian Psychiatry* 26(1): 88–91.

Grant BF, Chou SP, Goldstein RB, et al. (2008) Prevalence, correlates, disability, and comorbidity of DSM-IV borderline personality disorder: Results from the Wave 2 National Epidemiological Survey on alcohol and related conditions. *Journal of Clinical Psychiatry* 69(4): 533–545.

Gross R, Olfson M, Gameroff M, et al. (2002) Borderline personality disorder in primary care. *Archives of Internal Medicine* 162: 53–60.

Gunderson JG (2009) Borderline Personality Disorder: Ontogeny of a diagnosis. *American Journal of Psychiatry* 166: 530–539.

Hulbert C and Thomas R (2007) Public sector group treatment for severe personality disorder: A 12-month follow-up. *Australasian Psychiatry* 15(3): 226–231.

Kass F, Skodol AE, Charles E, et al. (1985) Scaled ratings of DSM-III personality disorders. *American Journal of Psychiatry* 142(5): 627–630.

Knaak S, Szeto A, Fitch K, et al., (2015) Stigma towards borderline personality disorder: Effectiveness and generalizability of an anti-stigma program for healthcare providers using a pre-post randomized design. *Borderline Personality Disorder And Emotional Regulation* 2: 9. Published online 2015 May 5 doi 10. 1186/s40479-015-0030-0.

Kullgren G (1988) Factors associated with completed suicide in borderline personality disorder. *Journal of Nervous and Mental Disorder* 176: 40–44.

Linehan M (1993) *Cognitive-Behavioral Treatment of Borderline Personality Disorder.* New York, NY: Guilford Press.

Linehan M, Armstrong H, Suarez A, et al. (1991) Cognitive-behavioural treatment for chronically parasuicidal borderline patients. *Archives of General Psychiatry* 48: 1062–1065.

McMain S, Links P, Guam W, et al. (2009) A randomized trial of Dialectical Behavior Therapy versus General Psychiatric Management for Borderline Personality Disorder. *American Journal of Psychiatry* 166: 1365–1374.

Meuldijk D, McCarthy A, Bourke ME, et al. (2017) The value of psychological treatment for Borderline Personality Disorder: Systematic review and cost-offset analysis of economic evaluations. *PLoS ONE* 12: e0171592.

National Health and Medical Research Council (2012) *Clinical Practice Guideline for the Management of Borderline Personality Disorder.* Melbourne, Australia: National Health and Medical Research Council.

Paris J, Brown R and Nowlis D (1987) Long-term follow-up of borderline patients in a general hospital. *Comprehensive Psychiatry* 28: 530–535.

Paris J and Zweig-Frank H (2001) A 27-year follow-up of patients with borderline personality disorder. *Comprehensive Psychiatry* 42: 482–487.

Rao S, Broadbear J, Thompson K, et al. (2017) Evaluation of a novel risk assessment method for self-harm associated with Borderline Personality Disorder. *Australasian Psychiatry* 25(5): 460–465.

Sansone A and Sansone L (2013) Responses of mental health clinicians to patients with borderline personality disorder. *Innovations in Clinical Neuroscience* 10: 39–43.

Stevenson J and Meares R (1992) An outcome study of psychotherapy for patients with borderline personality disorder. *American Journal of Psychiatry* 149: 358–362.

Yeomans F, Clarkin J and Kernberg O (2002) *A Primer of Transference-focused Psychotherapy for the Borderline Patient.* Northvale, NJ: Jason Aronson.

Zanarini MC, Frankenburg FR, DeLuca CJ, et al. (1988) The pain of being borderline: Dysphoric states specific to Borderline Personality Disorder. *Harvard Review of Psychiatry* 6(4): 201–207.

Zimmerman M, Rothschild L and Chelminski I (2005) The prevalence of DSM-IV personality disorders in psychiatric outpatients. *American Journal of Psychiatry* 162: 1911–1918.

29 Integrating trauma-informed care for Personality Disorders – The Project Air Strategy

Brin FS Grenyer

Introduction

Globally there are several challenges to the effective assessment and treatment of Personality Disorders, the most significant of which has been a lack of trauma-informed approaches to care. Patients, family members, carers and clinicians all report multiple sources of trauma, stress, and burden surrounding this group of conditions. Patients state that there are no sensitive models of recovery that include recognition of the "person within the illness". There is also a lack of understanding about the needs of individuals to grow, in both relationships and vocational outcomes that are personally meaningful, that goes beyond past history and symptoms (Ng et al., 2016). Carers feel excluded from participating in a patient's recovery, or report significant burden and stress in supporting a person with the condition (Bailey and Grenyer, 2014). Finally, clinicians report high sources of stress and conflict within the helping relationship, particularly if the clinician's workplace fails to provide collaborative and supportive models of care, including access to effective peer consultation (Bourke and Grenyer, 2013). All perspectives on the difficulties of providing and obtaining effective care for those with Personality Disorder need to be understood within a health care system that itself can sometimes present more challenges than solutions for this group.

It is also important to note that significant stigma and discrimination exist in health services against people with mental illness, but especially toward those with Personality Disorder (Grenyer et al., 2017). Estimates are that it takes at least 10 years for a person with a Personality Disorder to receive an accurate diagnosis, meaning they have many years of potentially iatrogenic harm from ineffective care not designed for their condition (Sulzer et al., 2016). There is widespread reluctance to diagnose the condition by health professionals and ongoing controversies about how to diagnose (Grenyer, 2018). Negative attitudes towards people with Personality Disorders reinforce stereotypes, and further entrench poor service delivery (Fanaian et al., 2013). Consumer and carer groups rightfully point out that a significant source of trauma comes from health services which fail to identify or treat the condition correctly, with subsequent years of poor functioning, loss of income, and failure to reach vocational goals (National Health and Medical Research Council, 2012).

Science is however transforming the understanding of Personality Disorder, in particular the category of Borderline Personality Disorder (BPD). There is now growing recognition of the underlying heritable precursors to this type of condition, including interpersonal hypersensitivity traits and underlying emotional dysregulation vulnerability (Gunderson, 2007; Amad et al., 2014). It is estimated that up to half of BPD vulnerability derives from such genetic factors (Amad et al., 2014), meaning that people with this condition are already more sensitised to experience ordinary interpersonal emotional events as traumatic. This has implications for models of early attachment and treatment (Leichsenring et al., 2011). People with BPD may also have co-morbid Posttraumatic Stress Disorder (PTSD), and it has been recognised since at least the 1970s that many people with BPD have significant histories of childhood neglect, abuse and trauma (Briere and Runtz, 1993). However, between 9 and 19 per cent of people with BPD report no history of overt trauma (Lewis and Grenyer, 2009), meaning that calls to re-name BPD a form of "Complex Trauma" may not be completely appropriate. It is also important to note that the majority of people who have suffered neglect, abuse and trauma do not have a Personality Disorder, and if a mental health condition is present it is more likely to be in the affective or anxious categories (Lewis and Grenyer, 2009). However, some types of trauma, including early attachment trauma, might not be recognised by either patient or clinician, and this might explain the genesis of some of those presenting with BPD.

It is also relevant to acknowledge that PTSD trauma-based treatments work in different ways from treatments for BPD (Grenyer, 2018). Treatments for PTSD primarily use exposure-based approaches focused on the desensitisation and reprocessing of the core trauma script or narrative, whereas BPD treatments seek to strengthen the sense of self, reduce emotional sensitivity and suffering, and improve interpersonal functioning (Lewis and Grenyer, 2009). An integrated approach is often necessary though, so that some trauma-based treatments can be used for some of the symptoms of patients presenting with BPD after the patient has achieved adequate self-esteem and trust to safely address trauma-related themes.

In response to the issues and challenges surrounding people who suffer with Personality Disorder, a new model of care, the Project Air Strategy, has been developed that aims to present an approach that is more compassionate and hopeful, and optimises access to research-informed psychologically-based treatments for patients and their carers (Project Air Strategy for Personality Disorders, 2011). The Project Air Strategy covers all Personality Disorders, and recognises that diagnosis is a current area of debate (Grenyer, 2018). The Project Air work spans mental health, drug and alcohol, justice, health, schools and young people, family and parenting support, workplaces and other community settings, where many different types of personality syndromes can be a focus of attention, including antisocial, narcissistic, dependent, depressive, masochistic, avoidant, obsessive-compulsive and paranoid. BPD is only one of the many Personality Disorders, however it is important as it has a high prevalence in mental health facilities and consequently a larger research evidence-base than many of the other Personality Disorders. It should also be recognised that some research suggests that the symptoms of BPD overlap with most other Personality Disorders, meaning it could be considered the "general" overarching disorder of which the others are specific features (Sharp et al., 2015). In addition, diagnostic methods have for many years recognised a "borderline personality organisation" (Lingiardi and McWilliams, 2017) that overarches many of the Personality Disorder subtypes, being on the "border-line" between neurosis and psychosis (Stern, 1938). This chapter provides an overview of some of the key strategies involved in this trauma-informed approach to the provision of effective treatment for Personality Disorders.

The Project Air Strategy

The Project Air Strategy seeks to improve the capacity of mainstream mental health services to manage and treat those with Personality Disorder, and to expand specialist treatment options, including improved referral pathways between generic and specialist services. This unique model uses a "whole of service" approach, with six key components: redesigning services; enhancing the quality of services; upgrading skills of mental health staff; connecting with families, carers and consumers; improving awareness and information; and evaluating outcomes. The six strategies and the 12 specific components are shown in Figure 29.1.

This model is operationalised through clinical guidelines which describe the pathway of a person through the health service, including assessment, diagnosis, formulation, and care planning, brief and longer-term therapies, the role of inpatient and community care, interaction with general practitioners, involvement of families and carers, and systemic issues for services (Project Air Strategy for Personality Disorders, 2015b). The implementation of the strategy requires a combination of leadership from senior management, training and support, clinical development within services by experienced staff, and the design of service models to enhance clinical pathways, using guidelines-based treatment to match patient need. Core to the strategy is the role of senior clinicians who coordinate the flow of people into both brief and more intensive treatments.

Also essential to the strategy is collaborative care planning to assist in the coordination and integration of services, including a core leadership role for mental health clinicians assisting physicians, public and private psychiatrists, community services, emergency departments, non-government agencies, community housing and other relevant services based on a collaborative assessment of needs. The approach uses clinical staging, including a stepped model of care (Grenyer, 2014). Brief interventions, and family and carer sessions and workshops (Grenyer et al., 2018a), complement more traditional individual and extended group therapies. The needs of the children of persons with a Personality Disorder are one example of how the model focusses on the broader social context of care through enhanced parenting interventions (McCarthy et al., 2016).

Project Air – individual treatment approach

Clinical guidelines and systematic reviews based on more than 33 randomised controlled trials support structured psychological therapy (psychodynamic or cognitive-behavioural) as the treatment of choice for BPD (Cristea et al., 2017). The National Health and Medical Research Council (2012) has also issued clinical guidelines for the treatment of BPD, with some core recommendations:

1. BPD is a legitimate diagnosis for healthcare services,
2. Structured psychological therapies should be provided,
3. Medicines should not be used as primary therapy,
4. Treatment should occur mostly in the community,
5. Adolescents should receive structured psychological therapies,
6. People should be offered a choice of psychological therapies,
7. Families and carers should be offered support,
8. Young people with emerging symptoms should be assessed for possible BPD.

Of the structured psychotherapies, there is evidence from the literature for several approaches, including cognitive-behavioural approaches, such as Dialectical Behaviour Therapy (DBT) and Schema Focused therapy (SFT), and psychodynamic approaches including Mentalization-Based Therapy (MBT),

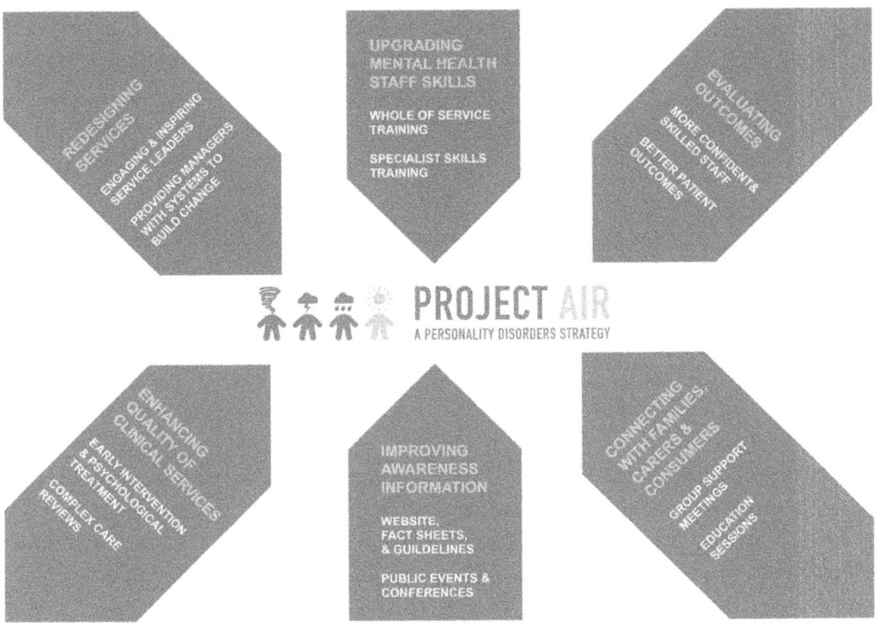

Figure 29.1. Six Project Air Strategies. Reproduced from Project Air Strategy for Personality Disorders (2015b). Treatment guidelines for Personality Disorders, with permission.

Transference-Focused Psychotherapy (TFP), Conversational Model therapy and Cognitive Analytic Therapy (CAT). Because there are little or no differences in efficacy between the different treatments evaluated (Cristea et al., 2017), clinical guidelines and researchers have proposed core components of therapy shared by all approaches as the essential ingredients of therapy. These include: a focus on the treatment relationship, an active therapist stance towards the patient, specific attention on affect, and the use of exploratory change-oriented interventions (Weinberg et al., 2011). The Project Air Strategy has synthesised the most important components into a set of key therapeutic attitudes and principles (Project Air Strategy for Personality Disorders, 2015b). The most important of these is to be compassionate. This means being able to see the world through the eyes of others, to understand their feelings, motives and behaviours – not to necessarily agree with their choices or behaviours – but to understand deeply and non-judgementally with empathy and respect. This requires the helper to be active, to listen intently to the person's current experience, and to note both verbal and non-verbal communications. Fostering trust allows strong emotions to be freely expressed, and attending to boundaries assists through being clear, consistent and reliable. Being human, it can also be appropriate to acknowledge both the serious and funny sides of life, remembering aspects of challenging behaviours have survival value given past experiences. The final key principle is to convey encouragement and hope about the person's capacity for change, while validating current emotional experience. The Project Air Strategy encourages all clinicians to uphold these core attitudes and principles, irrespective of whether the patients they are treating are engaged in long-term treatment or only have brief contact. Maintaining a focus on these shared values ensures a consistent and humane approach while minimising the potential for additional trauma being inflicted on patients receiving health-care.

Project Air – taking an active, planned approach that has patient engagement as a core principle

It is now known that an essential ingredient of the effective treatment for Personality Disorder is active engagement by both the patient and clinician in the tasks of psychotherapy (Bateman et al., 2015). By way of contrast, it has long been recognised that one of the most unhelpful approaches is unstructured, nondirective counselling. This is because the latter carries significant risks for the reinforcement of unhelpful past trauma narratives, and a lack of direction and structure may also lead to heightened regression and to more primitive forms of coping, including greater dependency, paranoia, and an increase in self-destructive behaviour. In contrast, many contemporary evidence-based approaches to clinical care use an active focus on current daily functioning, with specific and planned tasks between the patient and clinician to focus on understanding and changing core relational themes and patterns of behaviour (Grenyer, 2012). These tasks can include a focus on optimising a healthy mind in a healthy body by planning activities that bolster self-esteem, reduce sensitivity by titrating interactions that have toxic impacts, improving sleep cycles and healthy eating and exercise, and overcoming problematic relationship patterns by identifying better ways of fulfilling needs and wishes.

For the patient, this involves a recognition that sustained improvement in their life functioning can only occur if they take an active role in their rehabilitation. Lived experience stories by people recovering from Personality Disorder emphasise this "turning point" of moving from a passive ("things outside my control are to blame") to an active ("I can change my life by doing something for myself") attitude towards their difficulties. The example of Stephanie Leary demonstrates how daily effortful control can be utilised to maintain mental health (Leary, 2017). It should be acknowledged that this can take time to achieve and some people can find this difficult, even with the help of a trusting therapy relationship.

Being active can take many forms, including looking at how the diagnosis and symptoms are active within the patient's life; being curious to learn more about emotions and what they communicate; working with a clinician around setting goals that are specific, practical, and focused on the here-and-now; taking steps on a daily basis to change behaviours, thoughts, and assumptions to improve relationships with self and others; and ensuring ongoing engagement in life skills including working towards broader recovery goals (Ng et al., 2016).

Taking an active stance as a clinician can take a number of forms, including structuring the relationship and sessions to ensure there are clear goals focused on safety and trust; providing a place to think and feel difficult thoughts and emotions, knowing that these will be used to transform understanding; taking a curious stance within sessions focused on assisting the person to actively explore their appraisals of self and other; and putting in place practical strategies to ensure safety for the person (collaborative safety planning) and clinician (collaborative peer review sessions). These strategies go a long way towards humanising the care of people who meet the criteria for Personality Disorder and those that seek to help them on their journey.

The experience of new relationships within and outside of therapy fundamentally change internal working models of self and other, thereby modifying the patient's relationship to past trauma. These techniques also enhance skilful behaviours and positive coping approaches to conflict in the here-and-now. However, although the active engagement of the patient and clinician helps to ensure success, there are challenges. The relationship between the patient and clinician can also be conflictual and difficult to manage when intrusions occur, particularly of narcissistic, hostile or sexualised dimensions (Bourke and Grenyer, 2013). In addition, attention needs to be given to the clinician's own frame of mind and mental health, as the clinician's capacity to monitor internal thoughts and feelings can be clouded (mentalisation deficits) when confronted with very complex patients who may be dissociating, hostile or imposing unrealistic expectations in the treatment (Bourke and Grenyer, 2017). As a consequence, models of clinical supervision and consultation have been developed that focus in particular on relational complexities and competencies appropriate to the level of guidance needed (Calvert et al., 2016).

Project Air – focusing on improved access through stepped models of health care

Accessing clinical care for people with Personality Disorders remains a significant challenge (Grenyer et al., 2017), in part because of the high prevalence, and in part because of the scarcity of specialised treatment services (McCarthy et al., 2013). The population prevalence of Personality Disorder is estimated to be 6.5 per cent, with slightly higher estimates in men (6.83 per cent) compared with women (6.13 per cent) (Jackson and Burgess, 2000). Within mental health presentations to hospital, approximately 20.5% of emergency department and 26.6% of psychiatric inpatients have a primary diagnosis of Personality Disorder (Lewis et al., 2019). Despite their prevalence, clinical experience and information from health services show that there are significant challenges in accessing treatment (McCarthy et al., 2013). By way of example, data from the Project Air Strategy demonstrate gender biases in treatment allocation. Although the prevalence of Personality Disorder is equal between men and women at presentation to hospital, men are then underrepresented in referrals to a Personality Disorder service (30 per cent are men). Once places in specialist long term evidence-based treatment are considered, the proportion changes even further; only 15 per cent are men (Grenyer, 2014). Indeed, many treatment outcome trials have specifically excluded males from their trials in the first place, reinforcing such gender biases (Linehan et al., 1991).

Unfortunately, it is also important to note that "treatment as usual" often only involves the provision of crisis management services, that may include short-term admission for safety and de-escalation of distress. Longer-term service involvement has traditionally been regarded as counterproductive because of the possibility of potential reinforcement of helplessness and escalation of help-seeking behaviour through actions, for example, of increased self-harm. Frequent short admissions however often lead to an increasingly stigmatised response from mental health services and unconscious negative counter-transference responses from health professionals (Grenyer, 2014).

A report on mental health intake and emergency department data from a hospital system servicing a population of approximately 250,000 people demonstrated that about 16,250 people are estimated to have a diagnosable Personality Disorder (Grenyer, 2014). Of the 6,338 inpatients who presented at a given time within a four-year period, 1,584 people presented with difficulties associated with a Personality Disorder. This represents about 360 people per year, or one person per day. However, most specialist services in a catchment of this size operate only one or two programs per year, accepting only eight to 20 patients (McCarthy et al., 2013). Clearly, there is a need to provide better access for all 360 people with Personality Disorder presenting for help.

Project Air's stepped model describes clinical services using brief manualised interventions that specifically intervene when people present to services in crisis, thus creating an opportunity to divert patients from inpatient and emergency departments to rapid follow-up psychological care that services larger numbers of people (Wilhelm et al., 2007). The manualised brief intervention approach (Project Air Strategy for Personality Disorders, 2015a) also includes an opportunity to connect with family and partners, to provide psychoeducation, to reduce burden and increase positive models of coping in the family (Bailey and Grenyer, 2014). Providing easier access, greater capacity, rapid models of care, and further triage to community services has shown significant reductions in hospital and other health care costs (Grenyer et al., 2018b), but more importantly has gone some way to reduce the iatrogenic harm that can result from non-provision of a service (Grenyer, 2013). Indeed, a systematic review of all cost-benefit studies shows that providing evidence-based psychological care for those with Personality Disorder results in a saving of on average $USD 2,987 per patient per year (approximately $AUD 4,000), and providing psychotherapy is less expensive and more effective than inpatient treatment, irrespective of the differing funding arrangements between countries and jurisdictions (Meuldijk et al., 2017).

Project Air – taking a broader, whole of system family and community approach to care

The field also needs to move beyond an exclusive focus on the individual's intrapsychic difficulties, to an interpersonal focus, that includes health professionals, families, educators, employers and communities, within a broader recovery framework. Because, at their core, Personality Disorders are disorders of relationships (Grenyer, 2013), the Project Air Strategy has adopted a relational model to address this interpersonal need (Project Air Strategy for Personality Disorders, 2011), with particular focus on three key relationships: patient to self, patient to clinician, and patient to family and community. At present, all evidence-based treatments work to target the first relationship component (patient to self), some incorporate strategies to assist with the second (patient to clinician), but few address the third component including the broader context (patient to family and community). Working with families and communities is thus a much needed and neglected priority, and the Project Air Strategy has developed resources around working with families (Project Air Strategy for Personality Disorders, 2016), working with parents with Personality Disorder (McCarthy et al., 2015), working with teachers and schools for early intervention (Grenyer et al., 2016), and working with communities (Project Air Strategy for Personality Disorders, 2015b).

Similarly, the relationship between the patient, their family and community can be characterised at times by ambivalence in their capacity and willingness to provide adequate support (National Institute for Mental Health in England, 2003). The Project Air Strategy has therefore developed models of working with families and carers that focus on developing skilful relationship strategies, reinforcing staying calm during distress, ensuring carers attend to their own needs, set appropriate boundaries, and develop and use crisis plans (Project Air Strategy for Personality Disorders, 2016). This approach has recently been evaluated in a randomised trial with positive outcomes (Grenyer et al., 2018a).

Project Air – current status and future directions

The Project Air Strategy model was developed out of a recognition that mental health services needed a significant re-think of their whole approach to Personality Disorder. The Strategy itself began in 2010 within NSW Mental Health Services, Australia, where the status quo at the time involved widespread stigma and misdiagnosis. In addition, long-term therapy was only available for a very small number of patients, with very long waiting lists, such that most patients did not get access to treatment. With the support of the Minister for Mental Health, the NSW Chief Psychiatrist, and the governing Mental Health and Drug and Alcohol Program Councils and the state-wide Clinical Advisory Council, a whole of service approach was formulated based on the six strategies (Figure 29.1.), and the program is now being rolled out state-wide. As at December 2018, over half the state had been involved in implementation, with more than 5,000 staff trained, and more than 20 new Personality Disorder clinics running, with at least the same number being developed. Each local health district that has implemented the Project Air Strategy has opened between one and five clinics, accepting referrals from the acute care intake process for both adolescents and adults. Clinics follow the stepped care model of assessment, care planning, and brief interventions including connecting with families and carers, and integration of a variety of treatment options including longer-term therapies in the community (Grenyer, 2014). Analysis of longitudinal patient data has already demonstrated that people graduating from these clinics experienced significant improvement in symptoms, quality of life, and productivity in their daily activities, from initial assessment to follow-up at 12 months (Grenyer and Fanaian, 2015). They also report significantly lower ratings of suicidal ideation and attempts, and reductions in deliberate self-harm (Grenyer and Fanaian, 2015). Evaluation of the stepped care approach has also demonstrated significantly reduced presentations to emergency departments and significantly reduced admission numbers and lengths of stay in inpatient units, with the latter dropping from an average of 14 days to only four days per admission (Grenyer et al., 2018b). Using a hub and spoke design, the Project Air Academy connects the headquarters team with all clinic coordinators and leaders across implementation sites, to provide ongoing professional development, support, information exchange, complex care consultations and train-the-trainer resources, to ensure local sustainability. Along with the main implementation has been the provision of family and carer interventions, community forums, scientific conferences, parent intervention training, and whole of school early intervention models to raise awareness and provision of interventions to young people with emerging personality disorders, self-harm and suicidal behaviours.

Conclusion

There is much to be hopeful with respect to future developments in the treatment of Personality Disorder as a result of the wider availability of active strategies and approaches informed by research evidence. However, at present the predominant models are individually-focused, particularly for BPD (Cristea et al., 2017), and ignore the broader family and community surrounding the patient. Whole of service stepped models of care are only now becoming available, which may assist mental health services to provide more timely and adequate responses with broader benefits to the community (Grenyer et al., 2018b). The underlying stigma and negative attitudes towards Personality Disorder continue to reinforce the reluctance to diagnose (Grenyer, 2018), so people continue to live without the knowledge that evidence-based therapies are available for their condition. The comprehensive Project Air Strategy relational approach described here provides one model to integrate both individual consultation with broader social and emotional engagement and open dialogue with services, families, carers and the community. There is therefore new hope that the field of mental health can move to a more humane, responsive, efficient, and trauma-informed approach to mental health care for people meeting the criteria of Personality Disorder.

References

Amad A, Ramoz N, Thomas P, et al. (2014) Genetics of borderline personality disorder: Systematic review and proposal of an integrative model. *Neuroscience and Biobehavioral Reviews* 40: 6–19.

Bailey RC and Grenyer BFS (2014) Supporting a person with personality disorder: A study of carer burden and well-being. *Journal of Personality Disorders* 28: 796–810.

Bateman AW, Gunderson J and Mulder R (2015) Treatment of personality disorder. *The Lancet* 385: 735–743.

Bourke MB and Grenyer BFS (2017) Therapists' metacognitive monitoring of the psychotherapeutic process with patients with Borderline Personality Disorder. *Journal of Psychiatric Practice* 23: 246–253.

Bourke ME and Grenyer BFS (2013) Therapists' accounts of psychotherapy process associated with treating patients with borderline personality disorder. *Journal of Personality Disorder* 27: 735–745.

Briere J and Runtz M (1993) Childhood sexual abuse: Long-term sequelae and implications for psychological assessment. *Journal of Interpersonal Violence* 8: 312–330.

Calvert FL, Crowe TP and Grenyer BFS (2016) Dialogical reflexivity in supervision: An experiential learning process for enhancing reflective and relational competencies. *The Clinical Supervisor* 35: 1–21.

Cristea IA, Gentili C, Cotet CD, et al. (2017) Efficacy of psychotherapies for Borderline Personality Disorder: A systematic review and meta-analysis. *JAMA Psychiatry* 74: 319–328.

Fanaian M, Lewis K and Grenyer BFS (2013) Improving services for people with personality disorders: The views of experienced clinicians. *International Journal of Mental Health Nursing* 22: 465–471.

Grenyer BFS (2012) The clinician's dilemma: Core conflictual relationship themes in personality disorders. *ACPARIAN* 4: 25–27.

Grenyer BFS (2013) Improved prognosis for borderline personality disorder: New treatment guidelines outline specific communication strategies that work. *Medical Journal of Australia* 198: 464–465.

Grenyer BFS (2014) An integrative relational step-down model of care: The Project Air Strategy for personality disorders. *The ACPARIAN* 9: 8–13.

Grenyer BFS (2018) Revising the diagnosis of personality disorder: Can it be single, clinical and factorial? *Australian and New Zealand Journal of Psychiatry* 52(2): 202–203.

Grenyer BFS, Bailey R, Lewis KL, et al. (2018a) A randomised controlled trial of group psychoeducation for carers of persons with borderline personality disorder. *Journal of Personality Disorders* doi: 10.1521/pedi_2018_32_340.

Grenyer BFS and Fanaian M (2015) *Final Report on the Treatment of Personality Disorders Research Project (2010–2013).* Wollongong, Australia: University of Wollongong, Illawarra Health and Medical Research Institute.

Grenyer BFS, Gray AS and Townsend ML (2016) *Working with Young People with Complex Mental Health Issues: Understanding and Responding to Emerging Personality Disorder Trauma History, Self-harm and Suicidal Behaviour and Difficulties with Identity, Emotions and Relationships.* Wollongong, Australia: Illawarra Health and Medical Research Institute, University of Wollongong.

Grenyer BFS, Lewis KL, Fanaian M, Kotze B (2018b) Treatment of personality disorder using a whole of service stepped care approach: a cluster randomized controlled trial. *PLOS ONE* November, 13(11):e0206472 DOI: 10.1371/journal.pone.0206472

Grenyer BFS, Ng FYY, Townsend ML, et al. (2017) Personality disorder: A mental health priority area. *Australian and New Zealand Journal of Psychiatry* 51: 872–875.

Gunderson JG (2007) Disturbed relationships as a phenotype for borderline personality disorder. *The American Journal of Psychiatry* 164: 1637–1640.

Jackson HJ and Burgess PM (2000) Personality disorders in the community: A report from the Australian National Survey of Mental Health and Wellbeing. *Social Psychiatry and Psychiatric Epidemiology* 35: 531–538.

Leary S (2017) Stephanie Leary shares her daily recovery journey from BPD with Project Air Strategy. In: Project-Air (ed) *Lived Experience Stories.* Available at: youtube.com/watch?v=dqiz2TEUMjQ. Wollongong, Australia: Project Air Strategy for Personaity Disorders.

Leichsenring F, Leibing E, Kruse J, et al. (2011) Borderline Personality Disorder. *The Lancet* 377: 74–84.

Lewis KL and Grenyer BFS (2009) Borderline personality disorder or complex Posttraumatic Stress Disorder: An update on the controversy. *Harvard Review of Psychiatry* 17: 322–328.

Lewis LL, Fanaian M, Kotze B, et al. (2019) Mental health presentations to acute psychiatric services: 3-year study of prevalence and readmission risk for personality disorders compared with psychotic, affective, substance or other disorder. British Journal of Psychiatry Open 5: e1, 1–7. doi: 10.1192/bjo.2018.72.

Linehan MM, Armstrong HE, Suarez A, et al. (1991) Cognitive-behavioral treatment of chronically parasuicidal borderline patients. *Archives of General Psychiatry* 48: 1060–1064.

Lingiardi V and McWilliams N (2017) *Psychodynamic Diagnostic Manual (PDM-2), Second Edition*. New York, NY: Guilford.

McCarthy KL, Carter PE and Grenyer BFS (2013) Challenges to getting evidence into practice: Expert clinician perspectives on psychotherapy for personality disorders. *Journal of Mental Health* 22: 482–491.

McCarthy KL, Jarman H, Bourke M, et al. (2015) *Parenting with Personality Disorder Intervention: A Manual for Health Professionals*. Wollongong, Australia: University of Wollongong.

McCarthy KL, Lewis KL, Bourke ME, et al. (2016) A new intervention for people with borderline personality disorder who are also parents: A pilot study of clinician acceptability. *Borderline Personality Disorder and Emotion Dysregulation* 3: 10.

Meuldijk D, McCarthy A, Bourke ME, et al. (2017) The value of psychological treatment for Borderline Personality Disorder: Systematic review and cost-offset analysis of economic evaluations. *PLoS ONE* 12: doi:10.1371/journal.pone.0171592.

National Health and Medical Research Council (2012) *Clinical Practice Guideline for the Management of Borderline Personality Disorder*. Melbourne, Australia: National Health and Medical Research Council.

National Institute for Mental Health in England (2003) *Personality Disorder: No Longer a Diagnosis of Exclusion. Policy Implementation Guidance for the Development of Services for People with Personality Disorders*. London, UK: National Institute for Mental Health in England.

Ng FYY, Bourke ME and Grenyer BFS (2016) Recovery from Borderline Personality Disorder: A systematic review of the perspectives of consumers, clinicians, family and carers. *PLoS ONE* 11: doi:10.1371/journal.pone.0160515.

Project Air Strategy for Personality Disorders (2011) *Treatment Guidelines for Personality Disorders*. Sydney, Australia: NSW Health and Illawarra Health and Medical Research Institute.

Project Air Strategy for Personality Disorders (2015a) *Brief Intervention Manual for Personality Disorders*. Wollongong, Australia: University of Wollongong, Illawarra Health and Medical Research Institute.

Project Air Strategy for Personality Disorders (2015b) *Treatment Guidelines for Personality Disorders, Second Edition*. Wollongong, Australia: NSW Health and Illawarra Health and Medical Research Institute.

Project Air Strategy for Personality Disorders (2016) *Family, Partner and Carer Intervention Manual for Personality Disorders*. Wollongong, Australia: Illawarra Health and Medical Research Institute.

Sharp C, Wright AGC, Fowler JC, et al. (2015) The structure of personality pathology: Both general ('g') and specific ('s') factors? *Journal of Abnormal Psychology* 124: 387–398.

Stern A (1938) Psychoanalytic investigation of the theory in the border line group of neuroses. *The Psychoanalytic Quarterly* 7: 467–489.

Sulzer SH, Muenchow E, Potvin A, et al. (2016) Improving patient-centered communication of the borderline personality disorder diagnosis. *Journal of Mental Health* 25: 5–9.

Weinberg I, Ronningstam E, Goldblatt MJ, et al. (2011) Common factors in empirically supported treatments of borderline personality disorder. *Current Psychiatry Reports* 13: 60–68.

Wilhelm K, Finch A, Kotze B, et al. (2007) The Green Card Clinic: Overview of a brief patient-centred intervention following deliberate self-harm. *Australian Psychiatry* 15: 35–41.

30 Thirty-five years of developing, teaching and delivering a trauma-based relational psychotherapy – the Conversational Model

Michael Williamson

Introduction

In 1965 a form of psychotherapy emerged uniquely in England through the work of psychiatrists Robert Hobson and Russell Meares; it was later called the Conversational Model (CM). Their model of psychodynamic psychotherapy, its teaching, training and clinical delivery, has been further developed since 1983 by Meares, with the assistance of a faculty, in Sydney, Australia (Meares, 2004). Outcome studies and factor research have ensured that the CM is strongly evidence-based (Stevenson and Meares, 1992; Stevenson et al., 2005; Korner et al., 2006; Meares et al., 2011; Stevenson et al., 2015). In the UK Elspeth Guthrie also developed Psychodynamic Interpersonal Psychotherapy, based on the CM, primarily for patient stabilisation in a range of acute presentations, allowing the commencement of community mental health care with psychotherapy (Guthrie and Moghavemi, 2013).

The CM was originally designed to assist patients who were thought to be untreatable, those would now be usually diagnosed with Borderline Personality Disorder (BPD), in twice weekly therapy over several years. Over the course of time it was also found to be helpful for other Personality Disorders, Somatisation Disorder, as well as Treatment Resistant Depression. The principles of the CM have also been adapted to short term therapy and to assessment in emergency and other one-off situations. Based on one-to-one human interactions and conversation, the central theme of the model involves the damaging effects of interpersonal trauma on the development of Self, particularly early trauma, and the relevance of trauma to relationship.

Development of the model

It was evident that only a new theoretical model could provide successful therapy for those patients Hobson and Meares were attempting to treat. In the 1960s, while the Schizophrenia spectrum was still unclear, and as there were no adequate psychological explanations or treatments available for BPD, extremes of normality, neuroses and psychoses were all proposed to explain these types of presentations, namely, "pre-schizophrenic personality structure", "psychotic characters", "ambulatory schizophrenia", and so on (Kernberg, 1967). Stern had coined the term "borderline" to describe patients who were on the "border" between neuroses and psychoses (Stern, 1938). Kernberg agreed but saw BPD as a "psychopathological constellation" which connected a range of personality variables into "a rather specific and remarkably stable form of pathological ego structure" (Kernberg, 1967: p.641). The acceptance of this diagnostic term provided a focus for research into its complex symptom profile (Grinker, 1968). Increasing theoretical agreement led to publication of the first research-based diagnostic signs of borderline personality (Gunderson and Elliott, 1985). After BPD was more formally recognised in 1980 (American Psychiatric Association, 1980), diagnosis became increasingly possible, although effective treatment was not. Early use of medication was often an attempt to treat a proposed syndrome (Brinkley et al., 1979), whereas later and current treatments have aimed at symptomatic relief.

In his book, "Forms of Feeling", Hobson described his attempt with Meares to understand these patients (Hobson, 1985). They saw that personal relationship, valued over "diagnoses" and "treatments", was the primary principle. Most of all, they identified that it is the relational conversation that best transforms the traumatised Self. In 1983, Meares, in the Department of Psychiatry at Westmead Hospital, Sydney, began a treatment and research program which further developed psychotherapy for BPD. In "The Metaphor of Play: Origin and Breakdown of Personal Being", Meares explored the roles of play and trauma, and the "self as a self-organising system" (Meares, 2005). The development and elaboration of these concepts drew on the psychoanalytic traditions of Freud, Jung, Fairbairn, Winnicott, and the works of others such as William James, John Hughlings Jackson, and Heinz Kohut's Self Psychology. Meares invited professional colleagues, Bernard Brandchaft, Robert Stolorow, Edgar Levenson, Howard Bacal, Paul and Anna Ornstein, who worked in Self Psychology, and Charles Strozier, Kohut's biographer, to visit the program on various occasions (Meares, 2005). The purpose of these visits was to exchange views and to establish some means of qualitative estimation by other experts in the field of the work being done in the program. Kohutian Self-Psychology was however limited by its focus on narcissism, which did not further help clarify the nature of BPD (Kohut, 1989).

For an experience-near model of Self more relevant to the CM and BPD, Meares turned to the American psychologist-philosopher, William James. Years before the "radical-behaviourist purge" of the early twentieth century (Harter, 1983), when the concept of "Self" was unheard of in clinical discourse, James had explored the meaning of the Self; "What we mean by personal selves are thoughts connected as we feel them to be connected" (James, 1892: p.153). Although detailed analysis of the related development of the CM is beyond the scope of this chapter, it is outlined in the three following concepts: Self, trauma and dissociation.

The importance of the Self

Meares identified 12 main characteristics of a healthy Self (Meares, 2004).

1. Duality: Self has two poles, one that experiences, and the other that reflects on this experience.
2. Movement: Self lives, not in a static way, but with energy and progress.
3. Positive Feeling: despite negative and challenging experiences, Self maintains an overall positive feeling.
4. Non-linearity: while a person needs to be organised, Self has a life of flow, rather than a set agenda.
5. Coherence: despite conflicting pressures and responses, the wholeness of Self is maintained.
6. Continuity: Self does not live in a jerky, stop-start, or disconnected fashion, but with a flow of continuity.
7. Temporality: while it flows, Self is nevertheless measured and lives in a rhythm of time.
8. Spatiality: there is a sense of expansiveness, rather than a sense of contraction or diminishment.
9. Content beyond the present: the past and future are both represented.
10. Ownership: there is the sense of identity, of living a life which belongs to Self.
11. Boundedness: there is a sense of being comfortably enclosed.
12. Agency: Self is active and effective.

All 12 of these characteristics need to be present for Self to be truly healthy and vital, but they wax and wane, even in healthy individuals, depending upon circumstance and stress levels. It should also be noted that the term "Self" is seldom used in psychiatry, although the concept is of great significance with respect to mental health and those who have suffered trauma.

The effect of trauma and the need to adapt

Physical, sexual and emotional abuse, including emotional deprivation, can create an overwhelming traumatic system, affecting the development of the positive qualities of Self. Such trauma when severe and chronic can affect every part of an individual's life, emotional, physical, and social. Relationships may be particularly affected, as the trauma system, often laid down very early in life, involving unconscious traumatic memories of abuse, is likely to repeat itself within relationships. The traumatised Self also commonly struggles against fragmentation and dissociation. This new understanding of the relationship between the development of Self and trauma was fundamental to the CM and to the understanding of BPD. This also led to a revision of some traditional psychoanalytic concepts.

In earlier psychoanalytic models, unconscious attempts to avoid anxiety evoked by trauma were generally termed "defences", and "coping mechanisms" in later forms; there is an extensive literature that discusses the relationships between the two (Kramer, 2010). In Classical Psychoanalysis, resistance was traditionally seen as the patient's unconscious opposition to the therapist's efforts, and therefore an impediment to the therapy. In the CM, resistance is seen as the traumatised patient's unconscious fear of repetition of the trauma, or, in some cases, a fear of change and the acquisition of independence for which they feel ill-equipped (Meares, 2000, 2004). Defences previously regarded as unconscious factors contributing to resistance are seen in the CM as unconscious coping mechanisms and in fact adaptive strategies to deal with fearful, distressing and difficult early relationships that have become maladaptive over time. The CM emphasises "coping styles" or "coping mechanisms", over defences, as more representative of efforts by the traumatised Self to manage fragmentation and dissociation (Meares et al., 2012).

The relevance of dissociation

Dissociation is one of those early coping mechanisms used to deal with developmental traumata of physical, sexual, and emotional abuse and neglect that pervades the borderline condition (Meares, 2012). Dissociation involves pathological disconnection between thought and feeling, perception and awareness, behaviour and consciousness. In childhood, dissociation offers some protection from the harmful effects of abuse, as children are less likely than adults to be able to either "fight" or take "flight" in response to overwhelming stress. However, dissociation becomes pathological when habitual (Meares, 1999). Dissociation differs from day-dreaming or musing or distraction, or the distancing effects of intense concentration. Dissociation can involve significant memory lapses, loss of periods of time, unaccountable behaviour, and in some circumstances significantly different internal self-states. The more severe the traumatic system, the more severe the dissociation (Meares, 2012).

Therapy

"The aim of therapy is maturational. Specifically, it is to help the patient discover, elaborate, and represent a personal reality" (Stevenson and Meares, 1992: p.358.). Self-experience is fulfilled in language and in relatedness through conversation, "I can only find myself between me and my fellows in a human conversation" (Hobson, 1985: p.153). The development of Self in therapy involves the gradual development of awareness, thought, reflection and feeling. Through the therapeutic relationship, both separation and individuation are enhanced, and in Hobson's terms, a sense of "aloneness-togetherness" develops, a feeling that the therapist is neither too close, or intruding, nor too far away, or rejecting (Hobson, 1985), a critical development which generalises to other relationships.

Principle of therapy – listening

To potentiate the development of Self, a particular mode of listening and responding, or empathic resonance, is used to encourage the development of a special, but natural, form of conversation. The therapist does not control or redirect the conversation but aims to respond through an enlarged awareness to "what is there". Difficult feelings are acknowledged, given value, understood wherever possible, and, most importantly, not avoided. The most positive, vital elements in the patient's conversation are affirmed and amplified. As far as possible, the language of the patient is used, however, non-verbal communications must also be taken into account. Facial expression, body posture, behaviour, language, thought, feeling, imagery and speech tones must all be considered. For a therapeutic conversation, a listening, contemplative inner state, with a sort of relaxed, open, and thoughtful presence, or "quasi-meditative gaze," is maintained (Meares et al., 2012).

Principle of therapy – therapist awareness

Staying close to the experiences of Self requires the afore-mentioned empathic attitude. Avoiding "thinking about" content, but staying with feelings, expressed through the language of the right, more unconscious and more emotive, hemisphere of the brain is advocated. The therapist maintains an awareness of the drift and directions of the conversation, of the other person's unconscious needs and aims, reflects on the repetition of themes, narratives, disruption and repair of self-states in the conversation, and registers the increasing organisation of Self and its field of conscious and unconscious expectations. To do so it is important that the therapist not get caught up in the mainly negative, trauma-affected tone, and also focusses on his or her own conscious thoughts, feelings, and imaginative responses, as well as of his or her faint sense of things on the edge of awareness.

Principle of therapy – fostering the patient's awareness

The therapist aims to foster a developing self-experience and reflective awareness in the patient. Traditional analytic interpretations can impair this development and are not used. The therapist's natural conversational style includes coupling, representation, amplification, and linking. Coupling is an attempt by the therapist to align closely with the patient's words and to gently reflect them, or to re-iterate them to help the flow of conversation in the same direction. Representation involves an attempt to portray an understanding of what the patient is saying and feeling, by choice of words and tone of voice, from both a gentle and a tentative perspective, facilitating the patient's own efforts to represent or understand his or her experience. Representation is important, but it can heighten anxiety and be re-traumatising, so emotion needs to be monitored and kept at an optimal level. Importantly, the therapist also uses amplification to recognise a word that is emotionally charged, along with its associated affect, and reflects it back to the patient with an emphasis on the word or an inflection to which emotion is connected. The therapist does this to increase awareness of hidden or unexpressed affect, and to expand the patient's emotional range, and indeed their consciousness.

Transference and countertransference in the Conversational Model

The terms transference and countertransference have lengthy histories and both complex and varying meanings. Traditionally, the phenomenon of transference was thought to involve the unconscious transfer of experiences of early relationships on the part of the patient to the person of the analyst in the present, which, when brought to the attention of the patient served to help the patient explore significant relationships, particularly via any patterns that may become evident in the relationship with the analyst. In the CM, however, transference is always understood as a reflection of unconscious memories of early trauma and of relationships in which trauma occurred, where the therapist may be experienced by the patient much like an abuser from the past and nearly always in negative affective states (Meares et al., 2012). The transference in the CM is also referred to as the co-transference, as the therapist also makes a contribution to the transference, and therefore it is co-constructed.

The countertransference refers to the therapist's own feelings and attitudes toward the patient. Freud saw the countertransference as a problem to be overcome. More contemporary perspectives see the countertransference as an ongoing feature of the therapeutic relationship which includes the therapist's own unconscious reactions, emotional, physical and cognitive, to the patient's attitude and manner toward the therapist directly, or through activation of the therapist's own past (Haliburn, 2009; Meares et al., 2012). Maintaining awareness of the therapist's own reactions to the patient may increase understanding of what the patient is feeling, and thus serve as a source of invaluable data.

A growing conversation linking patient, therapist and history will be worked through in the co-transference and the countertransference. This will be strongest through the manifestations of unconscious traumatic memory and the trauma system, both obvious and subtle. Disjunctions or sudden fractures in the therapeutic relationship are intrinsic to the therapy of the traumatised Self and need to be repaired when they occur. This serves to reinforce the patient's trust in the therapist.

Linking replaces traditional psychoanalytic interpretations and is unique to the CM. Linking does not focus on meaning, but rather on connections between what the patient says and what the therapist says, in the context of the patient's history and repeating patterns, creating hypotheses which are speculative but integrating. Linking is an example of a transference intervention, replacing classical interpretation.

A vignette – "Andrew"

Andrew, a 30-year-old man, with a previous primary diagnosis of Major Depression, was unresponsive to several antidepressants and multiple courses of Electro-convulsive Therapy. His clinical notes were sketchy records of many presentations to his local Emergency Department (ED) with self-harm and unsuccessful suicide attempts. He was described by others as "absolutely nuts" and "the living dead". He described his own self-destructive behaviour with an empty, mechanical precision. Assessment by a female psychiatry trainee studying the CM found in Andrew's cold intellectualisation a barely concealed, and previously unrecorded, pattern consistent with childhood emotional trauma: a terror of abandonment, and a sense of meaninglessness, which could quickly reverse to a conviction that his perfect mother would come to the ED to rescue him. During an empathic first interview, he rapidly switched between grandiosity, identity confusion ("I don't know who I am"), sudden rage and suicidal hopelessness.

With a clear diagnosis of BPD, with significant dissociative features, Andrew commenced twice weekly, 50-minute sessions of psychotherapy in the CM. He had no memory of his childhood before the age of 10 years, after which he remembered his mother's affection towards his younger sister, but not toward him. His mother was a professional woman, who obsessively demanded extremes of "rational" behaviour. She punished any "childishness" (attempts to play or express feelings) by freezing withdrawal, and she rewarded "satisfactory behaviour" with hugs and kisses. His father was also a professional, and they saw little of him.

In therapy, Andrew initially asserted his intellectual superiority over the therapist with contempt, idealising his mother's abusiveness. Later, he curled up on the floor, crying in a toddler's voice, "I want my mummy". Through her consistent and empathic engagement with each of Andrew's presenting self-states, and through coupling with his expressed emotion, representation of his emerging traumatic memories, and amplification of any latent positive feelings, his cold perfectionism gradually faded, and was replaced by a more genuine ability to be himself and to acknowledge his therapist.

His disorganisation in his relationship with his therapist who, in contrast to his mother, was nonjudgmental, empathic and reliable, and able to withstand his powerful moods, was transformed. As a result, Andrew's terror of abandonment also gradually subsided. Though still impaired, after 12 months of therapy he had not taken an overdose, he had mostly stopped self-harming, and he had stopped presenting to the ED; he was no longer diagnosable as "borderline". Through the second year of therapy, he tentatively expressed an increase in positive feelings, and having achieved a stronger sense of self-cohesion and identity, throughout the third year he was able to gradually come to a realisation of his mother's cruelty. Over four years of a positive therapeutic relationship, his quasi-psychotic, dissociated Self had attained a new level of coherence and vitality, and a sense of identity and value.

Supervision

The renewal and growth of Self requires a positive therapeutic relationship, best supported by ongoing supervision, through which the trainee therapist's understanding and application of the model is continually reviewed. The aim of supervision is to clarify and help contain the therapist's conscious and unconsciousness anxieties, angers, fatigue, rescue fantasies and attractions.

Focused attention to the fluctuating conscious and unconscious exchange of self-states between patient and therapist, and the potential for previous traumas to be subtly re-enacted in therapy, are critical components of supervision in the CM. When the therapist is unconsciously placed in the role of an abusive other, referred to as a reversal (Meares, 2000), any persecutory tendencies must be recognised to enable the therapist to understand the dynamic and to respond accordingly (Meares, 1977).

The novel experience of learning a psychoanalytic, trauma-informed, relational therapy with seriously unwell patients may test a trainee's confidence. Regular individual and group supervision are both important components of CM training; this intensity of supervision acts as a container for the trainee, and this intensity contributes substantially to the optimal delivery of the CM, and to effective outcomes. Because of the complexities involved, personal psychotherapy for trainees is also encouraged in this training but is not compulsory.

Outcome studies

The first outcome study demonstrated the efficacy of the CM in the treatment of BPD (Stevenson and Meares, 1992; Meares et al., 1995). Trainee therapists under close supervision provided two sessions per week for 30 severely ill patients assessed to have BPD by clinician administered and self-report scales. Measures of functioning during the year prior to therapy, when compared with the same measures at the end of the first and second years, showed improved outcomes in most areas studied. These included significant reductions in the number of inpatient bed days, episodes of violence and self-harm, the use of illegal drugs, abuse of prescribed medications, and the number of visits to health professionals. In this study, at the beginning of treatment, 17 of the 30 patients met all eight of the criteria for BPD using the classification system of the day, the Third Edition of the Diagnostic and Statistical Manual of Mental Disorders (American Psychiatric Association, 1980). At the end of just 12 months of therapy, only 10 patients met the eight criteria, while 30 per cent of the study participants were no longer diagnosable with BPD at all. Improvement was also sustained five years after the completion of therapy (Stevenson et al., 2005). To avoid the unethical situation of severely traumatised patients being placed on waitlists and being deprived of therapy, the patients in the study served as their own controls. Without a more formal control group, however, the study findings have been questioned.

A replication study however confirmed the two previous studies and the clinical efficacy of the CM (Korner et al., 2006). Economic research has demonstrated significant savings for the Department of Health and the taxpayer by reduction in ED visits, hospital admissions and acute and ongoing community mental health care, of $8000 per patient in the first year of therapy (Stevenson and Meares, 1999). An independent University of Sydney study of the same cohort found a higher figure of $18,000 per patient (Hall et al., 2001).

Teaching and training

The first recipients of training were doctors concurrently completing their psychiatry studies at the Department of Psychiatry, Westmead Hospital, Sydney, in the early 1980s. Therapy patients were drawn from hospital admissions and community outpatients. The training faculty was drawn from senior psychotherapists and psychoanalysts in Sydney, all of whom were psychiatrists. Discussion of formative ideas and new research took place at Meares' weekly lectures, followed by training seminars, and individual and group supervision by the visiting consultants. The training was part-time, as it currently is, with assessments and essays required to be completed at regular intervals. Annual presentations of work towards a graduation thesis are required of all trainees, who are then encouraged to work their thesis towards publication.

The trainees saw, in once or twice weekly sessions, patients mostly with a diagnosis of BPD but with histories of severe physical, sexual or emotional abuse and neglect. These patients described receiving prior psychiatric treatments which had not been helpful, and on occasion had been re-traumatising; often they had undergone decades of treatment with no benefit. The trainees were challenged with learning and managing two related but essentially different models of treatment. Developing an ongoing therapeutic conversation with a person whose Self, relationships and living were dominated by an internal trauma system differed significantly from the general psychiatry model of patient assessment and management. In the latter model, symptoms and signs were of utmost importance, where there was little scope to attend to patients' trauma histories. While notions of consciousness in general psychiatry involved attention, concentration, cognition, memory, judgement and so on, they were not integrated into a total theory of Self or Self in Relationship. The trainees' successful integration of both models was evident in supervision and in ongoing assessments, in the way that trainees interacted with their patients, and from their own accounts.

Integral to the training was the use of supervision by audiotape, rather than presentation by process notes; the CM training was one of the first to use this technique. The trainees were taught to pay close attention to expression of feeling, to tone and to the use of language – to the process of therapy as opposed to the content – that the audio-tapes provided. The method emphasised attention to the "minute particulars" which Robert Hobson cited from the great English poet, William Blake, "He who would do good to another must do it in Minute Particulars" (Blake, 1908). It is only through working at this level of detail that a therapist can deeply understand the complexity of another and respond appropriately.

Individuals who had achieved fellowship as psychiatrists, and competence as psychotherapists, were later admitted to the Faculty of Psychotherapy, and fostered the further development of the training program. In 1988, a Masters' course was established at the University of Sydney, and the first trainees graduated in 1990 with a Master of Medicine degree. In 1990, the Australian and New Zealand Association of Psychotherapy (ANZAP) was developed. Faculty members from the Westmead program were founding members of ANZAP and its early presidents, and since the 1990s have provided teaching and supervision in NSW, Queensland, Victoria, Tasmania and New Zealand. ANZAP has always trained across disciplines, with medical, nursing and allied health staff completing a Diploma in the CM. The first Westmead program, in fact, consisted of a multidisciplinary cohort of trainees, but the introduction of a more formal university degree allowed only the admission of medical graduates for the first 10 years, when a Master of Medicine, Psychotherapy, was conferred on successful graduates. The introduction of a Master of Medicine in Science in 2007 changed this, and clinical psychologists, graduate nurses and social workers were admitted to training (Haliburn et al., 2008). A one-year certificate course in short-term psychotherapy based on the CM has become available since 2011, and planning for a university Graduate Certificate Course is also underway.

Delivering the model

In the 1980s, longer inpatient admissions for larger numbers of BPD patients presenting with suicidal behaviour, mood disorders and substance abuse allowed two or three weekly inpatient psychotherapy sessions which would be continued after discharge, allowing for continuity of care. Since the reductions in mental health funding in 1987, admissions of BPD patients have been much less frequent and of shorter duration, with an emphasis on community treatment. With increased demand and reduced resources ever since, the local health service has benefited greatly from an effective and essentially cost-free service to patients provided by trainees, patients who would otherwise utilise a broader range of resources across various government departments and the private sector.

Patients are regularly referred to the program from the local ED, inpatient and community mental health services, and from private practices. A CM-based exploration of how and why life may have turned out this way is completed, which is followed by psychoeducation on the model of therapy and reasons for its use, taking into account the patient's presentation. A series of research questionnaires are administered, and the patient advised as to the repetition of these questionnaires at different stages in the therapy. Care is taken that the patients are informed about the conduct of therapy, and consent is obtained for their participation in research and in presentations at seminars and conferences, assuring them of the maintenance of confidentiality and anonymity. They are then allocated to therapists in training. Since 2011, some patients have been offered a short-term version of the therapy of up to 25 weekly sessions (Haliburn, 2017), or long-term therapy, currently of one to three sessions per week for one training year, with subsequent ongoing referral. The patient is encouraged to have a case manager, drug and alcohol counsellor when applicable, and a General Practitioner. Most patients are on psychotropic medications which are generally continued under supervision.

Achieving competence in the successful treatment of patients presenting with BPD, Treatment Resistant Depression, chronic suicidality, and self-harm, and in the proper understanding of transference and countertransference, is positively regarded by the trainees. Having developed the capacity to engage with patients who tend to provoke anxiety, anger or dismissiveness or on the contrary, helplessness and pessimism in most clinical staff, graduate therapists report that their work, informed by the CM, has helped them withstand these pressures, enabled them to make a more fully informed diagnosis and to effectively manage these patients. Trainees working in EDs report remarkable changes in their attitudes and clinical efficacy with borderline and other challenging patients, which in turn assists both patients and other ED staff. They report in addition the ability to positively influence staff who have not trained in psychotherapy.

Research and academic development

Faculty members publish books and papers, both nationally and internationally (Meares, 1992; 2000; 2005; 2012; 2016; Meares et al., 2012). A book on short-term therapy based on the CM has also been recently published (Haliburn, 2017). Other faculty members, Janine Stevenson, Anthony Korner, Joan Haliburn, Loyola McLean, and Shaun Halovic maintain a wide range of research interests. These include neurophysiological studies involving P3a and right hemisphere function (Meares et al., 2011), linguistics (Butt et al., 2010), ongoing clinical outcomes studies, development of a Conversational Model Adherence Scale (Halovic et al., 2016), and the use of the CM in Group Therapy (Korner et al., 2014). In Newcastle, the Centre for Psychotherapy, directed by Nick Bendit, a graduate of the Westmead training program, provides and researches the use of both the CM and Dialectical Behaviour Therapy for BPD. In 2012, the first manual on the CM was written to present the essential therapeutic processes of the model (Meares et al., 2012). A manual had been resisted for many years out of concern about over-simplification, however the manual presents the clinical practice and complexities in a balanced and usable form to trainees, clinicians and the wider community.

A day conference on Complex Traumatic Stress Disorders is held annually at Westmead Hospital, where the major feature is the application of the CM. The model as taught and delivered has broadened from its initial focus on BPD to

Complex Traumatic Stress Disorders, Treatment Resistant Depression, Somatisation and other Personality Disorders. Faculty members regularly present papers to the Royal Australian and New Zealand Colleges of Psychiatrists (RANZCP) and its Psychotherapy Section annual conference, to overseas conferences, at regular ANZAP seminars and the annual two-day ANZAP conference. The CM Faculty holds memberships with a range of international associations and contributes to their leadership and functions.

In recognition of his research publications, the development of the CM and the success of the Westmead training program, Professor Meares was awarded in 2007 the title of, "Distinguished Psychiatrist of the Year" by the University of California at Los Angeles, and in 2012, the Meritorious Service Award by the NSW branch of the RANZCP. The influence of the CM on the interview process and the support of survivors has also been acknowledged as significantly contributing to The Royal Commission into Institutional Responses into Child Sexual Abuse (Ellis and Ellis, 2017).

Conclusion

The 35 years of developing, teaching and delivering a trauma-based, relational psychotherapy via the CM has been shown by repeated outcome studies to be successful. A key benefit of the CM is that it presents a way of being with and relating to our patients, a skill that all doctors, particularly psychiatrists, can benefit from, as it is truly trauma-informed, and offers an additional perspective to the biomedical paradigm. The CM training programs at Westmead continue to support the health services, clinically and financially, reducing repeated ED visits and utilisation of services for self-harming, emotionally dysregulated, and suicidal patients. The movement of graduates in CM training to other hospitals and to private practices has resulted in dissemination of most needed skills which provide therapeutic healing of patients in the wider community. Successful CM therapy improves not only the lives of patients but also helps reduce transgenerational trauma in families and society. A trauma-informed health policy and approach will recognise and maintain the unique contribution of this program.

References

American Psychiatric Association (1980) *Diagnostic and Statistical Manual of Mental Disorders, Third Edition*. Washington, DC: American Psychiatric Publishing.

Blake W (1908) Jerusalem [The Holiness of Minute Particulars]. In: Blake W (author) *William Blake (1757–1827) The Poetical Works*. London, UK: Macmillan.

Brinkley JR, Beitman BD and Friedel RO (1979) Low-dose neuroleptic regimens in the treatment of borderline patients. *Archives of General Psychiatry* 36: 319–326.

Butt D, Moore AR, Henderson-Brooks C, et al. (2010) Dissociation, relatedness, and 'cohesive harmony': A linguistic measure of degrees of 'fragmentation'? *Linguistics and the Human Sciences* 3(3): 263–293.

Ellis J and Ellis N (2017) Helping heal the sins of the past. *Law Society of NSW Journal* 37: 30–35.

Grinker R (1968) *The Borderline Syndrome: A Behavioral Study of Ego Functions*. New York, NY: Basic Books.

Gunderson JG and Elliott GR (1985) The interface between Borderline Personality Disorder and Affective Disorder. *American Journal of Psychiatry* 142(3): 277–288.

Guthrie E and Moghavemi A (2013) Psychodynamic-interpersonal therapy: An overview of the treatment and evidence base. *Psychodynamic Psychiatry* 41(4): 619–635.

Haliburn J (2009) Integration through relatedness in the conversational model: A case study. *Australasian Psychiatry* 17(1): 29–33.

Haliburn J (2017) *An Integrated Approach to Short-Term Dynamic Interpersonal Psychotherapy*. London, UK: Karnac Books.

Haliburn J, Stevenson J and Gerull F (2008) 25 years of a university training program on the treatment of patients with borderline personality disorder. *Australasian Psychiatry* 17(1): 25–28.

Hall J, Caleo S, Stevenson J, et al. (2001) An economic analysis of psychotherapy for borderline personality disorder patients. *Journal of Mental Health Policy and Economics* 4 (1): 3–8.

Halovic S, Komer A, McLean L, et al. (2016) *Using the CMAS to measure adherence to the Conversational Model: How expertise influences CMAS ratings*. Paper presented at The Society for Mental Health Research Conference. Sydney, Australia.

Harter S (1983) Developmental perspectives on the self-system. In: Mussen P (ed) *Handbook of Child Psychology, Volume Four*. New York, NY: Wiley, pp.275–385.

Hobson RF (1985) *Forms of Feeling: The Heart of Psychotherapy*. London, UK: Tavistock.

James W (1892) *Psychology: Briefer Course*. London, UK: Macmillan.

Kernberg O (1967) Borderline personality organisation. *Journal of the American Psychoanalytic Association* 15(3): 641–685.

Kohut H (1989) *The Analysis of the Self*. Madison, CT: International Universities Press.

Korner A, Gerull F, Meares R, et al. (2006) Borderline personality disorder treated with the conversational model: A replication study. *Comprehensive Psychiatry* 47(5): 406–411.

Korner A, Haliburn J, Stevenson J, et al. (2014) *Group Psychotherapy for Complex Traumatic Disorders: An Expansion of Service Delivery Through the Westmead Psychotherapy Program*. Sydney, Australia: Westmead Psychotherapy Program.

Kramer U (2010) Coping and defence mechanisms: What's the difference? Second act. *Psychology and Psychotherapy: Theory, Research and Practice* 83 (Pt 2): 207–221.

Meares R (1977) The persecutory therapist. *British Journal of Medical Psychology* 50: 340–359.

Meares R (1992) *The Metaphor of Play: Disruption and Restoration in the Borderline Experience*. New York, NY: Jason Aronson.

Meares R (1999) The contributions of Hughlings Jackson to an understanding of dissociation. *American Journal of Psychiatry* 156: 1850–1855.

Meares R (2000) *Intimacy and Alienation: Memory, Trauma and Personal Being*. London, UK: Routledge.

Meares R (2004) The Conversational Model: An outline. *American Journal of Psychotherapy* 58(1): 51–66.

Meares R (2005) *The Metaphor of Play: Origin and Breakdown of Personal Being, Third Edition*. New York, NY: Routledge.

Meares R (2012) *A Dissociation Model of Borderline Personality Disorder*. New York, NY: Norton.

Meares R (2016) *The Poet's Voice in the Making of Mind*. New York, NY: Routledge.

Meares R, Sara G, Stevenson J, et al. (1995) Outcome studies of psychotherapy in borderline personality disorder. *Directions in Psychiatry, Volume 15, Lesson Five*. New York, NY: The Hatherleigh Company Limited.

Meares R, Schore AN and Melkonian D (2011) Is borderline personality disorder a particularly right hemispheric disorder? A study of P3a using single trial analysis. *Australian and New Zealand Journal of Psychiatry* 45: 131–139.

Meares R, Bendit N, Haliburn J, et al. (2012) *Borderline Personality Disorder and the Conversational Model: A Clinician's Manual*. New York, NY: Norton.

Stern A (1938) Psychoanalytic investigation of therapy in the borderline group of neuroses. *The Psychoanalytic Quarterly* 7: 467–489.

Stevenson J and Meares R (1992) An outcome study of psychotherapy for patients with borderline personality disorder. *American Journal of Psychiatry* 149: 358–462.

Stevenson J and Meares R (1999) Psychotherapy with borderline patients II: A preliminary cost-benefit study. *Australian and New Zealand Journal of Psychiatry* 33: 473–477.

Stevenson J, Meares R and D'Angelo R (2005) Five-year outcome of outpatient psychotherapy with borderline patients. *Psychological Medicine* 35: 79–87.

Stevenson J, Haliburn J and Halovic S (2015) Trauma, personality disorder and chronic depression: The role of the Conversational Model in the treatment of resistant depression. *Psychoanalytic Psychotherapy* 2:135–148

Index

For Product Safety Concerns and Information please contact our EU
representative GPSR@taylorandfrancis.com
Taylor & Francis Verlag GmbH, Kaufingerstraße 24, 80331 München, Germany

www.ingramcontent.com/pod-product-compliance
Ingram Content Group UK Ltd.
Pitfield, Milton Keynes, MK11 3LW, UK
UKHW022213190926
475702UK00003B/333
9780367076580